Clinical Decision Making

This is a lucid series of essays in the nature of basic science essential to all the disciplines involved in medical care. It emphasizes critical thinking, reason, and analytic principles in the pursuit of valid solutions to the complex problems of modern practice.

William Weiss, MD
Emeritus Professor of Medicine
Hahnemann University

. . . tough-minded and fair.
John La Puma, MD
Director, Center for Clinical Ethics
Lutheran General Hospital

Worth reading. Dr Eddy calls a spade a "g.d. shovel."
George E Farrar Jr, MD, FACP
Past President Pennsylvania Medical Society

The most stimulating and provocative as well as informative of any of the current reviews and comments being made on clinical decisionmaking . . . considers a broad range of material and condenses it in a form that is readily understandable to the practicing physician . . . extremely relevant at a time when there is tremendous pressure for the practice of cost-effective medicine.

Howard H Kaufman, MD
Professor and Chairman
Neurosurgery, West Virginia University

Quite simply the best book yet written about how rational decisions can help shape the destiny of the US health care system.

James W Squires, MD
Chairman of the Board
Matthew Thornton Health Plan

Albert Einstein said, "The perfection of means and confusion of goals characterize the age." David Eddy gives us cause to look up from our work and more carefully determine those goals.

Frederik C Hansen, MD
Medical Director for InforMed

. . . invaluable to the practicing health law attorney.
Brenda T Strama, JD
Vinson & Elkins LLP

This work is so broadly applicable and the depth of resources provided by it are so remarkable, I can't conceive a simple phrase or uncomplicated sentence that would convey the extent of my appreciation for it . . . should make clinical and administrative decisions easier and more rational for any medical professional, from orthopod to ethicist.

David L Wishart, MD
Radiation Therapy Unit
Memorial Hospital

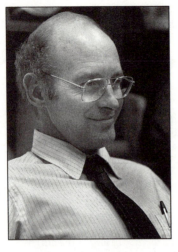

David Eddy, MD, PhD, trained in surgery and then received a PhD in engineering mathematics from Stanford. He has spent the last 20 years developing and applying methods for solving complex medical problems. He has written four books, more than 100 articles, and two commercially successful software programs. He has served on more than 40 national and international boards and committees, and has consulted for more than 50 groups ranging from medical specialty societies to insurance companies to foreign governments. He has won top national and international awards in several fields, including the Lanchester prize given by the Operations Research Society of America, the FHP prize given by the International Society for Health Technology Assessment, and the USQA prize for Quality of Health Care. He is an elected member of the Institute of Medicine, National Academy of Sciences. He has held full professorships and chairs at Stanford University and Duke University. He currently serves as Senior Advisor for Health Policy and Management at Kaiser Permanente Southern California.

Clinical Decision Making
From Theory to Practice

A Collection of Essays From
The Journal of the American Medical Association

DAVID M. EDDY, MD, PhD
Senior Advisor for Health Policy and Management
Kaiser Permanente Southern California

Jones and Bartlett Publishers
Sudbury, Massachusetts

Boston   London   Singapore

To Judy

Editorial, Sales, and Customer Service Offices

Jones and Bartlett Publishers
40 Tall Pine Drive
Sudbury, MA 01776
508-443-5000
1-800-832-0034

Jones and Bartlett Publishers International
Barb House, Barb Mews
London W6 7PA
UK

Library of Congress Cataloging-in-Publication Data
Eddy, David M., 1941-
    Clinical decision making : from theory to practice : a collection
of essays from The Journal of the American Medical Association /
David M. Eddy.
        p.   cm.
    Includes index.
    ISBN 0-7637-0143-2
    1. Medicine—Decision making.   2. Medical policy.   I. JAMA
II. Title.
        [DNLM: 1. Decision Making—collected works.   2. Health Services—
    collected works.   W 7 E21   1996]
R723.5.E33   1996
362.1'068--dc20
DNLM/DLC
for Library of Congress   96-4705
                                                                                CIP

Acquisitions Editor: Joseph E. Burns
Production Administrator: Anne S. Noonan
Senior Manufacturing Buyer: Dana L. Cerrito
Editorial Production Service: Ocean Publication Services
Typesetting: Ruth Maassen
Printing and Binding: Malloy Lithographing, Inc.
Cover Printing: Henry N. Sawyer Co., Inc.
Cover Design: Hannus Design Associates

Printed in the United States of America
00 99 98 97 96   10 9 8 7 6 5 4 3 2 1

❖ Contents

v

❖ Foreword

❖ Clinical Decisions: Practical, Economic, and Ethical Considerations

What is a good clinician if not an empathetic collector of observations who then decides whether to do something or nothing for a patient in need?

And how are these decisions made? By long habit, by intellect, by scientific deduction, by experience, by consulting books or journals, by interactive computer algorithms, by consulting colleagues, or by gut feel?

And what kind of decisions are there? To decide to listen carefully to the patient, to do a specific physical examination, to order diagnostic tests, to perform invasive techniques, to refer to a colleague, to prescribe drugs, to do surgery, to use a trial of therapy, or to let time pass?

And for what reasons are decisions made? To earn money, to save costs, to obey a law, to protect against a lawsuit, to buy time, to placate patient anger, to satisfy the payer, to relieve pain and suffering, to prevent disability and premature death, and to restore function?

No clinician ever has a complete database as a prelude for action. The difference between an outstanding clinician and an average one is the speed and focus that are used to draw the right conclusions and institute the best patient management with the minimum essential information, cost, risk, inconvenience, and delay.

This book by David M. Eddy, MD, PhD, is a jewel of insight into just how clinicians actually make decisions and a prescription for how they should make decisions for individual patients and for populations of patients. The product of five years of writing in *JAMA*, the chapters collected herein constitute an acclaimed source of fundamental information for every clinician.

GEORGE D. LUNDBERG, MD
Editor, JAMA

*   *   *

A fundamental principle of economics is that the production of anything should be expanded only if the *incremental* benefits from further production cover the associated *incremental* costs. Undergraduates grasp this point quickly, because it is so sensible. Alas, clinicians and patients always have had difficulty with it, for it implies that clinicians may refrain from "doing everything possible" for patients. Clinicians are not trained to practice that kind of benefit-cost analysis, and patients are loath to accept it as well—perhaps even economists, when they are patients.

In fairness, it must be conceded that economists usually offer their dictum in the abstract. Few of them have bothered to translate their hollowed principle into concrete guidelines that are useful at the patient's bedside. The American Economic Association, for example, would be hard put to field a toll-free telephone number to which practicing clinicians could call when confronted by the troublesome trade-offs implied by the principle. In the context of health care, the economist's principle has remained brave talk.

David M. Eddy, MD, PhD, is able to think and write like a physician and an economist. For years he has tried to bridge this glaring gap between principle and practice. The fruits of his labors are offered in this collection of his essays. The volume will undoubtedly be on the syllabus of every course on health economics, as many of his papers already have been, for they are not just models of decision analysis. They are also models of fine pedagogy.

Some of Eddy's essays (for example, his "Anatomy of a Decision") are lectures on clinical decisions at the individual patient's bedside. They offer a systematic approach to assessing the often subtle benefits and costs associated with particular treatment regimens. Here Eddy makes the important distinction between the two basic steps in clinical decisions: first, the clinician's *objective* estimate of the effect of a given treatment will have on the probability of particular outcomes and, second, the patient's *subjective* evaluation of these outcomes and their associated probabilities. While the second task may be beyond the mental acumen of many patients and their families, and often lands in the clinician's lap as well, it is nevertheless useful to reinforce that distinction in the clinician's mind.

Other essays in the volume address the perennial conflict between the individual's and society's perspectives on benefit-cost analyses. Eddy's "Connecting Value and Costs: Whom Do We Ask, and What Do We Ask Them?" and "The Individual and Society: Is There a Conflict?" are classics of this genre. These essays are useful reading not only for clinicians, but also for pollsters who regularly confuse the debate on health policy with surveys that ask the public entirely the wrong questions.

The tension between the individual's and society's perspectives in health care will be played out time and again within the walls of the so-called Accountable Health Plans (AHPs) that are to be the center stage of managed competition. A central tenet of managed competition is that the AHPs competing for enrollees should be held accountable on performance standards that are *averaged* over all of a plan's enrollees. These population-based *averages* necessarily trigger within each AHP trade-offs among individual patients. The trade-offs will be troublesome and may even attract the wrath of our tort system, because they entail *rationing* in the individual case to enhance the plan's reported *average* quality of health care.

Eddy offers a compelling logic for these trade-offs in several of his essays, notably in his "Rationing Resources Without Cutting Quality: How to Get More for Less." His prescription in these essays will remain controversial—certainly among libertarians—but his essays do constitute an answer to a decade-old dream had, first, by policy analysts on the left of the political spectrum (in the 1960s and 1970s) and now more vigorously pushed by analysts in the center and on the right of that spectrum. It is the dream to make our health system measurably accountable for the health of our entire population.

UWE E. REINHARDT, PHD
James Madison Professor of Political Economy
Woodrow Wilson School of Public
and International Affairs
Princeton University

* * *

Clinical decision making is notoriously subject to ungrounded assertions and facile generalization. The whole range of critical questions related to this central fact of the clinician-patient relationship has too long been sequestered from empirical examination. Yet, no topic is more crucial for the welfare of individual patients, the elaboration of public policy, and the ultimate utility and probity of any putative health care system reform.

The need to understand the structure of the clinical decision and to gather reliable data about effectiveness, benefits, harms, and outcomes of care should be obvious. Yet, the methodology for obtaining and validating reliable data is still imprecise and in need of development. Eddy's work employs a methodology and an interpretative format that has yielded useful data, applicable both to individual clinical decisions and to policy formulation.

Eddy's work shows just how far we are from ascertaining the reliability and precision of clinical decisional processes. His analyses emphasize the variability among and between clinicians in observations, perceptions of outcome, and reasoning processes. He has shown convincingly how these variations affect the outcome of diagnosis, prognosis, and treatment.

Eddy provides a basis for the design of practice policies and guidelines, as well as decisions concerning cost-benefit, cost-effectiveness, and cost-rationing. He pinpoints sources of error in data collection and clinical reasoning. Equally significant, he reminds us of the limitations of some of the more commonly used ways of measuring quality of care and outcomes. Given the probable irreversibility of current trends toward more organized, managed, and economically driven systems of health care, assessments of the kind Eddy has produced are indispensable. They help to grasp the nondollar as well as the dollar costs of any prepaid care system.

Ultimately, a viable health care system must be ethically as well as economically based. While Eddy's work is not analyzed ethically in any formal sense, it affords, nonetheless, an essential propaedeutic for reflection on the ethical impact of practice guidelines, policies, and regulations of proposed national health care policies. Eddy's data are crucial to answering the key ethical question: of all the things we *can* do, which *should* or *ought* we do? This question fuses the technical with the ethical aspects of the clinical decision. Without the anchor of empirical fact, health care ethics becomes speculation without moorings.

EDMUND D. PELLEGRINO, MD
Director, Center for Clinical Bioethics
John Carroll Professor of Medicine
and Medical Ethics
Georgetown University Medical Center

❖ Preface

In these chapters I have tried to lay out a unified theory of medical practice, and practical recommendations for applying the theory, that respond to the changing environment in which medical decisions are made. That environment is demanding something that seems impossible; we must simultaneously increase the quality of medical care while curtailing its costs. Indeed, the last quarter century has delivered two huge forces that are changing the way medicine is and will be practiced, forever. They both begin with the people who pay the bills—whether out of pocket, through insurance premiums or HMO dues, higher costs for goods and services (which pay for employee health benefits), or income taxes. The bill payers have said they will not continue to pay health care costs that rise twice as fast as the general inflation rate and incomes. Simultaneously they have begun to ask about the quality of the product they are receiving for their money. The latter is not a pretty sight: wide variations in practice patterns without any obvious medical justification; studies indicating that, according to expert panels, from one fourth to one half of the indications for which some major procedures are done are inappropriate or equivocal; studies showing that the experts themselves might not know what they are talking about; and exposés that major diseases are being treated on the flimsiest of evidence. Clearly, we need to rethink what we are trying to do and how we are doing it.

So that is "The Challenge" (Chapter 1). The remainder of the chapters try to solve this problem. They cover the central topics that have become buzzwords: guidelines, evidence-based medicine, explicit methods, conflict resolution, outcomes, patient preferences, costs, cost-effectiveness, the conflict between the individual and society, principles for making tough choices, responsibilities of practitioners, priority-setting, a formula for how to get more for less, and rationing (yes, rationing; we need to get used to that word).

To call the ideas I have described a unified theory is perhaps overblown. The unifying principle is actually quite simple; it is that we are in this business to serve people, and that means not only maintaining and restoring their health, but doing it without violating the budget they are willing to spend. We need to serve people not only when they are in our offices seeking care, but when they are in their living rooms writing out checks. A car salesman who sells a Lexus to a person who can afford only a Honda might have delivered higher quality, but has done the person a disservice. The unifying principle is that when we run into a tough choice, we should try to resolve it by reference to the people we serve: what is important to them and how they weigh the different consequences. But a theory is only half of a solution. The other half is implementation. In these chapters I have tried to be as practical as possible, consistent with the level at which these issues have to be discussed. I have tried to answer the question: What do we actually *do*? I mean, what do we do *tomorrow*?

The book has two parts. All but four of the chapters, the ones that weave through the ideas described above, were originally written for *JAMA* as part of a series. These chapters comprise Part I. Part II consists of four additional chapters that were not part of the series but were added to this collection to fill out the ideas. Chapter 28 is one of the original articles that described the existence and role of guidelines; chapter 29 discusses the importance of physician uncertainty; chapter 30 crosses the entire spectrum from our problems to the solutions. And I give the last word to my mother in chapter 31.

I have never liked articles that end up saying, "So these are important problems that society will have to address as we move into the 21st century." Society is us, or at least we are a very important part of it. There is no point in waiting for someone else to address these problems. What happens in the end will depend on how all of us respond to the forces at work. This book is a small push from a small tugboat against a very large battleship. But it does commit to a specific course of action.

❖ Acknowledgments

This is my opportunity to thank George D Lundberg, MD, *JAMA*'s editor, for giving me the opportunity to write for the world's largest and one of its most respected journals. His leadership has been invaluable. I also thank him for the wide latitude he has given me in writing styles. Through his editorial policies and aggressive pursuit of papers that address critical policy issues, he has become an important national force in health care.

I want to acknowledge the staff at *JAMA* and the American Medical Association for helping publish the original articles and this book. Specifically, I thank Mary Ann Lilly, Susan R Benner MLS, Brian P Pace MA, Norman Frankel PhD, and Annette Flanagin RN, MA, for their help in editing and publishing the collection of articles.

I also want to thank Joe Burns and his colleagues at Jones and Bartlett. Their contributions go far beyond the usual publishing chores. Through their commitment to health policy they have had a strong effect on the shaping of this terribly important national issue.

Finally, I want to thank my wife Judy, not only for all of her work in actually producing the articles and proofing the book, but for her help in developing the ideas.

❖ Part I

❖ CHAPTER 1
The Challenge

Medical practice is in the middle of a profound transition. Most physicians can remember the day when, armed with a degree, a mission, and confidence, they could set forth to heal the sick. Like Solomon, physicians could receive patients, hear their complaints, and determine the best course of action. While not every patient could be cured, everyone could be confident that whatever was done was the best possible. Most important, each physician was free, trusted, and left alone to determine what was in the best interest of each patient.

All of that is changing. In retrospect, the first changes seem minor—some increased paperwork, "tissue" committees, a few more meetings. These activities were designed to affect the presumably small fraction of physicians who, in fact, deserved to be scrutinized, and the scrutiny was an internal process performed by physicians themselves. But today's activities are aimed at all physicians, are much more anonymous, and seem beyond physician control. Now physicians must deal with second opinions, precertification, skeptical medical directors, variable coverage, outright denials, utilization review, threats of cookbook medicine, and letters out of the blue chiding that Mrs Smith is on two incompatible drugs. Solomon did not have to call anyone to get permission for his decisions. What is going on?

What is going on is that one of the basic assumptions underlying the practice of medicine is being challenged. This assumption is not just a theory about cholesterol, antiarrhythmics, or estrogens. This assumption concerns the intellectual foundation of medical care. Simply put, the assumption is that whatever a physician decides is, by definition, correct. The challenge says that while many decisions no doubt *are* correct, many are not, and elaborate mechanisms are needed to determine which are which. Physicians are slowly being stripped of their decision-making power.

❖ Challenging the Quality of Clinical Decisions

Why is the assumption that physicians' decisions are correct being challenged? At first thought, the challenge might appear to be a pernicious scheme launched by payers, motivated to save money, even at the expense of quality. Actually, while the rapid and apparently uncontrollable rise in health care costs might have been the initial pressure point, the challenge can be justified solely by a concern for quality. The plain fact is that many decisions made by physicians appear to be arbitrary—highly variable, with no obvious explanation. The very disturbing implication is that this arbitrariness represents, for at least some patients, suboptimal or even harmful care.

These are strong words that demand explanation. What is the evidence that decisions are arbitrary? The most impressive clues come in the form of variations across and within physicians with respect to observations, perceptions, reasoning, conclusions, and practices.

Observer variations have been recognized for decades, but the findings are still startling, and the problem has not been solved. A correct decision about an intervention requires that a patient's condition be diagnosed correctly. Substantial variations in what physicians see have been reported in virtually every aspect of the diagnostic process, from taking a history, to doing a physical examination, reading laboratory tests, performing a pathological diagnosis, and recommending a treatment. A 1985 bibliography listed more than 400 articles that describe this problem.[1] In general, observers looking at the same thing will disagree with each other or even with themselves from 10% to 50% of the time.

An example will provide the flavor. When four cardiologists were given high-quality coronary angiograms of representative patients and asked to estimate whether the percentage of stenosis in the proximal and distal left anterior descending artery was greater or less than 50%, they disagreed on 60% of the patients. If the distinction between proximal and distal stenosis is ignored and the question is reduced to whether there is 50% stenosis in any segment, they still disagreed on 40% of patients.[2] Another study evaluated the extent to which observers agreed with themselves on two successive readings of the same angiograms. The observers changed their minds from 8% to 37% of the time, depending on the vessel segment.[3]

The evidence of variations in perceptions is equally distressing. The crux of any decision is to estimate the consequences of the available options. It is easy to appreciate that if a physician's perception of the outcomes of alternative interventions is incorrect, the chance that he or she will choose the best intervention for a patient is severely threatened. Now consider the following true story. A specialty society, which by prior agreement will remain anonymous, convened a meeting to set a guideline about one of their most common and important practices. The 57 participants identified one particular outcome as being especially important. They agreed that a practitioner's belief about the magnitude of the outcome would largely determine his or her belief about the proper use of the practice and would determine his or her recommendation to a patient. The practitioners, all specialists in the field, were then asked to write down their beliefs about the probability of the outcome for a particular patient—who was described in considerable detail. The 57 respondents provided estimates that ranged from 0% to 100% (Figure 1.1).

It is tempting to speculate that nonspecialists would have a wider range of opinions, but the spread can hardly get any wider. Before anyone gets smug, understand that no specialty is immune. For example, after several meetings and a *unanimous* consensus, experts' estimates of the effect of colon cancer screening on colon cancer mortality ranged from 5% to 95%.[4] Fifty cardiovascular surgeons' estimates of the probabilities of various risks associated with xenografts vs mechanical heart valves ranged from 0% to about 50%. For one particular risk, the 10-year probability of valve failure with xenografts, the range of estimates was 3% to 95%.[5]

Even if decision makers' perceptions of the facts were always accurate, that information must be processed to draw conclusions applicable to individual patients. With rare exceptions, physicians depend on their judgment and intuition to do this. But it is easy to be misled. Rather than cite studies, I will ask a question. You have ordered a diagnostic test for a patient to rule out a relatively uncommon but serious disease that, given this patient's signs and symptoms, has a prevalence of approximately 1 in 100. The test, which has a sensitivity of 80% and a specificity of 80%, has positive results. You repeat the test and it has positive results a second time. What is the probability that the patient has the disease? Everyone should get the correct answer: this is one of the most straightforward and common problems encountered in medical practice, the problem has been simplified to the extreme, all of the ingredients have been presented, and the solution method (Bayes' theorem) was developed more than 200 years ago and has been described in scores of medical publications during the last 25 years. Yet, it is still a safe bet that at least 20% of physicians will get the wrong answer. (The correct answer is between 4% [if the tests are totally dependent] and 14% [if the tests are independent].) Our intuitions about problems like this are easily fooled by a variety of cognitive biases.[6] For other medical examples, see Berwick and colleagues.[7]

Given the variations in observations, perceptions, and reasoning, it is easy to imagine that when faced with the same information, different physicians can draw different conclusions. A study of second opinions illustrates the point. Surgeons given written descriptions of surgical problems have split down the middle regarding whether to recommend surgery—half recommending surgery, half not.[8] When surveyed again 2 years later, the same surgeons often disagreed with their previous opinions, with as many as 40% changing their recommendations.[9]

But the ultimate question is whether these uncertainties and variations cause patients to be treated differently. It appears that they do. For example, an analysis of procedure rates for Medicare patients in 13 large metropolitan areas in the United States showed that for more than half the procedures

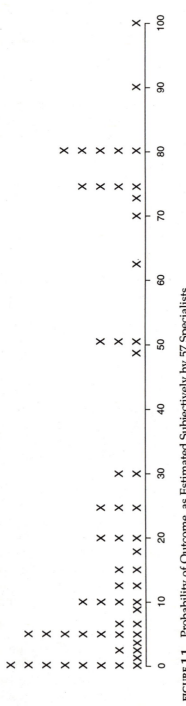

FIGURE 1.1 Probability of Outcome, as Estimated Subjectively by 57 Specialists.

studied, the rates varied more than 300% between the areas with high and low rates.[10] Another study that compared utilization rates in 16 large communities in four states found more than threefold differences between the highest and lowest rates for heart bypass, thyroid, and prostate surgery; fivefold differences for specific back and abdominal surgeries; sevenfold differences for knee replacements; and almost 20-fold differences for carotid endarterectomies (J. E. Wennberg, MD, oral communication, February 28, 1987). In Vermont, the chance of having one's tonsils removed as a child are 8% in one community and 70% in another. In Iowa, 15% of the men younger than 85 years in one region have had prostatectomies compared with more than 60% in another. In Maine, the chance of hysterectomy by the age of 70 years varies across communities from less than 20% to more than 70%.[11] While some of the variations might be explained by differences in disease incidence, available resources, and patient preferences, it is impossible to explain all of them.

These findings conjure up the image of a $650-billion tank rumbling down the road, with, depending on how you look at it, either no hands or a thousand hands on the wheel and the windows fogged over. To be fair, it must be understood that the evidence just given presents a caricature, highlighting the big nose, weak chin, and bald head. But it is undeniable that at least some decisions about important medical practices are subject to factors that are uncertain and variable. When so many people have such different beliefs and are doing such different things, it is absolutely impossible for everyone to be correct. There is a distinct possibility that many decisions made by practitioners are wrong—wrong in the sense that they are based on mistaken perceptions of the facts, and wrong in the sense that they are not in their patients' best interests.

The discovery that many of our decisions are vulnerable to error should not be surprising. The ingredients needed for accurate decisions are simply missing for many medical practices. The first ingredient is evidence—accurate, interpretable, applicable observations of the frequencies with which important outcomes occur with different practices. That type of evidence is not available for a large proportion of medical practices. When there is no formal evidence, practitioners have little choice but to turn to their personal experiences. However, these are notoriously misleading: the numbers of observations are small, there are no controls, patients' and physicians' decisions about interventions are not random, follow-up is incomplete and usually short-term, and memories are highly selective. The second ingredient is the ability to analyze the evidence. Even if good evidence were available, it is unrealistic, even unfair, to expect people to be able to sort through it all in their heads—especially people who were trained to provide medical care, not to analyze evidence and perform calculations.

❖ Implications for Clinical Practice

In summary, there is good reason to challenge the assumption that every individual practitioner's decision is necessarily correct. A failure of the assumption has immense implications for the quality of care. It implies that the same patient can go to different physicians, be told different things, and receive different care. No doubt some of the differences will not be important. However, some will surely be important—leading to different chances of benefits, different harms, and different costs. A failure of the assumption also has immense implications for informed consent, expert testimony, consensus development, the concepts of "standard and accepted" or "reasonable and necessary," malpractice, quality assurance programs that are based on statistical norms, and the cost of care.

It is for all these reasons that insurance companies, employers, and the government, as well as the medical profession itself, are aggressively seeking to understand the magnitude of the problem and find solutions. No responsible institution can sit still while patients are subjected to serious interventions and costs fly, knowing that there is such a large random component to the decisions. Without evidence that differences in the intensity of practices yield proportionate increases in value, these institutions are virtually forced to act. The mechanisms that have been developed during the last several years to assure quality and contain costs are not sinister attempts to save money by cutting quality or to seize control. They are conscientious responses to a real problem—a problem that is harming not just the cost, but the quality of care.

❖ Will Second-Guessing Physicians Solve the Problem?

At this point, it is reasonable to ask whether the mechanisms that have been put in place thus far will correct the problem. Can pre-guessing and second-guessing each physician's decision be counted on to make the ultimate choice correct? Unfortunately, no. While these mechanisms are well intentioned, while they are steps in the right direction, and while they might be the best we can do right now, they will by no means correct every error. There are three main problems. The first is that the mechanisms themselves depend on a questionable assumption. Virtually all of the current quality assurance and cost-containment mechanisms assume that there is not only "safety in numbers" but "accuracy in numbers." In other words, if the decisions of the individual physicians cannot be trusted, the collective decisions or actions of a larger number of physicians can be trusted. Second opinions expand the basis for a decision to two, precertification expands it to the number of people who defined the indications, searching for outliers expands it to everyone in the database, and so forth. The problem is that each of these mechanisms attempts to correct possible misperceptions of one physician by checking the decision, not against reality, but against the perceptions of other physicians. Why should we assume that the physician offering the second opinion knows the correct answer? Is there reason to believe that the manual used in a precertification program contains the revealed truth? Outliers are not necessarily bad. (Albert Schweitzer was an outlier.) Who can say that a guideline developed by an expert panel is correct? Indeed, what does a consensus of a group whose perceptions might vary from 0% to 100% even mean?

The second problem with current quality assurance and cost-containment mechanisms is that many medical decisions are inherently too subtle to be made at a distance. While these mechanisms vary in their flexibility, they all are based to some degree on a presumption that decisions fall in a definable number of categories that can be addressed in the abstract, and the answers can be applied to individuals. The problem is that the cliché about patients being individuals is true. While it is possible and even desirable to guide decisions, it can be dangerous to try to make them from a distance.

The third problem is that, even if these quality assurance and cost-containment mechanisms worked in the sense of "correcting" incorrect decisions, they are cumbersome, expensive, and demoralizing for both physicians and patients. They also create an adversarial atmosphere that can only harm patient care. In short, the current mechanisms are unlikely to solve the problem. If applied forcefully enough, these mechanisms will decrease variations in practices, which will decrease our sense of discomfort about the variations (although not our discomfort about being second-guessed). But there is no guarantee that the targets these recommendations construct are correct, or that the gains they make are worth the cost in time, money, and hassle.

❖ Four Conclusions

Where does this leave us? First, it must be emphasized that medicine is not practiced at random and is not a fraud. Physicians are not the Keystone Kops. Decisions might be variable but they are not whimsical or flippant. The variability occurs because physicians must make decisions about phenomenally complex problems, under very difficult circumstances, with very little support. They are in the impossible position of not knowing the outcomes of different actions, but having to act anyway.

Second, it is undeniable that many if not most medical practices are effective. My mother is fond of pointing out that she would be blind, deaf, bedridden, and depressed, were it not for her cataract surgery, lens implants, hearing aids, hip replacements, and amitriptyline. While there are undoubtedly some ineffective and unnecessary practices, the real questions pertain to which treatments work best and whether the costs and risks of more risky and expensive practices are matched by proportionate benefits.

A third point is that the problems just described are no one's fault. No one is questioning the sincerity, honesty, or diligence of physicians. Physicians face one of the most difficult social and intellectual problems. In addition to the mysteries of human biology and disease and continually expanding technologies, they must deal with a bewildering variety of other forces: expectations of patients and families; personal, professional, and financial goals; changing reimbursement systems; competition; malpractice; peer pressure; the press; politics; and incomplete information.

These three points, while encouraging, do not allow us to relax. A fourth conclusion is that we can do much better than we are doing now. For example, clinical research is extremely inefficient. Some questions are dissected beyond recognition, while others are virtually ignored. A tremendous amount of research energy is wasted on poor designs that yield unusable results. Even good designs are spoiled by poor coordination with other research and with clinical reality.

It is also possible to improve our ability to reason both collectively and as individuals. Our current approach to analyzing evidence, estimating the consequences of our actions, and determining the desirability of those outcomes is primitive. We are trying to solve in our heads problems that far exceed the capacity of the unaided human mind. There are tools, already in use in many other disciplines, to help us.

❖ Where Do We Go From Here?

Ideally, decisions about medical practices should be made between physicians and their patients, with each decision tailored to fit the patient's problems and desires. However, to achieve this ideal, physicians must have solid information about the consequences of different choices and must be able to process that information accurately. Currently, we lack both the information required for decision making and the skills needed to process the information. Quality assurance and cost-containment mechanisms that attempt to pre-guess and second-guess physicians' decisions from a distance suffer from the same problems. While well intentioned, these mechanisms create one more factor that distorts and strains the ideal process without offering a permanent solution for the problem.

The solution is not to remove the decision-making power from physicians, but to improve the capacity of physicians to make better decisions. To achieve this solution, we must give physicians the information they need; we must institutionalize the skills to use that information; and we must build processes that support, not dictate, decisions.

Challenges are healthy. This one goes deep, but promises great value.

❖ References

1. Feinstein A. A bibliography of publications on observer variability. *J Chronic Dis*. 1985;38:619-632.
2. Zir L, Miller S, Dinsmore R, Gilbert J, Harthorne JW. Interobserver variability in coronary angiography. *Circulation*. 1976;53:627.
3. Detre K, Wright E, Murphy M, Takaro T. Observer agreement in evaluating coronary angiograms. *Circulation*. 1975;52:979.
4. Eddy D. Variations in physician practice: the role of uncertainty. *Health Aff*. 1984;3: 74-89 (Chapter 29).
5. O'Connor G, Plume S, Beck J, Marrin CS, Nugent WC, Olsmtead FM. What are my chances? It depends on whom you ask: the choice of a prosthetic heart valve. *Med Decis Making*. 1988;8:341.

6. Kahneman D, Slovic P, Tversky A. *Judgement Under Uncertainty: Heuristics and Biases*. New York, NY: Cambridge University Press; 1982.
7. Berwick D, Fineberg H, Weinstein M. When doctors meet numbers. *Am J Med*. 1981;71:991-998.
8. Rutkow I, Gittelsohn A, Zuidema G. Surgical decision making: the reliability of clinical judgment. *Ann Surg*. 1979;190:409.
9. Rutkow I. Surgical decision making: the reproducibility of clinical judgment. *Ann Surg*. 1982;117:337.
10. Chassin M, Brook R, Park R, et al. Variations in the use of medical and surgical services by the Medicare population. *N Engl J Med*. 1986;314:285.
11. Wennberg J. Dealing with medical practice variation: a proposal for action. *Health Aff*. 1984;3:6.

❖ Source

Originally published in *JAMA*. 1990;263:287-290.

❖ CHAPTER 2
Anatomy of a Decision

The quality of medical care is determined by two main factors: the quality of the decisions that determine what actions are taken and the quality with which those actions are executed—what to do and how to do it. If the wrong actions are chosen, no matter how skillfully they are executed, the quality of care will suffer. Similarly, if the correct actions are chosen but the execution is flawed, the quality of care will suffer.

The importance of ensuring the quality of execution is well understood. In contrast, the medical profession has done much less to develop and evaluate its decision-making processes. If decisions are considered the command post and actions are considered the troops in the field, we have spent much more energy training and equipping the troops than providing intelligence and decision-support systems to the commanders. The place to begin is with the ingredients of a decision.

❖ Anatomy

In general, the goal of a decision regarding a health practice is to choose the action that is most likely to deliver the outcomes that patients find desirable. This identifies the two main steps of a decision (Figure 2.1). First, the outcomes of the alternative practices must be estimated; then, the desirability of the outcomes of each option must be compared. The first step involves collecting and analyzing whatever evidence exists regarding the benefits, harms, and costs of each option. Because the available evidence is virtually never perfect or complete, this step will also involve some subjective judgment. The estimates that result from this analysis then form the basis for the second step. Three types of comparisons are required in the second

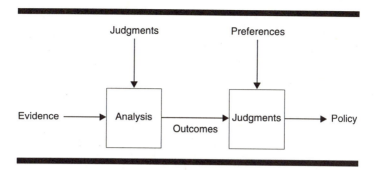

FIGURE 2.1   The Two Main Steps of a Decision.

step: (1) The benefits of a practice must be compared with the harms (such as risks, side effects, inconvenience, and anxiety). (2) The health outcomes must be compared with whatever costs will have to be paid. (3) If resources are limited and it is not possible to do everything, the amount of benefit gained and the resources consumed by a practice must be compared with other practices to give priority to practices that have the highest yield.

Explicitly or implicitly, consciously or subconsciously, correctly or incorrectly, each of these steps is performed every time a decision is made regarding a health practice. This is true whether the decision is made by an individual physician who is choosing an action for a particular patient, by a task force that is recommending a guideline to be applied to a group of patients, or by a third-party payer who is setting a coverage policy. To appreciate this, imagine trying to make a decision or design a guideline *without* giving any consideration to these issues. Imagine trying to advise a patient regarding the merits of a health practice without considering any evidence of its effects. Imagine not having any idea of the magnitudes of the benefits or harms of the practice, and imagine not caring whether the benefits outweighed the harms. Anyone who makes a responsible decision regarding a health practice must have some idea, however fuzzy, of the evidence that justifies its use, of its consequences, and of its desirability.

An example will solidify the concepts. Across from your desk is Mrs Smith, a 55-year-old, asymptomatic woman who is contemplating the pros and cons of being screened for breast cancer. The main benefit is that screening should decrease the probability she will die of breast cancer. Harms include the potential carcinogenic effect of the radiation; the chance of a false-positive result; and any inconvenience, discomfort, or anxiety associated with the examinations.

The first step in the decision for this woman is to estimate the magnitudes of these outcomes. Four prospective controlled trials[14] have observed decreases in the 10-year probability of breast cancer death resulting from approximately 5 years of screening. The actual decreases observed in the trials are 15 of 10 000, 9 of 10 000, 1 of 10 000, and 11 of 10 000. That is, of 10 000 women offered 5 years of screening in those trials, screening made the difference between life and death for 1 to 15 of the women. Three case-control studies[5-9] and one uncontrolled study,[10] because of their designs, cannot directly estimate how screening changes the actual probability of death from breast cancer, but their results are consistent with the four prospective trials. Combining all the results can be tricky, but for now let us assume the effect of 5 years of screening is to prevent a death from breast cancer for approximately 15 of 10 000 women. The probability of a false-positive result in this age group is approximately 2% per examination,[11] or approximately 10% for five annual examinations. Given modern techniques and radiation doses, the radiation should increase this woman's probability of developing breast cancer by less than 1 in 200 000. That completes the first step.

The second step is to weigh or compare these outcomes. Is a decrease in the probability of dying of breast cancer during the next 5 years of approximately 15 of 10 000 worth a 10% (1000 of 10 000) chance of a false-positive result, any inconvenience or anxiety associated with the five examinations, and a 1 in 200 000 chance of developing a new cancer?

It is important to separate the decision process into these two steps for several reasons. Specifically, the two steps involve different thought processes, have different anchors, and are performed by different people. In addition, we can expect different degrees of agreement about the results. The first step is a question of facts. The anchor is empirical evidence. The process is a scientific one that involves experiments, analysis of evidence, and forecasting. The required skills are analytic. Finally, assuming there is *some* evidence to evaluate, it should be possible to get reasonable, open-minded people to agree on the results of this step. There are rules of evidence and methods built up from axioms over hundreds of years that can be applied to the evidence. While there will always be some uncertainty and room for different scientific philosophies or schools of thought, there is at least the prospect that agreement can be reached. It is reasonable to imagine that there is a correct answer out there, and there is a scientific context and language for rational debate and resolution. In short, this is a job for the left side of the brain, and we turn to scientists to do it.

In contrast, the second step is a question not of facts but of personal values or preferences. The thought process is not analytic but personal and subjective—an appeal not to the left side of the brain, but to the right side of the brain, or even the gut. Different people can properly have different preferences. There is no single correct answer, and there is no obligation that everyone agree. To the extent that science is involved in this step at all, it is the science of discovering peoples' preferences—polls, questionnaires, and focus groups. Perhaps most important, the people whose preferences count are the patients, because they are the ones who will have to live (or die) with the outcomes. Others might intervene if an individual's decision is based on inaccurate information (eg, insistence on antibiotic therapy for a viral upper respiratory tract infection), is illegal (eg, drug abuse), or harms a public interest (eg, refusal of control measures for an infectious disease). However, assuming these complications do not apply, it is the patient's preference that should determine the decision.

With this in mind, revisit the example of screening for breast cancer. To estimate the possible benefits we look to the existing experiments, not to our imaginations, a coin, or what we hope will happen. The evidence is analyzed using accepted statistical techniques, and we should be able to reach agreement regarding the estimate of 15 of 10 000, or at least on a small range of uncertainty around it (eg, 10 of 10 000 to 20 of 10 000). If you disagree with my estimate, we can review the evidence (perhaps I overlooked an important experiment), review the statistical methods (perhaps I miscalculated), and in a scientific fashion seek to resolve the differences. The second step, however, should be handled differently. Ideally, you and I are not even in the picture. What matters is what Mrs Smith thinks. She might say the benefits are well worth the risks and inconvenience and whatever cost she has to pay; perhaps she is cancerphobic. On the other hand, she might find the benefits too small to be worth the trouble. Perhaps she is not concerned about cancer or dreads the possibility of a biopsy with a false-positive result. We can strive to make particular activities, such as being examined for breast cancer, agreeable and positive and can try to ensure that patients have accurate information regarding long- and short-term outcomes. However, in the end, it is the patient's preferences, not ours, that count. It is also quite possible that Mrs Smith's preferences will differ from Mrs Brown's preferences. If so, both are correct, because "correct" is defined separately for each woman. Assuming that both women are accurately informed regarding the outcomes, neither should be persuaded to change her mind.

Nancy Reagan's decision[12] to have a radical mastectomy for her early-stage breast cancer illustrates these points eloquently:

> At the time of my operation, there were some people, including doctors, who thought I had taken too drastic a step in choosing the mastectomy instead of a lumpectomy, which involved removing only the tumor itself and a small amount of tissue—but also weeks of radiation. I resented these statements, and I still do. This is a very personal decision, one that each woman must make for herself. This was my choice, and I don't believe I should have been criticized for it. For some women, it would have been wrong, but for me it was right. Perhaps, if I had been 20 years old and unmarried, I would have made a different decision. But I've already had my children and I have a wonderful, understanding husband.

❖ Pathology

Where can the decision process go wrong? The main sources of error correspond to the two main steps. A decision can be flawed either if there is a misperception of the outcomes or if there is a misperception of the values that patients place on the outcomes. Misperceptions of the outcomes can occur in many ways. Important outcomes might be ignored, extraneous outcomes might be included, the available evidence regarding an outcome might be incomplete, some of the existing evidence might be overlooked, the evidence might be misinterpreted, our reasoning might be incorrect, personal experiences (anecdotes) might be given undue weight, or we might simply succumb to wishful thinking. For example, some might have assumed that, because breast cancer is such a common cancer, that the benefits of screening must be high and not thought it necessary to review the actual evidence. Some might have heard that screening reduces mortality by approximately 30% and confused this *relative* reduction with an *actual* reduction in the chance of death. (Some might not even know the difference between a relative reduction and an actual change in an outcome.) A practitioner might have screened hundreds of women without ever finding a case and assumed the benefits were *smaller* than is actually the case.

Misperceptions of patient preferences can also occur. Patients might misunderstand an outcome, the measure of the effect might be misleading, the outcomes can be presented in different ways that lead to different conclusions, the patient might not be consulted at all, or physicians might project their own preferences onto their patients. In the example of screening for breast cancer, a woman might respond differently to hearing that "out of 10 000 women like you, screening during the next 5 years will make the difference between life and death from breast cancer for 15 women," compared with "screening will decrease your probability of dying of breast cancer by 15 of 10 000." People will respond differently if told that "screening will reduce your chance of dying of breast cancer by 30%," than if told that "screening will reduce your chance of dying of breast cancer from approximately 45 of 10 000 to approximately 30 of 10 000 (a reduction of approximately 30%)." Some people might misunderstand what a biopsy is, perhaps confusing it with a mastectomy or with a blood test. The word "radiation" might be so charged that it takes on an importance far beyond its actual impact.

❖ Treatment

Our goal is to avoid these pitfalls. Attention to three principles will help. First, decisions should be based on outcomes that are important to patients. These are the "health outcomes" that patients can experience and care about—pain, anxiety, death, disfigurement, and disability. It is important to distinguish health outcomes from intermediate outcomes, such as statistics (eg, the prevalence of a cancer), intermediate biological outcomes (eg, cell type of a cancer, serum cholesterol level), and test results. These "intermediate outcomes" may affect the effectiveness of an intervention, and can indicate the possible occurrence of health outcomes but by themselves cannot be experienced by a patient, and should not be the basis for a decision. The logic for this principle is straightforward; the ultimate purpose of all medical practice is to maintain and improve the health of patients. The only way to achieve this is to focus on the outcomes they can experience and care about—health outcomes.

Second, the effects of a practice on outcomes should be estimated as accurately as possible, given the available evidence. This implies that to the greatest extent possible, the estimates of outcomes should be anchored to evidence, all the pertinent evidence should be considered, the evidence should be interpreted accurately, any analytical methods should be appropriately chosen for the complexity of the problem, the estimates should not be affected by personal or professional biases, and the information should be presented in a form that is meaningful and intelligible to patients.

The third principle is that the preferences assigned to the outcomes of an intervention should reflect as accurately as possible the preferences of the people who will receive the outcomes—that is, patients. Patients should be encouraged to participate in the decisions to the extent they want. If a patient chooses to delegate the decision, the person chosen to act as the agent must understand that the values he or she expresses will be projected onto patients. That is, the agent's preferences will determine what will happen to another person. The responsibility obviously should not be taken lightly.

These principles might sound obvious, but it is easy to be misled. In the past, decisions have been determined by a variety of extraneous criteria. Some examples are instructive. Decisions have been based on the *type* of evidence available for an intervention (eg, "if there is no direct evidence from randomized controlled trials, you should not use the intervention"); the *degree of certainty* regarding the existence of an effect (eg, "the P value is only .1, which is not statistically significant; the intervention should not be used"); the actions of the *average* practitioner (eg, "if everyone is doing it, the intervention must be appropriate"); the *commonness* of the disease (eg, "if the disease is common, we have no choice but to use whatever treatment is available"); the *seriousness* of the outcome (eg, "if the outcome without treatment is very bad, we have to assume the treatment will work"); the *need to do something* (eg, "this intervention is all we have"); and the novelty or technical appeal of the intervention (eg, "if the machine takes a pretty picture, it must have some use").

Additional factors include pressure from the patient, the family, the press, the courts, the amount of paperwork, and personal financial interests. While each of these factors must be considered, and while some will continue to affect decisions regarding health practices, the ultimate purpose of the entire health care enterprise does not change—it is to improve the actual health outcomes of patients.

Given all these issues, what can we reasonably expect physicians to be able to do? Begin with the second step—the value judgments. If physicians are provided good information regarding how alternative practices affect the outcomes that are important to patients, physicians can discuss that information with their patients and either help them evaluate the options and make a decision for themselves, or, if patients choose to delegate the decision, make it for them. Obviously, we must be wary of imposing our own preferences or being swayed by extraneous factors and self-interest, but communicating with patients regarding their options is at the heart of the physician-patient relationship.

On the other hand, it is *not* realistic to expect physicians to be able to estimate the outcomes of different decisions accurately.[13] This task requires access to research results, analytical skills, and time, none of which are readily available to practicing physicians. The analysis of evidence and estimation of outcomes is a discipline in itself, requiring about as much training as is needed to train a physician. A physician who is trained to do surgery or read a CT scan can no more be expected to research scores of articles, analyze experimental designs, adjust for biases, and perform calculations, than a statistician can be expected to remove an appendix.

This seems to doom decisions to inaccuracy. Fortunately, during the last two millennia an ingenious solution has evolved. The solution is to analyze as many decisions as possible in advance, potentially taking whatever time, resources, and skills are needed to make the most accurate estimates of the outcomes of alternative practices, and then pass this information to practicing physicians. This is the role of practice policies or guidelines.

❖ References

1. Tabar L, Faberberg G, Duffy S, Day N. The Swedish two county trial of mammographic screening for breast cancer: recent results and calculation of benefit. *J Epidemiol Community Health*. 1989;43:107-114.
2. Andersson I, Aspergren K, Janzon L, et al. Mammographic screening and mortality from breast cancer: the Malmo mammographic screening trial. *BMJ*. 1988;297:943-948.
3. UK Trial of Early Detection of Breast Cancer Group. First results of mortality reduction in the UK trial of early detection of breast cancer. *Lancet*. 1988;2:411-416.
4. Shapiro S, Venet W, Strax P, Venet P. Current results of the Breast Cancer Screening Randomized Trial: The Health Insurance Plan (HIP) of Greater New York Study. In: *Screening for Breast Cancer*. Toronto, Canada: Sam Huber Publishing; 1988:chap 6.
5. Verbeek A, Hendriks J, Holland R, Mravunac M, Sturmans F. Mammographic screening and breast cancer mortality: age-specific effects in Nijmegen Project, 1975-82. *Lancet*. 1985;1:865-866.
6. Palli D, DelTurco M, Buiatti E, et al. A case-control study of the efficacy of a non-randomized breast cancer screening program in Florence (Italy). *Int J Cancer*. 1986; 38:501-504.
7. de Waard F, Collette H, Rombach J, Collette C. Breast cancer screening, with particular reference to the concept of 'high-risk' groups. *Breast Cancer Res Treat*. 1988;11: 125-132.
8. Collette H, Rombach J, Day N, de Waard F. Evaluation of screening for breast cancer in a non-randomised study (the DOM Project) by means of a case-control study. *Lancet*. 1984;1:1224-1226.
9. Verbeek A, Hendriks J, Holland R, Mravunac M, Sturmans F, Day N. Reduction of breast cancer mortality through mass screening with modern mammography: first results of the Nijmegen Project, 1975-1981. *Lancet*. 1984;1:1222-1224.

10. Seidman H, Gelb S, Silverberg E, La Verda N, Lubera J. Survival experience in the Breast Cancer Detection Demonstration Project. *CA*. 1987;37:258-289.
11. Baker L. Breast Cancer Detection Demonstration Project: five-year summary report. *CA*. 1982;32:19A-225.
12. Reagan N, Novak W. *My Turn: The Memoirs of Nancy Reagan*. New York, NY: Random House; 1989.
13. Eddy D. The challenge. *JAMA*. 1990;263:287-290 (Chapter 1).

❖ Source

Originally published in *JAMA*. 1990;263:441-443.

CHAPTER 3

Practice Policies and Guidelines

What Are They?

Practice policies are preformed recommendations issued for the purpose of influencing decisions about health interventions. As will be described below, practice policies come in a wide variety of forms. By far, the most common is the clinical practice guideline, or simply guideline, which is intended to help practicing physicians manage their patients.

The basic problem addressed by practice policies is that most health decisions are too complicated to be made on a one-by-one, day-to-day basis.[1] To make a health decision from scratch would involve identifying the options; identifying the possible outcomes of each option; evaluating the evidence that relates the options to the outcomes; estimating the consequences of each option; weighing the benefits of each option against its harms and costs; factoring in a variety of logistic, economic, legal, social, and personal considerations; and choosing the option that is in some sense the "best." If every practitioner attempted to do this for every decision, the result would be either mental paralysis or chaos.

Practice policies have been used for centuries to help solve this problem by enabling practitioners and researchers to analyze decisions before the fact, cast the conclusions as policies, and apply the policies to simplify future decisions. While many decisions can be addressed only on an individual basis, others recur frequently in similar forms. It is these "generic" decisions that are the targets of practice policies.

❖ Two Examples

The crucial role played by practice policies is illustrated by two examples. First, imagine a patient who sees a practitioner for frostbite of the foot. Several days have passed since the injury, dry gangrene has set in, and a black, wood-hard eschar has formed. The practitioner must decide how to treat it.

Compared with other decisions, this one is fairly straightforward. The patient is otherwise healthy, with no concurrent diseases or risk factors. The injury is well defined and limited. There are only a few outcomes to worry about, and they are easy to imagine. Surgery is unpleasant, could lead to infection, and if done too soon, might remove tissue that could have survived. On the other hand, if surgical debridement or amputation is necessary, the longer the delay the greater the chance of infection. It is also inconvenient for a patient to deal with dead tissue on his foot; if it will never recover, why not remove it? And if delay is chosen, for how long?

Ideally, the decision to operate would be determined by the practitioner's assessment of the probabilities of the various outcomes and their consequences. Questions include: What is the chance of infection? What is the chance I can save some tissue if I wait? How much tissue can I expect to recover?

The problem, of course, is that answers to these questions require observations of scores, if not hundreds of patients with this problem, some operated on immediately, some with delay. And because all patients differ in ways that could affect both the decision to operate and the outcome (eg, the extent of the frostbite), the cases, ideally, should be randomized between the two options. Our hypothetical practitioner has seen only five cases of frostbite, and three were fingers. The practitioner also knows that a handful of anecdotes can be very misleading. Even if all the practitioners in the area were consulted, they could not put together enough cases to draw meaningful conclusions. Nor do the textbooks describe the outcomes and probabilities needed to make a decision. Besides, our practitioner is not interested in starting a collaborative research project or building a decision tree; this patient is standing here now, waiting for an answer.

Fortunately, the answer exists. It is in all the textbooks: "Debridement and extirpation should be delayed until spontaneous amputation of the soft tissues is complete. This may take weeks or months."[2] (See also references 3 through 5.)[3-5]

For the second example, imagine a 51-year-old woman who was found, during a routine eye examination, to have ocular hypertension—29/27 mm Hg, 27/24 mm Hg, and 26/28 mm Hg on three separate readings. She has no other signs of glaucoma (eg, visual field defects or optical disc abnormalities) and has no special risk factors. Her ophthalmologist must decide whether to begin medical treatment. The main textbook on glaucoma[6] says the following:

> It is now clear that only about 0.5% to 1% of ocular hypertensive patients per year develop visual field loss as detected by kinetic perimetry. This creates a dilemma of what to do with these individuals who are at increased risk for developing primary open-angle glaucoma. On the one hand, ophthalmologists want to intervene as early as possible to prevent

optic nerve cupping and visual field loss. On the other hand, most ocular hypertensive individuals will lead their lives without developing substantial visual loss. Thus, instituting treatment in all patients does not seem reasonable taking into consideration the low incidence of ocular hypertension as well as the cost, inconvenience, side effects, noncompliance, and unproved efficacy of prophylactic therapy. . . . Most ocular hypertensive individuals do not require medical therapy. Treatment should be reserved for those patients who . . . are thought to be at high risk for developing glaucoma.

The authors then list about 100 risk factors, but do not state the actual increase in risk any of these factors implies. The authors also warn that "no parameter taken alone has proved to be a useful risk factor" and cite intraocular pressure as "the most obvious example of a single risk factor that fails to predict the development of primary open-angle glaucoma."

The authors have described the elements of the decision very well—the health outcomes that are the goal of treatment (prevent damage to the optic nerve and loss of visual field), the probabilistic nature of the outcomes, and the main drawbacks of treatment. Unfortunately, the text does not provide the probabilities that these outcomes will occur. For example, although the text gives the approximate probability a person with intraocular pressure greater than 20 mm Hg will develop visual field defects, it contains no information regarding how much the probability increases at various levels of intraocular pressure, how the probability is affected by any other risk factors, or how treatment can be expected to change the probability. In short, even if the ophthalmologist were inclined to try to analyze the decision, the most important information needed to do that is not presented. How then does an ophthalmologist decide to treat the patient? The authors of the text provide a guideline: "Many clinicians institute medical treatment if the intraocular pressure is 30 mm Hg or greater. . . . It may also be appropriate to recommend treatment for individuals with intraocular pressures in the middle to upper 20s who also have one or more risk factors."

Since this patient's pressures are all less than 30 mm Hg and she has no other risk factors, the ophthalmologist can apply the guideline to determine that treatment is not warranted.

❖ The Virtues of Practice Policies

Interest in practice policies and guidelines has exploded in the last few years. More than a dozen specialty societies, the American Medical Association, the National Institutes of Health, third-party payers, research groups, academic health centers, and commercial precertification and utilization review programs have all recently created programs to evaluate health practices and design practice policies. Government organizations such as the Health Care Financing Administration,[7] the Physician Payment Review Commission,[8] and the new Agency for Health Care Policy and Research (formerly the National Center for Health Services Research) have all identified the importance of practice policies, either by urging funding or by beginning research programs. Companion activities such as statistics, epidemiology, decision analysis, technology assessment, and health economics are feeding the effort. Perhaps most important, Congress has actually passed a bill to fund the design of guidelines and associated research.

This attention is entirely appropriate. Practice policies and guidelines present a powerful solution to the complexity of medical decisions. They free practitioners from the burden of having to estimate and weigh the pros and cons of each decision. They can connect each practitioner to a collective consciousness, bringing order, direction, and consistency to their decisions. Practice policies provide an intellectual vehicle through which the profession can distill the lessons of research and clinical experiences and pool the knowledge and preferences of many people into conclusions about appropriate practices. They provide a natural pathway to convey that information to practitioners. Practice policies are the central nervous system of medical practice.

Practice policies can have immense leverage. One well-designed policy—such as washing hands between deliveries—can improve the quality of care of hundreds of thousands of patients. Conversely, a poorly designed policy—such as performing lobotomies for the treatment of schizophrenia—can spoil the quality of care for just as many. A shift in a single policy—such as screening women younger than 50 years with mammography—can shift a billion dollars a year. Practice policies have the power to shape behavior for decades. A statement in 1916 by a single practitioner that "once a caesarean, always a caesarean"[9] based on a single patient still dominates that decision.

But along with this power is a remarkable delicacy. Practice policies can reach down to the finest level of detail. Mr Larsen has a carotid bruit. Should a carotid angiogram be done? If so, what views should be taken and how should he be positioned? What should be the radiation dose and exposure? What contrast material should be used? What medications should be on hand in case of an idiosyncratic reaction? There are practice policies for all of these and more. Practice policies have the potential to touch virtually every generic decision.

A final virtue of practice policies is that they provide the most natural mechanism for shaping physician behavior. They are an integral part of our individual and collective psychology, providing answers to questions that arise naturally as decisions are made. They can be finely tuned to fit the realities of clinical practice. As a mechanism for improving quality or containing cost, they can avoid the artificiality, inaccuracy, and imposition of more blunt approaches such as prepayment by diagnosis related groups, expenditure caps, and limits on lengths of stay. Practice policies are scalpels, not meat axes.

❖ Uses and Types of Practice Policies

Practice policies are extremely versatile. In addition to supporting individual decisions between practitioners and patients, practice policies can be used to specify who should perform a practice (eg, accreditation), how it should be performed (eg, performance criteria), where it should be performed (eg, inpatient vs outpatient), on whom it should be performed (eg, patient indications), and whether it will be paid for (eg, precertification criteria and coverage policies). They can be used prospectively to choose practices or retrospectively to judge the merits of practices after they are performed. They can be directed to structure (eg, the ratio of nurses and beds for an intensive care unit), process (eg, the need for institutional review for experiments that involve humans), and outcome (eg, an acceptable mortality rate for a surgical procedure). Their uses range all the way from the proper temperature for rewarming a frostbitten limb (40° C to 45° C), to guidelines for accepting gifts from drug companies.[10]

Practice policies are also the cornerstone of any effort to improve the quality and control the cost of health care. Practice policies are major determinants of what practitioners actually do. They are the comparison for judging the appropriateness of what is *about to be* done (eg, precertification and prospective utilization review) or what *was* done (eg, retrospective utilization review). Any quality assurance or cost-containment program that seeks to steer the behavior of practitioners will be using practice policies for its bearings.

❖ Flexibility of Practice Policies

Policies can accommodate a wide range of flexibility. A variety of terms have been introduced by different organizations to reflect different uses of practice policies. Examples are the American Medical Association's "practice parameters," the Joint Commission on Accreditation of Healthcare Organizations' "clinical indicators," and the American College of Physicians' "medical necessity guidelines." In general, the policies referred to by the different terms fall in one of three categories with respect to their intended degree of flexibility. "Guidelines" are intended to be flexible. They serve as reference points or recommendations, not rigid criteria. Guidelines *should* be followed in *most* cases, but there is an understanding that, depending on the patient, the setting, the circumstances, or other factors, guidelines can and should be tailored to fit individual needs. For example, "If vascular injury is the primary event (in frostbite), therapeutic measures to decrease vasoconstriction or blood clotting, such as sympathectomy or the administration of heparin should be of routine benefit."[4] "Standards," in contrast, are intended to be inflexible. They define correct practice, and should be followed, not tailored. (". . . A frostbitten part should never be exposed to hot water, an open fire, or excessively dry heat, as in an oven. . . ."[4]) The third category, "options" are so flexible as to provide virtually no guidance to a decision. Calling an intervention an option merely says that some practitioners use the intervention, while others do not, and there is little basis for determining which choice is correct. (". . . The use of fast-acting vasodilators such as papaverine [to treat frostbite] might be appropriate. . . ."[4]) The term "practice policy" covers the entire spectrum of uses and degrees of flexibility. However, because by far the most common use of practice policies is to assist physicians in their day-to-day decision making, and because by far the most common flexibility category is a guideline, the remainder of this chapter will focus on "practice guidelines" or simply "guidelines." In most contexts the terms "practice policies" and "guidelines" can be used interchangeably.

❖ Historical Role of Guidelines

The recent flood of attention to guidelines, while well deserved, tends to obscure the fact that they are neither new nor unusual. On the contrary, guidelines have been an integral part of medical decision making for centuries. Historically, they have appeared as statements in textbooks, indications and contraindications, drugs of choice, rules of thumb, recommended practices, essentials of diagnosis, standard practices, expert testimony, the correct answers to board examinations, and a wide variety of principles, maxims, rules, dicta, criteria, and axioms. If a decision is at all generic, the chances are someone has written a guideline for it.

To appreciate the ubiquity of guidelines, open any textbook, turn to any disease, find any section labeled "treatment," and begin reading. The text will be a series of guidelines. For example, "The immediate and basic care of frostbite, whether the tissue is blistered or discolored, is warming and cleaning followed by minimal debridement and watchful waiting for necrosis. After warming, the hand should be washed daily. (Some physicians use a Hubbard tank.) Blisters should not be debrided unless infected. Active motion should be encouraged and frequent washings continued. Amputation should be delayed until there is definite demarcation; this may require several weeks or a few months."[3]

Many guidelines have been in use for so long, they sound as though our grandmothers wrote them; in the Merck Manual the "adage" for treating frostbite is, "freeze in January, operate in July."[11]

❖ Recent Changes

However, several aspects of guidelines are new, and they have deep implications for the practice of medicine. Most important, there have been dramatic changes in the way guidelines are being produced and used. Until recently, virtually all guidelines were formed through an unplanned, highly decentralized, almost anonymous process and were addressed to individual practitioners to help them make individual decisions. During the last decade or so, a different approach to guidelines has been evolving. There are two main changes. First, the role of guidelines has been shifting away from serving as passive aids to decisions, available to practitioners for use as they see fit, to being used as active management tools. Practice policies in general and guidelines in particular now are being designed explicitly as instruments for quality assurance, precertification, utilization review, accreditation, coverage, and cost containment.

While this use of guidelines as a management tool might have a desirable impact on quality of care and health care costs, it has several undesirable effects for practitioners. One is that it puts a mechanism designed for internal use in the hands of "outsiders," such as utilization reviewers, the government, and insurers. Not only does this expose internal thoughts to external scrutiny, it opens those thoughts to manipulation. There is a concern that outsiders might write unnatural policies that do not match the instincts of practitioners. Another potential problem is misuse of a guideline. A practice policy intended to be a guideline or even an option might be misinterpreted as a standard, or a practice policy issued as a standard by a committee might not have wide support. But the greatest concern pertains to control. It is not stretching things too far to say that whoever controls guidelines controls medicine. That control used to lie exclusively, if diffusely, within the medical profession. However, as guidelines are designed and used as management tools, control could shift outside the profession. This possibility is a major force behind the surge of interest in guidelines. As nonphysician organizations develop guidelines to use as management tools, physician groups must race to develop their own guidelines, lest they lose control.

The second change affecting guidelines pertains to the methods by which they are being produced. The informal decentralized process is being replaced rapidly with formal programs. Guidelines used to evolve slowly over time, shaped by anonymous forces. Now they are made by committees and panels, with agendas, criteria, budgets, board approvals, and dissemination plans. This change in the methods used to design guidelines is critical to the future of medicine. This chapter has extolled the *potential* of practice policies and guidelines. Their actual performance, however, can vary tremendously, depending on how they are designed. The methods used to create guidelines will affect the number and types of practices that can be analyzed, the information and research required for the analyses, the skills needed to design policies, the cost and speed of the policy-setting process, the accuracy of the results, the credibility of the results, and the eventual impact of the entire exercise on patients. If the practice of medicine is largely determined by the practice policies and guidelines that guide it, the practice policies and guidelines themselves are largely determined by the methods used to create them.

❖ References

1. Eddy DM. Clinical policies and the quality of clinical practice. *N Engl J Med*. 1982; 307:343-347 (Chapter 28).
2. Shaw J. Frostbite. In: Rosen P, Baker F III, Barkin R, Braen G, Dailey R, Levy R, eds. *Emergency Medicine: Concepts and Clinical Practice*. St Louis, Mo: CV Mosby Co; 1988:chap 31.
3. Milford L. Special hand disorders. In: Crenshaw A, ed. *Campbell's Operative Orthopedics*. St Louis, Mo: CV Mosby Co; 1987:chap 9.
4. Imparato A, Riles T. Peripheral arterial disease. In: Schwartz S, Shires G, Spencer F, eds. *Principles of Surgery*. New York, NY: McGraw-Hill International Book Co; 1989: chap 21.
5. Demling R, Way L. Burns and other thermal injuries. In: Way L, ed. *Current Surgical Diagnosis and Treatment*. East Norwalk, Conn: Appleton & Lange; 1988:chap 15.
6. Hoskins H Jr, Kass M. *Becker-Shaffer's Diagnosis and Therapy of the Glaucomas*. 6th ed. St Louis, Mo: CV Mosby Co; 1989.
7. Roper W, Winkenwerder W, Hackbarth GM, Krakauer H. Effectiveness in health care: an initiative to evaluate and improve medical practice. *N Engl J Med*. 1988; 319:1197-1202.
8. Lee PR, Ginsburg PB, LeRoy LB, Hammons GT. The Physician Payment Review Commission report to Congress. *JAMA*. 1989;261:2382-2385.
9. Cragin E. Conservatism in obstetrics. *NY Med J*. 1916;104:1.
10. Chren MM, Landefeld C, Murray TH. Doctors, drug companies, and gifts. *JAMA*. 1989;262:3448-3451.
11. Berkow R, Fletcher A. *The Merck Manual of Diagnosis and Therapy*. 15th ed. Rahway, NJ: Merck Sharp & Dohme Research Laboratories; 1987.

❖ Source

Originally published in *JAMA*. 1990;263:877-878, 880.

CHAPTER 4

Guidelines—Where Do They Come From?

Recent changes in the methods used to create practice policies and guidelines have the potential to affect the quality and cost of medical care more profoundly than all the new treatments of the past or next decade. This potential comes from the fact that changes in methods for designing guidelines can be expected to change the content of guidelines, which in turn will guide hundreds of thousands of decisions about all interventions (preventive and diagnostic, as well as treatment), for decades to come. The changes currently under way in methods for designing guidelines represent a change in the intellectual basis of medicine.

The purpose of a guideline is to anticipate and simplify decisions that would otherwise have to be made on a one-by-one basis by individual physicians and their patients.[1] Thus, the tasks involved in the design of a guideline correspond to the two steps used by individuals for their decisions: estimation of the effects of a practice on outcomes important to patients, and comparison of the outcomes of the practice to determine whether its benefits outweigh its harms and whether its health outcomes are worth its costs.[2] The specific tasks are to (1) identify the important health outcomes, (2) analyze evidence for the effects of the practice on those outcomes, (3) estimate the magnitudes of the outcomes (benefits and harms), (4) compare the benefits and harms, (5) estimate the costs, (6) compare the health outcomes with the costs, and (7) compare alternative practices to determine which deserve priority. As with decisions made by individuals, all of these tasks are performed, explicitly or implicitly, every time a guideline is designed.

Note: This chapter was formerly titled "Practice Policies: Where Do They Come From?"

❖ The Traditional Approach

Guidelines have been used for centuries. Historically, their main role has been to summarize information regarding "standard and accepted" practices, not to change those practices. Thus, the traditional approach by which guidelines have been created is to identify practices considered to be standard and accepted, which in turn are defined by whatever practices are in common use.

Thus by the traditional approach, guidelines are not "designed." Rather, they evolve, continuously tracking practices in common use. The evolution occurs through textbooks, journal articles, speeches, letters to the editor, pronouncements by department chairpersons, and conversations in hospital cafeterias. The model is Adam Smith's 18th century marketplace.[3] The "invisible hand," which operates through individual decisions, can be counted on to sort everything out. Right ideas will thrive, wrong ideas will wither, and the collective medical consciousness will slowly converge on the correct guidelines.

An important feature of this approach is that the seven tasks for designing a guideline are never explicitly addressed. Instead, the tasks all occur implicitly, almost subconsciously, in the heads of practitioners and patients. Each participant in a decision has some perception of the outcomes and their desirabilities, but these perceptions are not explicitly described by anyone, much less analyzed by any formal techniques.

The guidelines for treating frostbite and ocular hypertension described in the previous chapter[1] are both good examples of the approach. Neither guideline is accompanied by any analysis of the consequences of the recommended practice or the relative merits of alternative practices. This information is not presented in the current textbooks, nor can the policies be traced back to any other reference that explicitly describes all the pros and cons of the recommended interventions or systematically nails them to experimental evidence. The guidelines are simply stated as the standard and accepted practice, with the implication that the fact that they are the common practice is sufficient justification. The actual wording of the policy for treating ocular hypertension illustrates this reliance on observed behavior: "Many clinicians institute medical treatment if the intraocular pressure is 30 mm Hg or greater."[4]

The traditional approach has a definite appeal. Because a guideline evolves from thousands of decisions, it potentially has a very large "sample size." Because a guideline is based on aggregate behavior, it pools the knowledge, judgments, and preferences of thousands of people. Wild ideas and unproved bursts of enthusiasm or disfavor will be resisted by the inertia of the average. To survive, a practice will have to stand the "test of time." The traditional approach also has logistic virtues. Because the approach requires no formal research or analysis, guidelines can be determined in minutes.

However, the traditional approach has two important drawbacks. The first is that it rests on a dangerous tautology. There are two issues involved: what people *should do* (guidelines) and what people *are doing* (standard practice). The purpose of the former (guidelines) is to define the latter (actual practices). But the guidelines themselves have to be anchored to something. Ideally, they should be anchored to reality—to the actual outcomes of the alternative practices and the actual desirability of those outcomes to patients. Placing this anchor, however, can be difficult. One option is to anchor the guideline to experimental evidence. Another is to anchor the guideline to the actual choices made by practitioners, on the assumption that practitioners' behavior is firmly anchored to reality—that practitioners have accurate perceptions of outcomes and preferences. The traditional approach takes the latter option and anchors guidelines to standard practice. This creates the tautology; guidelines for appropriate practices are determined by the collective actions of practitioners, but the actions of practitioners are themselves guided by the guidelines. In other words, everyone should do what everyone is doing. For example, if you asked someone to recommend a particular snow tire, the traditional approach would identify the brand that had the largest market share last year. The presumption is that, "Ten million buyers cannot be wrong." But when you and others follow that recommendation and buy that brand, it will quickly become this year's most popular tire. This will strengthen the recommendation to use it next year, and the cycle will be repeated.

A good medical example is the guideline for treating ocular hypertension. Lacking any better basis for a decision, most ophthalmologists, when they read about the 30-mm Hg cutoff point in the current textbook, will tend to follow that policy. This will reinforce the recommendation for the next edition. Why is the 30-mm Hg guideline popular today? It might well be because the previous edition said: ". . . Most ophthalmologists believe that persistent intraocular pressures over 30 mm Hg carry a sufficiently high risk of eventual field loss that therapy is warranted."[5] In fact, with slight variations in wording, the same statement can be found in the 1976, 1970, and 1965 editions.[6-8] A more general example of the tautology is any quality assurance program that uses statistical tests to look for outliers. The assumption is that the average is correct; the effect is to consolidate the average.

The danger of this tautology, of course, is that it requires that the average behavior be firmly anchored to reality. In fact, the entire cycle can float free from reality. Perhaps the most popular tire last year was not the best; it was only the most popular tire last year because it was the most popular tire the year before, which in turn could have been due to a onetime discount or an advertising blitz. If we make our decisions each year based on peoples' choices from the previous year, we might never scrutinize the actual merits of different tires. Perhaps a more appropriate cutoff for treating ocular hypertension is 35 mm Hg, or 25 mm Hg, or perhaps we should not treat it at all until visual field defects appear. The traditional approach will work properly only if the individual decision makers—physicians and their patients—have accurate understandings of the actual consequences of the alternative practices.

This introduces the second problem. The success of the traditional approach rests on a crucial assumption—that decision makers can accurately perceive the consequences of a practice and determine its appropriate use *sub-*

jectively, without explicitly examining the evidence that supports its use; estimating its outcomes; or comparing its benefits, harms, or costs.

This assumption pervades medical reasoning to this day. Pick up any medical textbook, open to any page, and read about a diagnostic test or treatment. You are unlikely to find an explicit (eg, quantitative) description of how the practice will affect even the most important health outcomes, and even more unlikely to find a systematic comparison of its benefits and harms. You will rarely find a discussion of the cost of the practice and virtually never find a comparison of its cost-effectiveness with that of alternatives. The tradition in medicine holds that decisions can be made and guidelines can be written without this information.

The guideline for the treatment of ocular hypertension again provides a good example. The 30-mm Hg cutoff point for medical therapy has evolved without any explicit analysis or even conjecture of the actual probabilities that people with intraocular pressures of various levels will develop visual field defects, or of the extent to which treatment will decrease those probabilities. There is no way to determine from anything written in any edition during the last 30 years, the actual consequences of initiating treatment at any level of intraocular pressure. The first (1961) edition described a therapy threshold of 24 mm Hg.[9] The next (1965) edition[8] changed the threshold to 30 mm Hg, but did not draw attention to the change, much less describe the impacts of the two options for patients. All subsequent editions[4-7] continued to use 30 mm Hg, still with no comparison of the merits of different thresholds. The notion that information regarding actual outcomes is pertinent is reflected in statements such as, "when the risk is sufficiently high," and references to "risk-benefit ratios," but the references are purely conceptual. If no information is provided regarding the actual magnitudes of the risks or benefits, a statement about a risk-benefit ratio is operationally meaningless. (During the last few months, two small trials of treatment for ocular hypertension have been published.[10,11] Now, 30 years after the first edition recommended treatment and almost 100 years after the medical treatment of ocular hypertension was introduced, it might be possible to answer some of the questions about this treatment.)

The assumption behind the traditional approach is that the outcomes of a medical practice can be sensed intuitively, without explicit analysis or description.[12] At some time in the past, this assumption might have been true. Decisions might have been sufficiently simple that they could be made by clinical judgment and intuition alone. Compared with today, interventions were fewer and conceptually more straightforward. Health problems were fairly immediate, and outcomes were short-term. The pace of new interventions was much slower—providing ample time for outcomes to occur and results to sort themselves out. There might have been few enough alternatives, a wide enough margin between benefits and harms, and a wide enough margin between benefits and costs, so that precise estimates and explicit descriptions were not necessary.

Whatever the validity of the assumption in the past, it is seriously threatened today. New interventions are appearing at an increasing rate, increasing the number and complexity of choices. The margins between benefits and harms and between benefits and costs are narrowing. As new interventions push further against the frontiers, the added benefits tend to get smaller, while the costs, risks, and inconveniences tend to get higher. There is increasing uncertainty about the effects of interventions, both from the increased complexity of new interventions and from new questions about old interventions. The evaluation of evidence is becoming more complicated.

It is simply unrealistic to think that individuals can synthesize in their heads scores of pieces of evidence, accurately estimate the outcomes of different options, and accurately judge the desirability of those outcomes for patients. Wide ranges of uncertainty among practitioners, wide variations in beliefs among experts, and wide variations in actual practices all confirm what would be expected from common sense: the complexity of modern medicine exceeds the inherent limitations of the unaided human mind.[12] The ultimate clue that the traditional approach has floated free from reality is that "standard" practices can vary by factors of 2, 3, 5, even 20, across county lines.

❖ New Approaches

In the last decade or so, several new approaches to designing guidelines have begun to develop. These approaches are the result of two main forces. One is a need to serve the increasing demand for practice policies and guidelines as management tools, such as precertification and cost containment. The second force is a growing recognition that the assumptions underlying the traditional approach do not hold. All the new approaches are "organized," in the sense that some group consciously sets out to develop a guideline. This group might be a task force of a specialty society, an advisory panel of a third-party payer, a consensus panel, a Food and Drug Administration committee, or any other group convened to create a guideline. The groups have different structures (eg, number of people, mixture of skills, and geographic diversification) and use different processes (eg, commissioned papers, Delphi methods, rating systems, and late-night vigils until a consensus is reached). But far more important than the structure and process are the *methods* used to perform the specific task of a guideline-setting exercise, because it is the methods that determine the *content* of a guideline. Four main methodological approaches can be distinguished on the basis of the explicitness with which various tasks are performed: "global subjective judgment," "evidence based," "outcomes based," and "preference based."

Global Subjective Judgment

In a global subjective judgment, those who are designing the guideline (hereinafter called "policymakers") perform all of the tasks subjectively. As the term implies, the guideline is the result of the opinions ("judg-ments") of individuals who attempt to consider all the important factors at once ("global") in their heads ("subjective"). There is no explicit identification of the important outcomes, no analysis of the evidence pertaining to those outcomes, no estimation of the effect of the practice on the outcomes, no as-sessment or description of patient preferences, and no description of the ratio-nale for the guideline. The guidelines are simply announced as the judgments of the policymakers.

This approach is very much in the spirit of the traditional approach. The only real difference is that it is organized—a specific group uses some prede-fined process to identify the guideline instead of allowing the guideline to manifest itself gradually through the behavior of practitioners and sentences in textbooks. However, the role of the group is not to explicitly *analyze* the problem, but to give their *beliefs* about what is, or what in their opinions should be, the "standard or accepted" practice. The policymakers are not so much analysts as interpreters or observers. Examples of this approach are the Diagnostic and Therapeutic Technology Assessment project of the American Medical Association (AMA), which polls a panel of experts for their views; the current policy-setting programs of many specialty societies, which de-scribe the collective beliefs of the task force members; and many consensus programs. The identifying feature of this approach is that when the guide-lines are issued, they are not accompanied by any comprehensive analysis of supporting evidence or estimation of outcomes.

The global subjective judgment approach is by far the simplest, fastest, least expensive, and most accessible method for setting a guideline. The rea-son for all these virtues is that it requires no analysis of evidence or estimation of outcomes. The main expense is to convene the panelists. The main techni-cal problem is to schedule the meeting. No analytic skills are required, so any-one can contribute an opinion. The reports are usually easy to write, because there is no analysis or rationale to be described. The only time limit is the time required for panelists to reach agreement. Guidelines can be set by this method in hours, for a few thousand dollars.

Evidence-Based Guidelines

The evidence-based approach explicitly describes the available evidence that pertains to a guideline and ties the guideline to evidence, but does not explicitly estimate the magnitudes or compare the benefits and harms. Like the traditional and global subjective judgment approaches, the evidence-based method relies on the subjective judgments of the policy-makers for the latter tasks.

This approach is a major advance over global subjective judgment because it openly acknowledges the possibility that the invisible hand might not work, and consciously anchors a guideline, not to current practices or the beliefs of experts, but to experimental evidence. Examples of this approach are the Technology Evaluation Center program of the Blue Cross and Blue Shield Association, the Clinical Efficacy Assessment Project of the American College of Physicians, the recommendations of the US Preventive Services Task Force, the reports of the Congressional Office of Technology Assessment, and the reports of the AMA's Council on Scientific Affairs. The hallmark of this approach is that it makes a commitment to evidence—the policy must be consistent with and supported by evidence. The usual question is whether the practice under consideration has been shown to be effective in improving the most important outcomes. Merely providing evidence as background material or peppering a guideline with occasional references to support particular positions do not count.

The evidence-based approach is considerably more demanding than global subjective judgment. The pertinent evidence must be identified, described, and analyzed. The policymakers must determine whether the guideline is justified by the evidence. A rationale must be written. Knowledge of experimental design is required. Designing a guideline by this method can take several months and cost several thousand dollars.

Outcomes-Based Guidelines

The outcomes-based approach not only anchors the guideline to available evidence, but explicitly estimates the outcomes of alternative practices. This additional step represents another major advance in methods because it shifts the basis for the guideline from *qualitative* reasoning to *quantitative* reasoning. The evidence-based method focuses on the qualitative question of whether evidence exists that the practice is effective and/or is safe. It does not require a quantitative analysis of the *magnitude* of the benefits or the magnitude of the harms. The explicit estimation of outcomes, on the other hand, does require this information.

The outcomes-based approach has two subcategories, depending on the specific method used to estimate the magnitudes of the outcomes. One method is to estimate the outcomes subjectively. This requires little additional work. The policymakers need only write down what they are thinking when they make their judgments. The other method is to estimate the outcomes objectively, using formal quantitative techniques. This method requires additional skills (eg, statistics and mathematics), time, and resources. Designing guidelines by the latter method can cost tens of thousands of dollars and require several months.

Currently there are no policy-setting programs that systematically estimate the magnitudes of the outcomes of the practice that is the subject of the policy, even subjectively. Most of the examples are from research programs, although some policy-setting programs such as those used by the Congressional Office of Technology Assessment, American College of Physicians, Blue Cross and Blue Shield Association, the AMA's Council on Scientific Affairs, and the Centers for Disease Control have applied this approach to some problems. The identifying feature of this approach is that the guideline is accompanied not only by a description of the supporting evidence, but also by a description of the important outcomes, the magnitudes of those outcomes, and the method used to derive the estimates.

Preference-Based Guidelines

The preference-based approach performs all of the tasks explicitly, including the assessment of patient preferences for outcomes. This is the most complete approach, presenting a full description of the reasoning behind a policy. At present, the only examples of this approach are from research programs, and they are rare. Adding this element to an outcomes-based approach requires skill in the psychology and science of assessing and combining preferences (eg, interviews, questionnaires, polls).

As the examples indicate, dozens of programs are already in place, creating guidelines by different methods. At one end of the spectrum, a group of specialists can meet for an hour, agree on a policy, and write up a bulletin. At the other end of the spectrum are multiyear projects that involve dozens of investigators and million-dollar budgets. The great differences in approaches raise an obvious question: Is the additional effort worth it?

❖ References

1. Eddy DM. Practice policies—what are they? *JAMA*. 1990;263:877-878, 880 (Chapter 3).
2. Eddy DM. Anatomy of a decision. *JAMA*. 1990;263:441-443 (Chapter 2).
3. Smith A. *An Inquiry Into the Nature and Causes of the Wealth of Nations*. 1776.
4. Hoskins H Jr, Kass M. *Becker-Shaffer's Diagnosis and Therapy of the Glaucomas*. 6th ed. St Louis, Mo: CV Mosby Co; 1989.
5. Kolker A, Hetherington J Jr. *Becker-Shaffer's Diagnosis and Therapy of the Glaucomas*. 5th ed. St Louis, Mo: CV Mosby Co; 1983.
6. Kolker A, Hetherington J Jr. *Becker-Shaffer's Diagnosis and Therapy of the Glaucomas*. 4th ed. St Louis, Mo: CV Mosby Co; 1976.
7. Kolker A, Hetherington J Jr. *Becker-Shaffer's Diagnosis and Therapy of the Glaucomas*. 3rd ed. St Louis, Mo: CV Mosby Co; 1970.
8. Becker B, Shaffer R. *Diagnosis and Therapy of the Glaucomas*. 2nd ed. St Louis, Mo: CV Mosby Co; 1965.
9. Becker B, Shaffer R. *Diagnosis and Therapy of the Glaucomas*. St Louis, Mo: CV Mosby Co; 1961.
10. Epstein DL, Krug JH Jr, Hertzmark E, Remis LL, Edelstein DJ. A long-term clinical trial of timolol therapy versus no treatment in the management of glaucoma suspects. *Ophthalmology*. 1989;96:1460-1467.
11. Kass MA, Gordon MO, Hoff MR, et al. Topical timolol administration reduces the incidence of glaucomatous damage in ocular hypertensive individuals. *Arch Ophthalmol*. 1989;107:1590-1598.
12. Eddy DM. The challenge. *JAMA*. 1990;263:287-290 (Chapter 1).

❖ Source

Originally published in *JAMA*. 1990;263:1265, 1269, 1272, 1275.

❖ CHAPTER 5

Guidelines—How Should They Be Designed?

Your Office, 10:35 AM

Your investment counselor calls you up.

"Boy, have I got a deal for you. We're opening up a limited partnership to develop some property in the Midwest. The price is $50 000 a unit. Can I sign you up?"

"Sounds exciting. Send me the business plan."

"We don't have one."

Click.

Washington, DC, 1:30 PM

The senator knocks the table with her gavel.

"Will the hearing please come to order. Thank you very much, Dr Evans, for agreeing to appear before our committee to help us with this most important social problem. We understand that your organization has recently issued guidelines for the prevention of egophilia. We would be most appreciative if you could provide us with the results of your study."

"Thank you, senator. The organization I represent is composed of the great majority of the practitioners in this field. As you know, egophilia is a common and pernicious disease—most of the people who have it don't know it. As a consequence, more and more of our practitioners are vaccinating their high-risk patients. To address the appropriateness of this practice, we con-

---

Note: This chapter was formerly titled "Practice Policies—Guidelines for Methods."

vened an expert panel and used a modified-qualified-intensified Delphi process to develop a vaccination policy. The policy described in exhibit 1 received the highest possible score."

"Most impressive, Dr Evans. May I begin the questions by asking the number of people in the country who currently suffer from egophilia?"

"Pretty much all of us."

"Yes, I know what you mean. Now, you indicate that people in seven particular occupations—I see that physicians, lawyers, and politicians are all on the list—are especially susceptible to this disorder. You recommend that everyone in these seven occupations should be vaccinated every 6 months. How many people does that represent?"

"I'm sorry, senator. We never actually estimated that figure."

"Um. Well, can you tell us the probability that an individual in any of those occupations will develop the disease in the coming year and how the vaccine you recommend will change that probability?"

"Those numbers are hard to come by."

"Yes, Dr Evans, we understand. You can just give us the best estimates used by your committee in developing its policies."

"Actually, we never tried our hand at making those estimates."

"I see. . . . Well, I suppose the vaccine has some risks. Can you tell us about that?"

"Yes, indeed. Exhibit 2 is a table of 53 possible risks and side effects of the vaccine."

"Wonderful! . . . Oh, I notice that the table is just a list. What are the probabilities of the various risks?"

"We don't have information on that."

"Oh. . . . Well, then, let's turn to the costs. What would be the annual cost of implementing the program you recommend?"

"We didn't go into that. But now that you ask, I expect it's in the billions."

"Will there eventually be some savings? Might they offset the costs?"

"We like to think so."

"Help me, Dr Evans. I'm trying to understand the basis for your recommendation so that we can consider what role, if any, we should play in implementing it."

"Of course, senator. I did point out, didn't I, that this is rapidly becoming a standard practice among our practitioners, and our panel of experts strongly believes its policy is correct."

"Yes, you did. . . . Thank you, Dr Evans. Next witness."

Dozens of programs have been created during the last few years to design guidelines for medical practices, and more are being created every month. They use very different methods and produce very different documents. Some programs convene experts for a day, cost a few thousand dollars, and issue guidelines on a single sheet of paper; others involve international teams, cost a million dollars, and will generate 200-page reports. Obvious questions arise: Is there a "correct" method for designing a guideline? Are there any minimal requirements for a guideline? In general, what standards should we require our guidelines to meet?

"Standards for standards" must address both the substance and form of a guideline—both how a guideline should be constructed (methods), as well as how a guideline should be described (the policy statement or rationale). This chapter will examine the qualities we want our methods to have and will propose guidelines for methods. It is appropriate to begin with methods, because unless a guideline is designed correctly, it does not matter how well it is described.

❖ What Are We Trying to Accomplish?

The choice of a method should be determined by what we want the method to accomplish. Five objectives seem reasonable. First, the method should produce guidelines that are accurate: The outcomes actually caused by the guidelines should be the outcomes the people who designed the guidelines ("policymakers") think they are causing. Second, the method should be accountable, enabling others to review the reasoning behind the guideline. Third, it should enable people to anticipate the health and financial consequences of applying the guideline, both to an individual and to a population. Fourth, the method should facilitate resolution of conflicts across guidelines. Finally, it should facilitate the application of the guideline, both to individual patients and to populations. In essence, these objectives attempt to ensure that a guideline is accurate, accountable, predictable, defensible, and usable.

The reasons for each of these objectives seem obvious—to belabor them might appear condescending. They need to be reviewed, however, because of an important fact: few guidelines that are currently being set meet any, much less all, of these objectives. As obvious as these objectives might seem in the abstract, for one reason or another they are not pursued in actual practice. If the methods for designing guidelines are to be brought up to the desired standards, there must be a clear understanding of why these objectives are important and what they imply in terms of practical requirements for a method.

The first objective is that the method be accurate. You would not want to recommend a treatment thinking its success rate is 80% when in fact its success rate is 10%. To achieve accuracy, policymakers must have accurate perceptions of how the important outcomes are affected by the practice they are recommending. They can try to accomplish this subjectively, but at great risk of incomplete or inaccurate information, errors in reasoning, and personal and professional biases.[1] The best protection against these cognitive problems is to evaluate the evidence explicitly and to analyze that evidence using formal, axiom-based techniques (such as statistics and probability theory). The use of explicit and formal methods is never worse than a subjective approach, and is usually vastly superior. To appreciate this, think of trying to estimate your income tax in your head.

The objective that a method should be accountable addresses a tremendous potential problem. Anyone can issue guidelines—all you need is a pencil and paper. The groups that write guidelines have different backgrounds, skills, and incentives. Each is asking practitioners and administrators to accept and apply its recommendations. The consequences of these requests can be enormous; single guidelines, if implemented, could easily affect tens of thousands of patients and hundreds of millions of dollars. Given the variety of sources and the high stakes, it would be very unwise to simply accept every guideline at face value—no questions asked. Even if you wanted to, the presence of conflicts across guidelines would make it impossible to accept them all. How do you decide? By asking questions. For example, what factors did the policymakers take into account? What evidence did they consider? How did they estimate the pros and cons of the recommended practice? Questions like these place several practical requirements on the method used to produce the guideline. The most obvious is that the method must leave a record or trail that describes the facts, assumptions, and logic that led to the policy. An ability to review the reasoning behind a guideline is essential to its credibility and acceptability.

The third objective, to understand the consequences of a guideline, responds to several needs. Practitioners will want to be able to answer patients' questions about why a particular practice is being recommended and what patients can expect if they comply. (In theory, informed consent makes this a legal requirement.) Even if patients do not ask, practitioners want to know the effects of what they are being told to do. If they are to apply the practice intelligently, practitioners need to know how important the practice is, how forcefully to push it, and the consequences of not performing it.

The practical consequence of this objective is that the method for producing a guideline must provide information regarding the actual magnitudes of the outcomes of the recommended practice. Statements such as "It will decrease the chance of death" are of little help. The pertinent questions are, "What is the actual decrease in probability of death? One out of 1000? One out of two? How many fewer deaths will we see in the population 5 years from now? 50? 5000?"

The fourth objective is that the method should provide the information needed to resolve conflicts. Many guidelines are already in conflict, and the frequency of conflicts can be expected to increase as more programs issue guidelines. The initial step in resolving a conflict is to identify the sources of disagreement (see Chapter 9). For example, different policymakers might be focusing on different outcomes, might be using different evidence, might be interpreting the evidence differently, might have different estimates of the outcomes, or might have different ideas about patient preferences. The second step is to address the areas of disagreement, correct any errors of fact or analysis, and probe differences in assumptions and preferences. Resolving conflicts requires that the methods used to design the guidelines describe how they addressed each task of the policy-setting process.

The last objective addresses the need to apply the guideline. Even if practitioners and administrators are willing to accept a guideline without being able to review its logic or understand its consequences, they will need some information if they are to apply it intelligently. The basic problem this objective addresses is that patients do not come in neat packages. There is too much variety with respect to specific features of the disease, concurrent diseases, risk factors, lifestyles, preferences, and other factors. It is rarely possible to capture all the possible variations in a finite number of categories and policies. In practice, guidelines can be written for the most common health problems and types of patients ("generic" problems), but these guidelines must be tailored to fit individual circumstances. Indeed, tailoring a guideline to fit an individual patient is the essence of clinical judgment.

To be able to tailor a guideline intelligently, practitioners must be given information about how the outcomes of the recommended practice vary with different patients' characteristics. For example, how do the probabilities of particular outcomes differ for different risk groups? Would the guideline be different if the patient were highly cancerphobic? The practical consequence of this objective is that the method used to produce a guideline for a generic problem should not only estimate the consequences of the guideline for the generic case, but should produce information regarding how the outcomes vary with different patient characteristics.

❖ How Well Do Different Methods Perform?

With these concepts in place, it is instructive to revisit the four main approaches for setting guidelines.[2] With global subjective judgment, the guideline is simply announced. There is no explicit description of evidence, description of how the guideline is derived from the evidence, estimation of outcomes, or any other aspects of a rationale. The method is entirely subjective, which, for all but the most straightforward problems, is a severe threat to accuracy. The threat of inaccuracy is compounded because there is no way to review any of the ingredients of the guideline. The expected consequences of the guideline are not described, there is no basis for identifying sources of conflict, and there is no information regarding how to tailor the guideline.

The evidence-based approach describes the evidence and ties the guideline to the evidence. This enhances the accuracy of this aspect of the policy-making process and opens it to review. However, the estimation of outcomes and other aspects of the policy-making process are still subjective. This threatens the accuracy of these tasks and prohibits their review. Because this method does not explicitly estimate outcomes, it provides little information regarding the expected consequences of applying the guideline. If there are conflicting guidelines, the evidence can be compared, but other potential sources of conflict, such as differences in estimates of outcomes or differences in beliefs about preferences, are invisible. Guidelines set by this method are also difficult to tailor to individual cases—that requires information about how the outcomes vary with patient characteristics.

Because the outcomes-based approach describes the evidence and estimates the outcomes, it comes much closer to satisfying the objectives. Both the evidence and methods used to estimate outcomes can be reviewed, the consequences of the guideline are described, the main sources of potential conflict are exposed, and the information needed to tailor a guideline is available. The accuracy of the outcomes-based approach will depend primarily on the particular method used to estimate the outcomes. If the outcomes are estimated subjectively from the evidence, the accuracy will depend on the simplicity of the clinical problem, the clarity of the evidence, and the mental powers of the policymakers. If the outcomes are estimated using formal techniques, the accuracy of the estimates will be enhanced accordingly.

The preference-based approach adds to the strengths of the outcomes-based methods by incorporating explicit information regarding patient preferences for outcomes. This increases the accuracy of that aspect of the policy-setting process, opens it to review, and exposes it as a potential source of conflict. Explicit information regarding patient preferences is also extremely valuable for tailoring a guideline—providing practitioners with information regarding the range of preferences across patients and the sensitivity of a guideline to the range of preferences.

❖ Recommendations for Methods

The practical implications of these objectives can be summarized as the following six points:

1. Separate the two main steps of the policy-making process[3]—first estimate the outcomes of the proposed intervention, *then* make judgments about the desirability of the outcomes.
2. Estimate explicitly the effect of the intervention on all of the outcomes that are important to patients.
3. To the extent necessary to tailor a policy, estimate how the outcomes vary with different patients' characteristics.
4. To the greatest extent possible, base the estimates of outcomes on experimental evidence.
5. To the extent necessary to estimate outcomes accurately, use formal methods to analyze the evidence and estimate the outcomes.
6. To the extent necessary to understand patient preferences accurately, use actual assessments of patient preferences to determine the desirability of the outcomes.

These points are tantamount to an outcomes-based approach, with the addition of an explicit assessment of patient preferences as needed. The recommendations are firm in specifying that the methods produce particular types of information—such as estimates of the important outcomes—and that they be powerful enough to deliver that information accurately. However, they recognize that different evidence exists for different problems and that different evidence is needed for different problems. They are also flexible in not dictating specific methods for specific tasks, such as how to estimate outcomes. For example, the recommendations do not dictate particular outcomes that must be considered, evidence of a particular type (eg, at least two statistically significant randomized, controlled trials), particular measures for outcomes (eg, Sickness Impact Profile[4]), a particular type of model (eg, decision tree), or particular statistical methods. These decisions are left to the policymakers.

This flexibility is necessary for two reasons. First, methods change, and it is not appropriate to lock in particular methods that might become outdated. Second, different methods will be appropriate for different problems, just as different research designs are appropriate to answer different research questions. The applicable motto is, "One size does not fit all." In general, the formality of a method will depend on four factors: the importance of the health problem (eg, number of patients, severity of the outcomes, cost), the potential for harm that could be caused if a policy is incorrect, the simplicity of the clinical question, and the nature of the available evidence. For an extreme example, if the clinical question is whether to put a finger on a bleeding artery or the merits of keeping a frostbitten limb clean and dry, no controlled trials or formal quantitative methods are needed. On the other hand, if the question is whether all male smokers 50 years or older with low-density lipoprotein levels greater than 4.40 mmol/L and high-density lipoprotein levels less than 1.29 mmol/L should be treated with a lipid regulator, powerful techniques will be required to analyze the existing evidence, estimate outcomes, and assess preferences.

Because the recommendations for methods leave it to policymakers to choose methods capable of delivering the information needed for intelligent decisions, it is essential that policymakers expose their methods to review. The vehicle for this is the guideline.

❖ References

1. Eddy DM. The challenge. *JAMA*. 1990;263:287-290 (Chapter 1).
2. Eddy DM. Practice policies—where do they come from? *JAMA*. 1990;263:1265, 1269, 1272, 1275 (Chapter 4).
3. Bergner M, Bobbit R, Carter W, Gillson B. The Sickness Impact Profile: development and final revision of a health status measure. *Med Care*. 1981;19:787-805.
4. Eddy DM. Anatomy of a decision. *JAMA*. 1990;263:441-443 (Chapter 2).

❖ Source

Originally published in *JAMA*. 1990;263:1839-1841.

❖ CHAPTER 6

Recommendations for Guidelines

The Explicit Approach

The first obligation of a policymaker is to design a guideline that, if accepted and applied correctly, will improve patients' lives. The second obligation is to present the guideline in a way that ensures it will be accepted and applied correctly. The first obligation is addressed through the choice of methods for designing a guideline.[1] The second obligation is addressed through the guideline itself.

❖ Objectives

The objectives for guidelines are similar to the objectives for methods: accuracy, accountability, predictability, defensibility, and usability.[1] The pertinence of these objectives to guidelines can be appreciated by viewing the guideline from the perspective of the people who will be affected by it—practitioners, patients, and payers.

Begin with the primary audience of a guideline—practitioners. The purpose of a guideline is to modify the behavior of practitioners to steer their decisions toward actions that the policymakers consider desirable. Needless to say, this has important implications for the practitioners whose decisions are being influenced—what they subject their patients to, how they administer their programs, how they spend their time, what new skills they need to learn, what income they receive, what costs they generate, and their exposure to malpractice. If an organization issues a guideline that all patients with a

---

Note: This chapter was formerly titled "Guidelines for Policy Statements: The Explicit Approach."

particular problem must be treated in a particular way or that a particular test will not be paid for, and the practitioners disagree, they're stuck. Practitioners can continue to follow their instincts and buck the policy, but the cost in patient relations, peer relations, reimbursement, and lawsuits, not to mention personal discomfort, could be extreme. If practitioners acquiesce and simply accept the new guideline, they must live with the personal tension of doing something that contradicts their beliefs.

The threat of discordance between a practitioner's current practices and a new guideline is real. Many guidelines are created by individuals or organizations that have narrower or different perspectives than the people who will eventually have to implement the guideline. For example, the government might design a guideline with an eye toward cost control; investigators might let their enthusiasm for an intervention spill over into a premature or inappropriately aggressive guideline; specialists might forget that their selective practices distort the apparent frequencies of diseases and outcomes; organizations that focus on single diseases might try to load practitioners with guidelines that are unrealistic in a busy general practice; one specialty society might write a guideline that restricts the role of another specialty.

Given the stake practitioners have in any guideline, it is important to ask what information they would need to accept the guideline and implement it correctly. In essence, they will want to review the reasoning behind the guideline. What are the expected consequences (benefits and harms) of applying the guideline? How were the benefits and harms estimated? What evidence supports the estimates? And so forth.

Patients and payers have similar concerns. While individual patients will rarely see the inside of a guideline, they most certainly want the guidelines to be designed, communicated, reviewed, and executed correctly. As for payers, they are generally happy to pay the bill for a service, provided the service is in the best interests of the people on whose behalf they are making the payments—their subscribers, members, employees, or taxpayers. What payers are unwilling to do is pay money for a service whose value is unknown, or worse, nil.

The only people who have conflicting interests with respect to the standards their guidelines should meet are those who design the guidelines. On one hand, they want to minimize the cost and inconvenience of producing a guideline. That argues for the loosest possible standards. On the other hand, they have an overriding interest in producing a guideline that is in the best interest of patients, that will be implemented accurately, and that can be defended. They also want other policymakers who issue competing guidelines to justify their choices. These concerns argue for rigorous standards.

To summarize, with the exception of the policymakers' natural desire to simplify their work load, the interests of all parties point in the same direction: a policy statement should not only describe the recommended action, but should describe the rationale for the recommendation and the consequences of following it.

❖ Recommendations for Guidelines

These objectives lead naturally to recommendations for guidelines. The specific elements of a guideline and the appropriate degree of detail will depend on the importance of the clinical problem, the complexity of the analytical problem, and the type of guideline (eg, guidance to practitioners vs retrospective quality review). However, the main elements that should be included in any guideline are well illustrated by the particular case of a guideline that recommends a specific intervention for an important and difficult clinical problem. Such a statement should contain the following information:

1. Summary of the Guideline. This is the one- to three-line statement that everyone will remember and quote. It should be as concise, clear, specific, and operational as possible. It should describe the guideline in sufficient detail that, if taken out of context, the guideline will still be applied accurately. That description should include the intended use of the policy and the intended degree of flexibility (eg, "standard," "recommendation," or "option").[2]

2. Background. The guideline should include any background information needed to understand the problem addressed by the guideline and to interpret the guideline effectively. The background will answer the broad question, "Why is this guideline being written?" For example, it might describe basic information regarding the frequency of the disease, a sudden growth in use of a device, or a particular quality problem that motivates the guideline.

3. Health Problem. This section will define the clinical question in sufficient detail to eliminate any ambiguity about the target of the guideline. It will describe the health problem being addressed (eg, the specific disease or diagnostic problem), the intervention that is the object of the guideline, the alternative intervention(s) with which it was compared, the patients to whom the guideline will be applied (eg, specific patient indications), any restrictions on the type of practitioners who should provide the intervention (eg, training, experience, certification), and any restrictions on the setting in which the intervention can be applied (eg, facilities, equipment, ancillary personnel). This section answers the question: "Exactly what are we talking about?"

4. Health and Economic Outcomes. This part is the easiest to write. It simply asks the policymakers to list the health outcomes (eg, 5-year survival, pain relief, impotence, nausea, the need for a colostomy) and economic costs that they considered in the design of the guideline.

5. Evidence. One of the most important aspects of a guideline is a description of the evidence about the effect of the intervention on the important outcomes. This section will describe what evidence was considered, how it was interpreted, and what subjective judgments were used to supplement the experimental evidence.

6. Effect on Health and Economic Outcomes. This is the core of the guideline. It should provide *quantitative* estimates of the magnitudes of the health and economic outcomes, including, when appropriate, a range of uncertainty. This section answers the questions: "What effect do the policy-makers think this guideline will have? What can I expect if I apply the guideline? What should I tell my patients?"

7. Methods Used to Derive the Estimates of Outcomes. In this section, the authors of the guideline will describe how they made the estimates given in the previous section. This part will describe such things as statistical meth-ods used to interpret experimental evidence and any models used to analyze indirect evidence.

8. Preference Judgments. This section will describe the judgments made about the desirability of the outcomes. It will compare the benefits and harms, compare the health outcomes and economic costs, and describe the spectrum of preferences (eg, degree of unanimity). It will also describe the sources of the preference judgments (eg, a survey of patients, subjective impressions of the policymakers).

9. Instructions for Tailoring Guidelines. For guidelines that are in-tended to be flexible (ie, recommendations), the policymakers can describe any factors that should be considered when applying the guideline (eg, patients' characteristics, setting, provider) and instructions for tailoring the guideline to fit different circumstances. This section will include estimates of outcomes for different patients' characteristics or settings.

10. Conflicts With Other Guidelines. If another organization has issued a different guideline for the same health problem, the conflict should be explained and, if possible, reconciled. If the authors of the conflicting guide-line have not described their reasoning, it might not be possible to reconcile the conflict.

11. Comparisons With Other Interventions. Ideally, guidelines for any intervention should be set in the context of other interventions. For example, when discussing the merits of screening for breast cancer, it would be in-structive to compare that activity with screening for cervical cancer or colo-rectal cancer. This is rarely done at present but will be done more frequently as the limits on resources tighten and the need to consider alternative uses of resources grows. This section would describe any other interventions with which the intervention of interest has been compared and would give the results of any cost-effectiveness analyses.

12. Caveats. No guideline is final. This section will describe any ex-pected technical developments or new information (eg, research in progress) that could modify the guideline and will suggest dates for reviewing the guideline.

13. Authors of the Policy. The guideline should include the authors of the guideline, their expertise, and any conflicts of interest.

This list is similar in spirit to the suggested format for a research article (introduction, methods, results, etc) or a history and physical examination (chief complaint, present illness, review of symptoms, etc). It is important to emphasize that the specific elements and format will be different for different types of guidelines. For example, consider the format for a guideline that recommends an acceptable operative mortality rate for a surgical procedure. The guideline will obviously be restricted to that particular outcome (item 4); the estimated effectiveness of the intervention on outcomes (item 6) will not apply, and so forth. Similarly, the degree of detail for a guideline will vary with the complexity and importance of the problem being addressed. A guideline that a frostbitten foot should be kept clean will require much less documentation than a guideline that recommends lifelong treatment for uncomplicated ocular hypertension.

❖ Observations

Several observations are important. First, the key to these recommendations is explicitness. The recommendations ask policymakers to be explicit in describing the evidentiary basis, methods, and expected consequences of a guideline. Thus, a guideline that follows these recommendations will be said to be "explicit."

Second, although the recommendations ask policymakers to provide considerable information regarding evidence and outcomes, the intention is not to burden practitioners with unwanted details or to force them to second-guess the application of the guideline to every patient. Indeed, that would defeat the purpose of the guideline, which was to simplify decisions for practitioners. The reason for requesting all the information regarding evidence and outcomes is to enable practitioners and others to review the merits of the guideline for the generic case.

Third, the form of a guideline is distinct from the methods used to create the guideline.[1] The recommendations for the guideline only ask the policymakers to describe the *results* of their thinking; they do not specify any particular methods that must be used. For example, an estimate that a treatment should increase the probability of 1-year survival from 3% to 10% could be based on the subjective judgment of a single practitioner, the pooled beliefs of a panel of experts, or a statistical analysis of five randomized controlled trials. Clearly, the source of the estimate will strongly affect the credibility of the guideline, but the method used to derive an estimate is addressed by the recommendations for methods,[1] not by these recommendations for guidelines. The reason for this leniency is to make it possible for all policymakers to follow the recommendations for guidelines, no matter what methods they used. If there are deficiencies in the methods, they will be exposed through descriptions provided in the guideline, and the credibility of the guideline will be determined accordingly.

Fourth, because these recommendations do not specify any particular methods, policymakers who for one reason or another do not choose to use formal methods can still supply the information called for by the recommendations for guidelines. Stated another way, lack of hard data or use of purely subjective methods do not decrease the need for or the ability to adhere to these recommendations. All the recommendations require is that policymakers describe whatever evidence and reasoning went into their guideline. Thus, the spirit behind the recommendations is "tell it like it is." For example, the following (abbreviated) rationale would satisfy the recommendations just presented.

> We considered the effect of [the proposed treatment] on 5-year survival, but ignored the risks, side effects, and financial costs (item 4). There are no controlled experiments that compare the proposed treatment with any alternatives (item 5). Despite this, we estimate that the treatment should increase the probability of 5-year survival by about 3% (from about 20% to about 23%) (item 6). This estimate is subjective, based on observations of about 20 patients followed for about 3 years in our personal practices (item 7). Concerning patient preferences, we assumed that for virtually all patients, even a small increase in chance of survival is worth whatever risks and side effects the treatment might have. This belief is based on our conversations with our patients (item 8). . . . Our guideline is in conflict with that of the Surgeon General's Task Force, which did not recommend the treatment due to lack of evidence of effectiveness, and what it considers to be substantial side effects (item 10). . . .

The fifth observation is that compliance with these recommendations does not ensure that the guideline itself will be correct, any more than a researcher's description of methods ensures that the methods were correct, or a description of a physical examination of the heart with normal findings ensures that a subtle murmur was not missed. These recommendations for guidelines only specify the information policymakers should provide in support of their guideline and only ensure that those who want to review the guideline have the information they need to perform that review.

Finally, at first thought, both the recommendations for guidelines and the recommendations for methods might appear stiff. Anchoring a guideline to evidence, explicitly estimating the outcomes of a guideline, and explicitly addressing patient preferences will require more work and cost than many groups are used to. The following three facts help justify the burden: (1) The principles behind these recommendations are already widely accepted. They are the same principles that call for excellence in research, excellence in provision of care, and peer review of proposals and publications. (2) The actual amount of work required to follow these recommendations, while large in comparison to simply announcing a guideline, is small compared with the costs of other activities that have much less impact. Compare the cost and importance of a guideline with the million-dollar cost of conducting a single experiment that might never affect a decision, or with the multi-thousand-dollar cost of just providing an intervention to a single patient. (3) The recommendations were derived from the five objectives of accuracy, accountability, predictability, defensibility, and usability. If we want our guidelines to have these qualities, we must be willing to take the steps necessary to achieve them.

The design of a guideline is the final step in a long process that begins with a research idea and ends in actual changes in peoples' health. It is the step that converts all the accumulated research, development, and experience into practical recommendations that largely determine what happens to patients. In this pivotal position, the design of a guideline deserves whatever effort is required to ensure that all the work that preceded it is put to the best effect.

❖ References

1. Eddy DM. Practice policies—guidelines for methods. *JAMA*. 1990;263:1839-1841 (Chapter 5).
2. Eddy DM. Practice policies—what are they? *JAMA*. 1990;263:877-878, 880 (Chapter 3).

❖ Source

Originally published in *JAMA*. 1990;263:2239-2240, 2243.

❖ CHAPTER 7

Comparing Benefits and Harms

The Balance Sheet

The central elements of a decision about a medical activity, and therefore the central elements of a guideline, are the consequences of the interventions that are being considered—their benefits, harms, and costs. The estimates of health and economic outcomes condense the information from clinical research and clinical experience into a form suitable for decisions and provide the basis for judgments about the desirability of the intervention.

A simple but powerful way to present information on the outcomes of an intervention is the balance sheet. The idea is old and familiar; when you are trying to decide between two or more options that are complex and important, such as whether to buy a new car, make a list of the pros and cons of each option. The overall goal of the balance sheet is to help decision makers develop an accurate understanding of the important consequences of the different options. The balance sheet helps accomplish this in two main ways. First, it condenses all the important information into a space that can be grasped visually (and, it is hoped, mentally) at one time. This decreases the tendency to ignore important outcomes or to vacillate between outcomes. Second, by formalizing the description of outcomes, the balance sheet increases the prospects that decision-makers will gain an accurate perception of the effects of different options. An additional virtue of the balance sheet is that the act of constructing it is a helpful mechanism for organizing thinking, structuring the analysis of evidence, and focusing debates.

❖ An Example

The use of the balance sheet for clinical decisions is well illustrated with the case of screening high-risk people for colorectal cancer. The

US Preventive Services Task Force recently published recommendations for screening asymptomatic people for colorectal cancer.[1] It concluded that although "there is insufficient evidence to recommend either for or against fecal occult blood testing with sigmoidoscopy as effective screening tests for colorectal cancer in asymptomatic persons, [it] may be clinically prudent to offer screening to persons age 50 and older with known risk factors for colorectal cancer. These patients should receive current information regarding the benefits, risks and uncertainties of both fecal occult blood tests and sigmoidoscopy. The optimal interval for screening is uncertain and is left to clinical discretion."

This statement leaves the burden of the decision squarely on the shoulders of the practicing physician. The basis for the decision is clearly indicated— "information regarding the benefits, risks and uncertainties" of the different options. What is now needed is a description of those benefits, risks, and uncertainties, so that clinicians will have something to think about when they apply their "prudence" and "discretion."

Consider the particular question raised by the Task Force—the value of screening a high-risk person older than 50 years with fecal occult blood tests and sigmoidoscopy. To make the analysis more specific, I will tell you that I fit this description; I am 48 years old and my father died of colorectal cancer. What are the "benefits, risks and uncertainties" of screening a person like me with annual fecal occult blood tests and 3-year 60-cm flexible sigmoidoscopies, from age 50 years through, say, age 75 years?

❖ Development of a Balance Sheet

The first step in developing a balance sheet is to identify the health outcomes—the outcomes that are important to people who will receive the intervention. In this example, there are two main benefits: screening should decrease the probability a person ever gets an invasive colorectal cancer (because premalignant adenomas can be detected and removed), and screening should decrease the probability a person dies of colorectal cancer (by decreasing the probability of getting colorectal cancer, and by detecting invasive cancers in earlier stages, when survival rates are higher). Another benefit that someone might consider is reassurance from a negative screening test. The main harms of screening are the possibility of having a false-positive result leading to a workup, with its attendant anxiety, discomfort, and cost; the possibility of perforating the colon, with its morbidity, mortality, and cost; and the sheer discomfort, inconvenience, and anxiety associated with the delivery of the tests. The financial costs include the cost of screening (which the patient might have to pay), the cost of workups for any false-positive results, the cost of perforations, and potential savings in treatment costs.

The next step in the development of a balance sheet is far more difficult; it is to estimate the magnitudes of each of these outcomes. For this example, I have used evidence and methods published elsewhere to estimate the outcomes.[2] To keep the focus on the balance sheet, I will not describe them herein. However, the evidence and methods used to estimate outcomes for a balance sheet are extremely important, and a complete guideline would describe them.[3] One important fact to keep in mind for this particular problem is that there is not yet any direct evidence from randomized controlled trials that screening with any test decreases mortality from colorectal cancer. Rather, the available evidence is all indirect—based on information about such factors as incidence rates of colorectal cancer, the anatomy and natural history of colorectal cancer, and the accuracies of various screening tests.

Once the magnitudes of the outcomes have been estimated, the last step is to design the balance sheet. Important issues are the choice of words to describe the outcomes, the ordering of the outcomes, and the layout of the information. While these issues might appear trivial, they can have an important impact on a person's decision. For an extreme example, imagine putting the benefits in bold print at the top of the page and the harms in small print at the bottom, or vice versa.

❖ A Balance Sheet for Colorectal Cancer Screening

A balance sheet for the colorectal cancer screening problem is shown in Table 7.1. Without screening, a high-risk 50-year-old man (like me) has about a 10.3% probability of developing colorectal cancer sometime in the rest of his life and about a 5.3% probability of dying of colorectal cancer. If such a person is screened with the proposed strategy, the probabilities of getting and dying of colorectal cancer are decreased to about 7.3% and 2.9%, respectively. Thus, the effect of this screening strategy is to decrease the actual probability of getting or dying of colorectal cancer about 3.0% and 2.4%, respectively. Stated another way, of one thousand 50-year-old men who have family histories of colorectal cancer but who are *not* screened, we would expect about 103 of them to get colorectal cancer and 53 to die of colorectal cancer sometime in the rest of their lives. If the 1000 men *are* screened, the expected number who will get colorectal cancer decreases to 73 (a decrease of 30), and the expected number who will die of colorectal cancer decreases to 29 (a decrease of 24).

The main harms of screening are that there is about a 40% chance of having a false-positive fecal occult blood test during the 26-year period of screening (age 50 years through age 75 years) and about a 0.3% (3/1000) chance of perforating the colon (either by the sigmoidoscopic examination or during the workup of a false-positive fecal occult blood test). Patients will also suffer the discomfort and anxiety of sigmoidoscopic examinations nine times during the 26-year period (every third year), as well as whatever inconvenience and anxiety the fecal occult blood test causes each year for 26 years.

Notice that there is a wide range of uncertainty around these estimates. It is possible that there is no benefit at all. On the other hand, the benefit could be twice as great as the "best guess." The sources of uncertainty and the

TABLE 7.1 Benefits, Harms, and Costs of One Colorectal Cancer Screening Strategy*

Outcomes	No Screening	FOBT Every Year and Scope Every 3 y	Difference Caused by Screening	Range of Uncertainty About Difference
Benefits				
Probability of getting colorectal cancer	10.3% (103/1000)	7.3% (73/1000)	-3.0% (30/1000)	0%-6%
Probability of dying of colorectal cancer	5.3% (53/1000)	2.9% (29/1000)	-2.4% (24/1000)	0%-5%
Probability of harboring a hidden cancer†	0.1% (10/10000)	0.03% (3/10000)	-0.07% (7/10000)	0.05%-0.09%
Harms				
Probability of a false-positive FOBT	0%	40% (400/1000)	+40% (400/1000)	20%-60%
Probability of perforation‡	0%	0.3% (3/1000)	+0.3% (3/1000)	0.1%-1.0%
Inconvenience/anxiety/discomfort				
FOBT, No. of tests	0	26	26	...
Scope, No. of tests	0	9	9	...
Financial costs, $$				
Screening	0	643	643	...
Treatment	1155	1106	-49	...
Net	1155	1749	594	...

*FOBT indicates fecal occult blood test; and scope, 60-cm flexible sigmoidoscope.
†This is the probability that the patient has a cancer that will develop signs or symptoms in the coming year.
‡This is the probability of perforation due to workup of false-positive fecal occult blood test or sigmoidoscopy.
§These are present values, discounted at 5%. A $4 fecal occult blood test and $135 60-cm flexible sigmoidoscopy are assumed. Costs of screening and treatment vary widely in different settings.

assumptions that lead to different estimates would be described in the guide-line that accompanies the balance sheet. (In this case, they are discussed in another publication.[2])

The screening procedures themselves will cost about $1050, spread over 26 years, for a present value of $643. The expected costs of working up false-positive test results and treating perforations are almost exactly offset by expected savings in initial treatment costs; the net effect of screening on these costs is a decrease of about $50 (present value). All these cost estimates will vary in different settings.

Some important outcomes are difficult to describe succinctly. The benefit of reassurance is a good example. People who seek the reassurance of a nega-tive examination want to hear that they do not have colorectal cancer. Unfor-tunately, the actual meaning of a negative examination is not that simple. In the first place, without any screening examination, the chance an asympto-matic person harbors a hidden invasive colorectal cancer that will become apparent, say, in the next year is already small; for a high-risk 50-year-old man, the probability is about 0.1% (10/10 000). In the second place, if an exam-ination with fecal occult blood testing and 60-cm flexible sigmoidoscopy is done and is negative, the probability the person is still harboring a colorectal cancer does decrease, but not to zero. (There is a chance the tests will fail to defect an existing cancer.) In this example, the probability that a high-risk man who tests negative still harbors a cancer that will become apparent in the com-ing year is about 0.03% (3/10 000). Thus, the "reassurance value" of the negative examination is to decrease the chance the man will develop a colorectal cancer in the coming year from about 0.1% to about 0.03%, or an actual decrease of about 0.07% (7/10 000). The probability a person will receive whatever reassur-ance this provides is the probability the tests will not detect a cancer, which is about 99.5% (9950/10 000). This concept is difficult to describe; you can see my attempt in Table 7.1.

❖ Properties of a Balance Sheet

The balance sheet has several important properties. First, it should include all the outcomes that are important to patients. A balance sheet that omits some important harms, for example, is obviously mislead-ing. It is particularly important to resist the temptation to include only out-comes for which there is good experimental evidence. If the evidence for an outcome is poor, that can be described explicitly in the guideline and can be indicated in the balance sheet by stating a wide range of uncertainty.

The flip side of the first property is that the balance sheet should include *only* health outcomes that are meaningful to decision makers. In particular, interesting but irrelevant facts should be excluded. Examples are "Colorectal cancer is the second most common cause of cancer" and "The incidence of colorectal cancer has been decreasing gradually over the last several decades." While interesting as background information, these statements provide no information about the effect of the proposed guideline on the intended targets of the balance sheet (patients).

A third property is that the measures used to describe the outcomes should be intuitively understandable to the intended audience. Consider the effect of screening on mortality. Three different ways of describing this outcome are as follows: the expected length of life (the life expectancy of a 50-year-old high-risk man is about 74.75 years without screening, and about 75 years with screening), the probability of surviving 5 years after diagnosis of colorectal cancer (about 55% without screening vs 67% with screening), and the probability of ever dying of colorectal cancer (about 5.3% without screening vs 2.9% with screening). Of the three, the probability of ever dying of colorectal cancer is the most intuitive and perceptually accurate. Life expectancy is easily misunderstood; many people think of adding some days (in this case, about 90) to the end of one's life. Five-year survival after diagnosis does not take into account either the fact that screening changes the probability a person will ever get a diagnosis of colorectal cancer or the fact that screening changes the timing of diagnosis, which can affect 5-year survival independently of any effect on chance or time of death ("lead time").

Fourth, the measure used to describe the *effect* of the intervention on the outcomes must also be clear. An especially important distinction is between an *absolute* or *actual* change in outcomes and a *relative* (or *percent*) change. The actual change caused by screening in the chance of dying of colorectal cancer is from 5.3% to 2.9%, an actual decrease of 2.4%. The relative or percent change in chance of death is 2.4% ÷ 5.3%, or about 45%. A relative or percent change always makes the effect of an intervention appear larger than it really is. Furthermore, to call the effect of screening "45%" begs the question, "45% of what?"

Many outcomes have no direct numerical measures. The anxiety of a false-positive fecal occult blood test, the discomfort of a sigmoidoscopic examination, and the reassurance of a negative screening test are good examples. For these outcomes, the best that can be done is to name the event, describe it in words if it is not already familiar, and provide information on the frequency with which the event is expected to occur with each option. Even if a physical or psychological impact cannot be measured, the balance sheet will at least remind decision makers that these outcomes occur.

A fifth property of a balance sheet is that it should describe the range of uncertainty about an estimate. This is most easily done with probability distributions or 95% confidence ranges (calculated formally or subjectively). A sixth observation is that a balance sheet *cannot* include *all* the factors that affect an individual's decision. Most important, it cannot include information about the expectations, fears, and resources of individual patients. In this particular example, such factors as the cancerphobia, stoicism, curiosity, and financial resources of particular patients must be considered in the decision to screen.

A seventh point is that a balance sheet does not stipulate any specific type of evidence or methods. The accuracy and credibility of a balance sheet will obviously depend on the quality of the evidence and methods used, but for many problems the evidence is weak, and the methods will be subjective. Because the bases for estimates can vary so widely, people who produce balance sheets must describe their evidence and methods to help decisionmakers interpret the balance sheet.

Finally, it is important to understand that the design of a balance sheet is an art. There is no single set of outcomes, methods, or layouts that is best for all problems. The objective is to describe the information needed to make decisions in as simple, understandable, and neutral a fashion as possible. The principles are to include all the pertinent information, exclude all irrelevant and misleading information, choose measures that are intuitively understandable, and present the information in a balanced way.

❖ Using the Balance Sheet

If a decision is fairly straightforward, a balance sheet can simply be handed to patients. For most problems, however, physicians will need to act as interpreters, counselors, and agents. In this particular case, physicians and patients can examine Table 7.1 and discuss whether decreasing the chance of getting colorectal cancer by an actual 3%, and decreasing the chance of dying of colorectal cancer by an actual 2.4%, is worth the discomfort of nine sigmoidoscopies, a 40% probability of a false-positive fecal occult blood test, and an additional cost of about $600—all spread over 26 years. A complete decision would require consideration of other options that involve different screening procedures (eg, colonoscopy and barium enema examination) and different frequencies. That information is summarized in Table 7.2.

❖ Strengths and Weaknesses

Balance sheets have several virtues. Perhaps greatest is their usefulness to practitioners; balance sheets provide the information that forms the basis for clinical "prudence," "judgment," and "discretion." Without the balance sheet, practitioners must perform two tasks.[4] First, they must determine the consequences of the different options. Then they must make the value judgments about the desirability of the outcomes. The first task is extremely difficult, and it should be no surprise that the perceptions of individual practitioners, even experts, vary widely.[5] The balance sheet provides a vehicle through which the practitioners and experts can consolidate their knowledge, taking whatever time and methods are necessary to maximize the accuracy of the estimates. Practitioners are then free to focus on the second step—tailoring and balancing that information for individual patients.

A second virtue is that balance sheets help both policymakers and decision makers organize their thinking. Policymakers can address each outcome, one at a time, examine the evidence and methods for estimating that outcome, and summarize their knowledge and benefits in explicit terms. Decision makers can see all the important outcomes at once and are encouraged to appreciate

TABLE 7.2 Best Estimates of Benefits, Harms, and Costs of Colorectal Cancer Screening Strategies*

Outcomes	No Screening	F1 and S3	S3	B5	C5	F1 and B5	F1 and C5
Benefits							
Probability of getting colorectal cancer, %	10.3	7.3	8.4	4.7	3.8	4.2	3.5
Probability of dying of colorectal cancer, %	5.3	2.9	4.0	2.0	1.5	1.5	1.2
Harms							
Probability of a false-positive FOBT, %	NA	40	NA	NA	NA	40	40
Probability of a false-positive barium enema examination, %	NA	NA	NA	16	NA	16	NA
Probability of perforation, %†	NA	0.3	0.3	0.09	0.9	0.09	0.9
Inconvenience/anxiety/discomfort							
FOBT, No. of tests	NA	26	NA	NA	NA	26	26
Scope, No. of tests	NA	9	9	6	6	6	6
Financial costs, $‡							
Screening	NA	643	584	568	1418	647	1476
Treatment	1155	1106	1069	672	548	775	676
Net	1155	1749	1653	1240	1966	1402	2152

*F indicates fecal occult blood test; S, 60-cm flexible sigmoidoscope; B, air-contrast barium enema examination; C, colonoscopy; 1, every year; 3, every 3 years; 5, every 5 years; and NA, not applicable.
†This is the probability of perforation due to endoscopy, barium enema examination, or a workup of a false-positive fecal occult blood test.
‡These are present values, discounted at 5%. A $4 fecal occult blood test, $135 60-cm flexible sigmoidoscopy, $200 air-contrast barium enema examination, and $500 colonoscopy are assumed.

the trade-offs in a balanced fashion. A third virtue is that the act of creating balance sheets will stimulate better habits. Gaps in evidence and widely varying perceptions will be exposed. Debates will be targeted. Research needs will be obvious.

The main danger of a balance sheet is that the use of numbers might falsely imply that outcomes are known with greater precision than is in fact the case. This can be guarded against by stressing the uncertainty, describing it explicitly, and describing the quality of the evidence. The main barrier to using balance sheets is the poor quality of evidence. This, however, is not a reason to discard balance sheets. Whatever the quality of evidence, policymakers who recommend an intervention (or recommend against an intervention) must have *some* perception of the outcomes. The balance sheet conveys those perceptions to the people who are asked to implement the guideline or who will have their lives affected by it. The balance sheet also exposes the beliefs, evidence, and methods to review. To a great extent, we do not have good information to fill out balance sheets today, because we did not ask the right questions yesterday. To have the information we will need for decisions tomorrow, we must ask those questions today. An important goal for the next 5 years is to develop balance sheets for the 1000 most important clinical decisions.

❖ Designing a Guideline

This chapter has focused on the use of balance sheets by individual physicians and patients. The next questions concern the design of a guideline. Suppose we accept the estimates in Tables 7.1 and 7.2 as reasonable? Should we recommend (1) that 50-year-old high-risk men *be* screened, (2) that they *not* be screened, or (3) that they not be given any advice at all? Whichever choice we determine to be the most desirable, should it be a *standard* (physicians *must* recommend it for *all* patients), a *guideline* (physicians *should* recommend it for *most* patients), or an *option* (physicians are totally free to choose)? Answering these questions requires converting a balance sheet into a guideline.

❖ References

1. US Preventive Services Task Force. Screening for colorectal cancer. *Am Fam Physician*. 1989;40(5):119-126.
2. Eddy DM, Nugent FW, Eddy JF, et al. Screening for colorectal cancer in a high-risk population: results of a mathematical model. *Gastroenterology*. 1987;92:682-692.
3. Eddy DM. Guidelines for policy statements: the explicit approach. *JAMA*. 1990;263: 2239-2240, 2243 (Chapter 6).
4. Eddy DM. Anatomy of a decision. *JAMA*. 1990;263:441-443 (Chapter 2).
5. Eddy DM. The challenge. *JAMA*. 1990;263:287-290 (Chapter 1).

❖ Source

Originally published in *JAMA*. 1990;263:2493, 2498, 2501, 2505.

Designing a Practice Policy

Standards, Guidelines, and Options

Designing a practice policy is similar to making a decision for an individual patient. In both cases, one must identify the available options, estimate the consequences of the different options, and determine the desirability of those outcomes to patients. Practice policies can be thought of as generic decisions—recommendations intended for a collection of patients rather than for a single patient.

Beyond these similarities, however, are some important differences that make practice policies considerably more difficult to design. In the case of a decision, the outcomes and preferences apply to a particular patient. There might be a range of uncertainty about the outcomes, the comparisons might be difficult, and there will be varying degrees of conviction about which is best, but, in theory at least, there is a single choice that is best for that patient. Practice policies are inherently more difficult because they attempt to make decisions for a collection of patients. This additional dimension adds several types of complexity. First, it increases the stakes. If an individual physician and a patient make a wrong decision, that patient will be harmed, but the damage will stop there. In contrast, practice policies are intended to influence thousands, even millions, of decisions. If a guideline is wrong, the harm can be huge. The second type of complexity is a spin-off of the first: the higher stakes increase the effect of uncertainty. Uncertainty is the main cause of mistakes. As the effect of a mistake increases, the importance of uncertainty also increases. The third source of complexity is variability. Ideally, the group of patients to whom a guideline is directed will be entirely homogeneous, with no important differences among the individuals in the group. In practice, however, inevitably there will be some differences in the patients and the settings that will cause individuals within the group to have slightly different outcomes as well as different preferences for the outcomes.

❖ The Need for Flexibility

The high stakes, uncertainty, and variability introduce a new factor into the policymaking process: flexibility. When the outcomes of an intervention are uncertain or variable, and/or when patient preferences for those outcomes are uncertain or variable, practitioners must be given flexibility to tailor a policy to individual cases. This need is addressed by having three types of practice policies according to their intended flexibility: standards, guidelines, and options.

Standards are intended to be applied rigidly. They *must* be followed in virtually all cases. Exceptions will be rare and difficult to justify. Violation of a standard should trigger thoughts of malpractice, and the defense will be difficult. A standard tells a practitioner, "you don't have to ponder this one, just do it." Other terms for standards are "rules," "strict" indications or contraindications, "strict criteria," and "clearly" appropriate or inappropriate practices.

Guidelines are intended to be more flexible. They *should* be followed in *most* cases. However, they recognize that, depending on the patient, setting, and other factors, guidelines *can* and *should* be tailored to fit individual needs. Deviations from guidelines will be fairly common and can be justified by differences in individual circumstances. Deviation from a guideline by itself does not imply malpractice. A guideline tells a practitioner "the majority of your patients will want this, but some won't. For important interventions, you must discuss the pros and cons." Other terms for guidelines are "relative" indications and contraindications, "relative criteria," "generally" appropriate or inappropriate practices, and drugs and procedures "of choice."

Options are neutral with respect to recommending the use of an intervention. They merely note that different interventions are available, and different people make different choices. Options leave practitioners free to choose any course.

❖ Determining the Flexibility of a Practice Policy

It is easy enough to define these flexibility categories; a more difficult issue is to operationalize the definitions. Specifically, how do we determine whether a particular practice policy should be a standard, a guideline, or an option? Placement of a practice policy for an intervention in one of these categories is determined by three things: the extent to which the outcomes of the intervention are known, the extent to which the preferences of individuals for the outcomes are known, and the spectrum of preferences among individuals. To say that outcomes are known implies more than an ability to list them; outcomes are considered known if their magnitudes (eg, the probabilities the outcomes will occur) can be estimated within a narrow enough range of uncertainty to permit decisions.

Standard

To write a standard for or against the use of an intervention, the main health and economic consequences of the intervention must be known sufficiently well to permit decisions and there must be virtual unanimity among patients about the overall desirability (or undesirability) of the outcomes. An indication that outcomes are sufficiently well known is that policymakers should be able to fill out a balance sheet.[1] Filling out a balance sheet does not require that the magnitude of outcomes be known precisely; a range of uncertainty can be described. The notion behind "virtual unanimity" of preferences is that at least 95%, perhaps even 99%, of people who are candidates for the intervention should agree on the desirability of its outcomes. The reason for these rather strict requirements is that once a standard is issued it will be applied rigidly to all patients. If policymakers are unclear about the outcomes, or if there are many patients who would disagree with the standard, great harm could be done.

Guideline

To write a guideline, at least some of the important outcomes of an intervention must be known, and what is known about the outcomes must be preferred (or not preferred) by an *appreciable but not unanimous* majority of people. Such a majority might be said to exist if 60% to 95% of people agree on the overall desirability (or undesirability) of the outcomes. Ideally, for a guideline all the important outcomes will be known, at least within a narrow enough range of certainty to permit decisions. If only some of the outcomes are known, the preference questions become more difficult. In general, if harms have been documented but there is no evidence of benefit, a guideline against the intervention can be written.

Option

Everything else will be an option. Thus, an intervention will be considered "optional" if (1) none of the important outcomes are known (outcomes unknown), (2) its outcomes are known but the desirability of the outcomes to patients is not known (preferences unknown), (3) patient preferences are known and patients are indifferent about the outcomes (preferences indifferent), or (4) patient preferences are known and are divided evenly (preferences split). Preferences might be considered to be divided evenly if about half (say, 40% to 60%) of the patients prefer one intervention, with the other half preferring an alternative. It is important to distinguish the four types of options because they have different implications for the responsibilities of practitioners when applying an option to individual patients, as well as for quality of care and for research.

Option, With Outcomes Unknown. If an intervention is considered an option because its outcomes are not known, the decision to use the intervention is arbitrary. There is no way to discuss the pros and cons of this type of option with patients, except to warn them that the pros and cons are unknown. This lack of knowledge and arbitrariness might or might not be causing harm; there is no way to tell. Notice that while this classification leaves practitioners free to use the intervention or not, there are good reasons not to use interventions for which the outcomes are unknown. To the extent that such interventions are actually used, they are obvious targets for research, first to estimate outcomes and then to assess preferences.

Option, With Preferences Unknown. If the outcomes of an intervention are known but the desirability of the outcomes is not known, the physician has an obligation to explain the outcomes to patients and help them determine their individual preferences. If this type of option is handled properly, it poses little threat to the quality of care. Options with preferences unknown are good candidates for research on patient preferences.

Option, With Preferences Indifferent. If the outcomes and preferences for an intervention are known but patients express no strong preferences either for or against the intervention, use of the intervention again becomes arbitrary. However, unlike options with outcomes unknown, it makes little difference which option is chosen. There is no need to explain the outcomes to patients because they will be indifferent. Quality of care will not be affected by the choice, and there is little need for additional research.

Option, With Preferences Split. In contrast to the previous case, if patients are divided about the desirability of an intervention, it is crucial for practitioners to describe the outcomes to their patients and to elicit their preferences. If patient preferences are elicited, this type of option poses little threat to quality of care and does not require additional research.

❖ Application to Colorectal Cancer Screening

These definitions can be applied to determine a practice policy for colorectal cancer screening with annual fecal occult blood tests and 3-year 60-cm sigmoidoscopy for high-risk men (due to a first-degree relative with colorectal cancer) age 50 through 75 years.[1] (To isolate the issues involved in the design of a practice policy, assume that there are only two choices: to screen with this strategy or not to screen at all.)

The first question is whether the outcomes are known. In this case, there is no direct evidence but considerable indirect evidence. Putting myself in the place of a policymaker, I believe the indirect evidence supports estimates of the benefits, harms, and costs of screening, albeit with wide ranges of uncertainty. This also seems to be the conclusion of the US Preventive Services Task Force ("[High-risk] patients should receive current information regarding the benefits, risks and uncertainties . . . ").[2]

The next question is whether patient preferences for the outcomes are known. To answer this, imagine 100 randomly selected 50-year-old high-risk men. We then present them with the balance sheet.[1] If they are screened with the proposed strategy, each of them can expect to decrease the actual probability he will ever get invasive colorectal cancer by about 3% and to decrease the actual probability that he will ever die of colorectal cancer by about 2.4%. However, he also can expect a 40% probability of a false-positive fecal occult blood test result, a 0.3% probability of perforating a colon, and the discomfort and anxiety of nine sigmoidoscopic examinations. He also will have to write out a check for about $650 (assuming the costs of screening are not covered). How many would say they want to be screened? Unfortunately, this question has never been asked. If the outcomes were clear-cut and obviously desirable or undesirable, there would be no need for a formal survey. However, in this case it is easy to imagine that different people could have very different feelings.

The lack of information on the desirability of the outcomes to patients means that colorectal cancer screening is an option. The preferred course is for physicians to discuss the balance sheet with their patients. An important research priority is to present the balance sheet to potential candidates for this intervention and see what they say. Such a study would be inexpensive compared with the health and economic implications of screening.

❖ Observations

This classification of practice policies has several important implications. First, because we lack information on outcomes and preferences relating to many interventions, there will be few standards. People who hope for a long list of rigid criteria that can be used in quality assurance and cost-control programs will be disappointed. People who fear losing their freedom to make decisions will be pleasantly surprised. Second, it is dangerous to call something a standard unless the outcomes are truly known, the preferences are truly known, and the preferences are truly virtually unanimous. To do so would imply we know more than in fact we do, would stifle research, would impede adaptation of practices to new information, and would expose practitioners to inappropriate professional, legal, and economic sanctions. When in doubt, downgrade the rigidity of a practice policy. Third, even if we end up calling most interventions options, there is still value to conducting the analyses and issuing those practice policies. It is honest, it alerts physicians and patients to the lack of information, it helps keep patients' expectations more realistic, it decreases the threat of malpractice, and it stimulates research.

Fourth, for practitioners the most difficult judgments will involve interventions for which some important outcomes—either benefits or harms—are unknown. Unfortunately, this is a large class of interventions. Traditionally, our responses have varied widely, from denouncing some treatments that are "unproved" (eg, laetrile), to embracing a huge number of diagnostic tests and procedures that have never been examined explicitly (and therefore are also "unproved"?). Furthermore, different decision makers can exercise their choices in different ways—practitioners may choose to use an optional intervention whose effects are poorly understood, while a third party may refuse to pay for it. Factors that affect the decisions include whether the procedure is new or old, how familiar it is, whether its use will impede the use of an alternative intervention that is known to be effective, the magnitudes of the harms (not only risks but inconvenience, discomfort, and anxiety), the cost and potential for misallocating resources, and the desperateness of patients. The interplay between these issues is subtle, complex, and important and will be discussed in a future chapter.

Finally, we are somewhat schizophrenic about how much flexibility practitioners want. On one hand, life is much simpler if there are clear lines (standards) that define the correct use of each intervention. It is difficult and time-consuming to discuss outcomes and preferences with patients. On the other hand, there is a strong tradition of individual decision making, and most practitioners bridle at the notion of being mere technologists who follow preformed rules. Discussing options with patients might be difficult, but it is the heart of the patient-physician relationship. For better or for worse, we have no choice about how much flexibility practitioners should have. The plain fact is that uncertainty, variability of outcomes, and variability of preferences exist, and practice policies must be responsive to those realities.

❖ References

1. Eddy DM. Comparing benefits and harms: the balance sheet. *JAMA*. 1990;263:2493, 2498, 2501, 2505 (Chapter 7).
2. US Preventive Services Task Force. Screening for colorectal cancer. *Am Fam Physician*. 1989;40:119-126.

❖ Source

Originally published in *JAMA*. 1990;263:3077, 3081, 3084.

❖ CHAPTER 9

Resolving Conflicts in Guidelines

As more and more organizations begin to develop guidelines, some are bound to be in conflict, recommending different things for the same patients. It is important to resolve conflicts in policies for several reasons. First, the differences in recommended actions can lead to differences in health outcomes; the existence of conflicting policies implies that at least some patients will be mistreated (unless neither recommendation has any effect on health outcomes). Second, differences in policies cause confusion. Practitioners will be advised to do different things, and will not know the standards to which they will be held. Patients will get conflicting messages, third-party payers will get the sense that decisions are arbitrary, and quality assurance programs will use different criteria. A third reason to resolve conflicts is that they harm the credibility not only of the guidelines in question, but also of the organizations that issued them. In general, conflicts in guidelines give everyone—practitioners, patients, the public, the press, the courts, the government, and third-party payers—the impression that the medical profession does not have its act together.

When the guidelines of two or more organizations are in conflict, some method is needed to at least explain, if not resolve, the differences. The current approach is to leave the choice between competing guidelines to individual decision makers, buffeted by whatever pressures the competing organizations place on them. The drawbacks of this approach are that the resolution can take a long time (decades) and the "winner" can depend more on the lobbying skills of the organizations than on the merits of the guidelines. This approach avoids none of the problems just described.

A preferred approach is to identify conflicts quickly, address them before they become embedded or cause damage, and resolve them through an orderly process according to the merits of the conflicting guidelines. The key to this approach is to break the conflict resolution process into two parts. First, identify the specific sources of disagreement that led to different guidelines ("make the diagnosis"). Then try to resolve the disagreements that are identified ("treat the problem").

❖ Diagnosing the Sources of Conflict

There are three main places to look for sources of disagreement: the targets of the guidelines, the objectives of the guidelines, and the rationales for the guidelines.

The first step should be to confirm that there really is a conflict—that the guidelines really do recommend different things for the same health problem. The most likely place for a misunderstanding to arise is confusion about the intended target of the guideline. The target is defined by five main factors: the health condition (disease or diagnostic problem), the patients (the specific indications), the intervention, the people who are to provide the intervention, and the setting (available resources). Guidelines that seem to be in conflict might in fact be intended for slightly different health conditions, patient indications, interventions, providers, or settings. The conflict might only be apparent, due to an incomplete or ambiguous description of the intended target. If this is the case, the conflict can be resolved quickly by rephrasing the guideline to clarify the intended target.

The second place to look for differences is the objective of the guideline. Most guidelines are written for the purpose of improving patient care. To be more precise, let us say that the main objective of most guidelines is to "maintain or improve the outcomes of patients to the maximum extent possible with the available resources." This objective recognizes that there might be a tension between the desire to maximize the care of an individual patient and the fact that pouring too many resources into a small number of patients can harm the care of other patients. While this is the presumed objective of most guidelines, it is possible that some guidelines have other objectives. Examples are to save money (regardless of the effect on patient outcomes), to protect the territory of a particular specialty, to promote a technically appealing device, or to achieve personal financial gain. The remainder of this chapter will assume that the conflicting guidelines have the same objective: to improve patient outcomes to the greatest extent possible with the available resources.

The third place to look for sources of disagreement is the rationale. Depending on the method used to design the guideline, the authors of a guideline ("policymakers") might or might not have described the rationale for their guideline. If both organizations have described their rationales through policy statements[1] and balance sheets,[2] the conflict resolution process can move immediately to a comparison of these documents. If one or both of the organizations have not described the rationale for their guideline, they must do so if they want their guideline to be considered in the conflict resolution process. The type of information needed for a rationale has been described previously.[1] Briefly, it consists of a list of the outcomes considered, a description of the evidence for the outcomes, estimates of the effect of the proposed guideline on the outcomes (as described in a balance sheet), a description of the methods used to make the estimates, and a description of patient preferences for the outcomes. These are the minimum elements needed to review the merits and expected consequences of a guideline. If an organization declines to describe the rationale for its guideline, that fact can be noted, and the conflict resolution process can be terminated. However, any organization that cannot explain its guideline must understand that decision makers will be unlikely to take its guideline seriously. Announcing a guideline without describing its origins or impact is analogous to announcing that an experiment demonstrates the effectiveness of some intervention, without describing the methods or results.

Organizations that have not yet written a rationale but that do want to participate in a conflict resolution process might fear that producing a rationale is too difficult or that the evidence is too weak to support any precise statements. It is important to understand that describing the rationale for a guideline should not require any new research or analysis, and the statements need not (indeed, cannot) be any more precise than the evidence permits. All that is required is for the policymakers to describe the thinking and evidence that led to the guideline—whatever that thinking and evidence was. Unless the guideline was arbitrary, which is rarely the case, the authors must have had some beliefs about how their recommendation would affect patients and some basis for those beliefs; they need only to describe those beliefs and the thinking that led to them. If the evidence is poor, if the estimates are subjective, if the range of uncertainty is wide, simply say so. The applicable maxim is, "tell it like it is." The remainder of this chapter will assume that both organizations are able to describe the rationales for their guidelines.

The rationale has many elements, and a comparison of rationales can become confusing unless a well-marked path is followed. The objective of improving patient outcomes suggests an obvious starting point. Begin by comparing the authors' estimates of the effects they expect their policies to have on patient outcomes (the balance sheet). If there is agreement there, it should not be necessary to review all the technical aspects of the policy-making process, such as the evidence and statistical and analytical methods.

The first question to ask about the balance sheets is whether the policymakers considered the same outcomes. For example, one group might have been concerned about an important harm that was overlooked by the other group. If the policymakers considered different outcomes, the merits of expanding or contracting the lists can be debated.

The second question to ask is whether the policymakers' estimates of the magnitudes of the outcomes are similar. Just as estimating the magnitudes of outcomes is the crux of the policymaking process, differences in these estimates will be the primary source of disagreement. People's perceptions of the effect of an intervention on an outcome can vary across a wide range.[3] Frequently, differences in guidelines will be traced to differences in perceptions of outcomes—one group might think the effect of the intervention is tiny, while another group could think it is huge.

If differences are discovered in the estimates of outcomes, additional questions are triggered. The questions will examine the evidence considered in making the estimates (perhaps one group was aware of unpublished research results), the interpretation of the evidence (perhaps the groups used different statistical methods or had different perceptions of the biases affecting a study), and the methods used to synthesize the evidence (one group might have used subjective judgments, while the other used statistical models). Any differences in the evidence, assumptions, or methods that led to the estimates should be identified and discussed.

When there is agreement about the outcomes of the intervention but there still is disagreement about the guideline implied by the outcomes, the next set of questions should examine the policymakers' assumptions or beliefs about the desirability of the outcomes to patients (patient preferences). For example, policymakers might agree that screening high-risk men for colorectal cancer with annual fecal occult blood tests and 3-year 60-cm flexible sigmoidoscopy from age 50 to 75 years will decrease the probability such a man will die of colorectal cancer by about 25%, that there is about a 40% probability the fecal occult blood test will cause a false-positive result during that time, and that sigmoidoscopic examinations are uncomfortable.[2] But the policymakers might disagree on how men feel about that. One group might believe that virtually all high-risk men will find the benefit well worth the risk, discomfort, and inconvenience; the other group might believe that a high proportion (say, one third) of such men will find the benefits too small to justify those harms. If it is determined that policymakers have different beliefs about the desirability of the outcomes to patients, the bases for their beliefs can be explored. Typical questions would address the policymakers' sources of information about patient preferences (eg, policymakers' personal impressions, patient interviews, a poll) and the methods used (eg, the representativeness of patients surveyed and the framing of questions).

❖ Treating the Differences

Once the source(s) of disagreement are identified, the second step is to try to resolve them. If the difference in guidelines is only apparent, and can be traced to differences in the intended targets, the resolution is to clarify the description of the health problems the guidelines are intended to address. If the difference in guidelines is due to different objectives, the merits of different objectives can be discussed. One or both organizations might modify its objective to align the guidelines. If this is not possible, the different objectives should be made an explicit part of the guideline, and decisionmakers should be invited to review the objectives and choose the guideline that corresponds to their own objective.

When differences are identified in the balance sheets, they can be more difficult to resolve. Policymakers should be able to reach agreement on the pertinent outcomes and pertinent evidence. (If there is disagreement about what outcomes are important to patients, the simplest solution is to ask some patients.) However, it might be more difficult to reach agreement on the interpretation and synthesis of evidence. There are well-established and widely accepted practices that make it possible to identify and correct oversights, oversimplifications, and errors in calculation. But there are also philosophical issues about which there are no uniform views. The prime example is the amount of evidence required to support a guideline. One school of thought holds that for an intervention to be promoted, there must be direct evidence from randomized controlled trials showing the intervention has a statistically significant beneficial effect. Another school of thought allows the use of indirect evidence. A third school of thought might permit a policy to be based on the perceptions of practitioners with no evidence at all. The objective of this aspect of the conflict resolution process is to identify existing differences, determine which are due to oversights or errors and therefore can be corrected, and determine which remain. The goal is to agree at least on a range of uncertainty for the outcomes. Ideally, new research might be conducted to settle a debate, but this will not be feasible for most problems.

If there is agreement about outcomes, but disagreements about patient preferences for outcomes, the reasons for different beliefs can be discussed. If agreement cannot be reached, the most straightforward solution is to agree on a representative group of patients and ask them what they think. Unlike research on outcomes, which usually is expensive and time-consuming, research on patient preferences is relatively simple and inexpensive.

Two temptations should be avoided: "copping out," and giving everyone what they want. Suppose one group believes that a particular treatment should be done, and another group believes it should not. Copping out would recommend that the treatment "might be a useful adjunct in certain cases," without specifying the cases or the criteria. This approach merely shifts the burden of resolving the conflict to practitioners; in essence it says, "we can't figure it out, you do it." This is unrealistic and unfair to practitioners. For an example of the second temptation, imagine that one group recommends a barium enema for a particular diagnostic problem, while another group recommends colonoscopy. It is tempting to resolve the conflict by recommending that patients get *both* a barium enema and colonoscopy. If there is a difference in the outcomes of the two procedures, that should be determined and the recommendations rewritten accordingly. If there is no difference, the "both . . . and . . ." should be "either . . . or . . . ."

The presence of a conflict is a valuable signal that important issues might have been overlooked by one or both groups. Conflicts should not be run away from, but engaged as valuable learning opportunities.

❖ Options

If after good faith discussion some unresolvable differences remain, there are three main options. One is to ignore the conflict and carry on in the traditional manner, letting practitioners, patients, third-party payers, and the courts deal with the confusion. The second is arbitration. The opposing organizations can agree on a forum, a process, and neutral judges and present their cases. The format for the debate would follow the process just described for identifying differences. The additional element would be an agreement to abide by the conclusions of the judges. This option has the virtue of resulting in a single guideline (that might or might not correspond to one of the original guidelines).

The third option is to agree to disagree. In this option, both organizations agree to rewrite their policy statements to describe the existence of the opposing guideline (with references) and the sources of disagreement. They also invite readers to review the different objectives, assumptions, evidence, and methods that underlie the conflicting guidelines and to choose the guideline that matches their own belief.

❖ References

1. Eddy DM. Guidelines for policy statements: the explicit approach. *JAMA*. 1990;263: 2239-2240, 2243 (Chapter 6).
2. Eddy DM. Comparing benefits and harms: the balance sheet. *JAMA*. 1990;263:2493, 2498, 2501, 2505 (Chapter 7).
3. Eddy DM. The challenge. *JAMA*. 1990;263:287-290 (Chapter 1).

❖ Source

Originally published in *JAMA*. 1990;264:389-391.

❖ Chapter 10

What Do We Do About Costs?

As a society we have conflicting views about the financial cost of health care. On one hand, virtually everyone is concerned about paying for health care. Health care expenditures now exceed $600 billion, an increase of 700% just since 1970, twice the rate of increase for other goods and services. At current rates, expenditures will reach $1 trillion by 1995 and $1.5 trillion by 2000. Health care, which was only 5% of the gross national product in 1940, is now more than 11%, and if current trends continue, it will reach 15% by the end of the century.[1] Everyone is affected. For industry, the average cost per employee increased 18.6% in 1988 (to $2354), more than twice the rate of increase seen the previous year.[2] Employers' future obligations for retiree health benefits is in the range of one-quarter trillion dollars.[3] Five years ago, states spent about 8% of their general revenues on Medicaid; in 1988 most states spent 15%.[4] (Recall that states pay less than half the Medicaid bill.) In 1980, employees had about $8 deducted from their paychecks for health care each month; by 1988, the amount had increased 400%.[5]

These increases would be fine if people were willing to pay the bills. Unfortunately, they are not. Everyone is trying to pass the costs on to someone else. Medicaid payments are small. Hospitals and physicians shift the costs to private insurers and businesses and sue states for more money.[6] The government wants industry to pay for its retirees before it kicks in with Medicare.[4] Industry is trying to restrict its benefits for retirees and is being sued in return. In the "spin the bottle" game of who should pay for the uninsured, the bottle is now pointing at small business. In 1989, the major issue in labor strikes was health benefits; for 78% of striking workers, the primary target was health benefits.[7] When individuals do end up paying some bills—because of exclusions and deductibles—they are shocked. Most of these problems could be solved by raising taxes and premiums, but the public refuses. At one time or another virtually everyone has cried out that health care is too expensive and something must be done.

That is one side of our conflict. The other side is symbolized by the cry, "Doctor, spare no cost." Patients expect the latest and best technologies, no matter how expensive and no matter how small or uncertain the benefit. Many people consider it unethical to take costs into account when deciding what tests or treatments a patient should receive. If an insurance company tried to justify not covering an intervention by pleading cost control, it would be skewered. Rather than assisting attempts to control costs, most practitioners see it as their duty to run interference for their patients to fight such efforts. The word *rationing* has come to symbolize an inhuman attitude and is used only by the most courageous speakers. Attempts by states to control costs by reducing the use of expensive interventions are far more likely to be called a scandal than a victory. Put simply, we want to have our cake and eat it too.

❖ Guidelines and Costs

Our conflicting views about costs take their most tangible form in the design of guidelines. Whether a guideline is intended to serve as advice to practitioners and patients, to determine if a procedure will be paid for by a third party, or any other purpose, it contains an implied judgment about costs and has a direct effect on costs. Depending on how costs are addressed, guidelines can serve either of our two desires. On the one hand, guidelines can consider cost an integral part of a medical decision and recommend a practice only if its health outcomes (benefits minus harms) are deemed to be worth its costs. On the other hand, guidelines can recommend a practice simply if its benefits outweigh its harms, without asking whether those health outcomes are worth the cost that will have to be paid to obtain them. The former position will help control costs, but will result in some beneficial practices not being recommended because they are considered too expensive. That's rationing. The latter position will not withhold any beneficial practices, but will drive up costs.

The majority of programs for designing guidelines have evolved from our second desire. While cost might be in the background, guidelines that explicitly and systematically consider costs are rare. For example, the appropriateness method developed by the RAND Corporation explicitly excludes costs.[8] The Consensus Conferences of the National Institutes of Health, the US Preventive Services Task Force, the Office of Health Technology Assessment in the Agency for Health Care Policy and Research, and most specialty societies do not systematically incorporate costs or cost-effectiveness into the design of their guidelines. Even the criteria used by the Blue Cross and Blue Shield Association to design its coverage policies do not include costs. Examples of programs that are beginning to consider costs are the Congressional Office of Technology Assessment and the Health Care Financing Administration. The

Office of Technology Assessment calculates the costs for some, but not all, of the options it analyzes for Congress. The Health Care Financing Administration is developing new regulations that will include cost-effectiveness as a criterion for coverage. This aspect of the regulation has drawn heavy fire and will be applied cautiously.

A useful way to focus the debate about costs is to determine how they should be handled in practice policies. This requires answering the following questions: (1) What are we trying to achieve? (2) Why are we not achieving it? and (3) What must we do to correct that?

❖ What Are We Trying to Achieve?

First, it is worthwhile to state the obvious: costs are real and people care about paying them. To appreciate this we can examine not only our own behavior, but there is empirical evidence as well.[9-14] If any more evidence is needed, consider the fact that all the strain caused by costs could be eliminated immediately just by increasing insurance premiums and taxes. Our strenuous avoidance of these most obvious solutions documents that people do care about costs.

Next, we have to convince ourselves that there is no way to make costs disappear. Whether through out-of-pocket expenses, insurance premiums, health maintenance organization fees, smaller benefit packages, lower salaries, the cost of automobiles, stock losses, recessions, higher interest rates, or taxes, all the costs will eventually be paid by people. Our attempts to rearrange the payments can launder, disguise, and hide costs, but cannot make them go away.

Consider an example. Several states have laws requiring insurance companies to pay for screening mammograms. When a woman walks in for an examination, she pays no bill. That sounds good. However, the screening center will send a bill to the insurance company. The insurance company will pass the cost of the mammogram on to its subscribers through increased premiums. Some of the subscribers are individual policyholders, who will immediately pick up part of the tab. Other subscribers have group contracts through their employers. Employers might reduce personnel costs (lowering employee benefits or raises), raise the costs of its products (passing the costs to consumers), or see lower profits (passing the costs to stockholders). Because business contributions to health plans are deductible, part of the increased premium will be passed to the government through lower tax payments. If the government raises other taxes to cover the deficit, taxpayers will pick up that tab. If the government covers the deficit by cutting back on some other service (eg, education, transportation, or housing), people who would have been helped by those services will help pay for the mammogram. If the government does not try to cover the deficit, it will go further into debt. The debt will cause the government to borrow, which will drive up interest rates, which effectively passes the costs to people who use loans. The net effect is to spread the cost of the mammogram across virtually everyone in the country. Now, each person's share of that single mammogram is only $0.0000002 (about $50 divided by about 250 million people). If that were the only activity being shared, nobody would feel it, and there would be no problem. Indeed, it is this tremendous dilution that creates the illusion that the cost has disappeared. However, by the time we finish tracking all the costs of all medical activities (about $600 billion) for 250 million people, we find that every man, woman, and child in the country ends up paying an average of about $2500 every year. That amounts to about $10 000 for a family of four.

Once we recognize that all costs will eventually be paid by people, we can set aside the fantasy that there is a magic financing formula that can somehow make health care free, and focus on the real problem, which is to ensure that the costs that inevitably must be paid are matched by the value of the health outcomes that are received in return. "What we are trying to achieve" is not the disappearance of cost, but an equilibrium between cost and value.

❖ Why Are We Not Achieving It?

A basic principle of our society is that, to the greatest extent possible, the equilibrium between cost and value should be achieved through individual choices in a free marketplace. When people have information about the value of a product or service (in economic terms, a "good"), and when they have to pay the bill for whatever goods they buy, they can compare the value they expect to receive against the cost they will have to pay and determine if one is worth the other. The virtue of this approach is that the "worth" of something is determined not by bureaucrats or planners, but directly by the people who pay the cost and receive the value. In such a system, wonderful things happen. Ideally, people spend their money only on goods that to them have equal or greater value. They automatically allocate their resources to goods that maximize their happiness. Producers compete to produce the goods as efficiently as possible and to develop new goods to serve people's tastes. The delicate tradeoffs between benefits vs costs occur naturally and continually at the level of individual decisions. If decisions in medicine worked this way, there would be no question about costs. We would be no more concerned about the proportion of the gross national product consumed by health care than we are about the proportion of gross national product spent on transportation, housing, or shoes.

Unfortunately, in medicine the conditions required for a market-based system of this type either are distorted or do not exist at all. Several conditions are essential for an efficient market: (1) that decisions be made by consumers, (2) that they know the value and cost of the goods they are contemplating buying, and (3) that they pay the full cost and receive the full value of the goods they choose to receive. All three fail in medicine. Because of "third-party payment," the people who are receiving the value of a health activity pay only a fraction of its costs, or none at all. Because of the specialized knowledge required and the emotional nature of medical decisions, many decisions are either strongly influenced by or made entirely by practitioners (let us call this "third-party advice"). And because of incomplete evidence and analysis, we are uncertain about the value of most medical activities.

Each of these features of the medical marketplace distorts decisions, with a strong net bias toward overconsumption. Begin with third-party coverage. Under most circumstances, insurance is a highly desirable economic tool. It allows people to avoid the cost of a rare but potentially devastating event in return for a certain, but far smaller, fee. However, a requirement for the efficient use of insurance is that insured individuals must not be able to control the events they are being insured against; a good example is an earthquake. Unfortunately, in medicine people have considerable control over the events that are insured. While few people will choose to contract a disease, physicians and patients have a great deal of control over which tests and treatments patients receive.

When insurance is applied to events that are under the control of the insured person, there is great potential for distortion. It is well known that people consume more when they do not pay the full cost of something than they would consume if they did pay the full cost. If they are the only ones overconsuming, that is a good deal for them (although it is a bad deal for whoever gets stuck with the difference). What needs to be emphasized is that *collectively* when *everyone* overconsumes, the result in the *aggregate* is not a good deal for *anyone*. Collectively, the costs people end up paying for health care exceed the value of what they are receiving in return.

This problem is compounded by the second failure of the medical marketplace: poor information about the outcomes of many medical practices.[15] If a practitioner or patient wanted to see a systematic description of either the health outcomes or costs of a particular medical practice, there is virtually no place to find it. Assessing a medical technology is a major research problem. The main problem with balance sheets[16] is that the data needed to fill them out are so poor.

The third failure of the medical marketplace is that many decisions are made by practitioners, not patients. Without debating here the appropriate roles of patients and practitioners in medical decisions, when practitioners make decisions for patients, the possibilities of distortions increase. To the extent that a practitioner's advice is influenced to do "more" because of professional incentives, pressure to "do something," wishful thinking, and income, this feature of the medical marketplace also will be biased toward overconsumption. In summary, the reason we are not achieving the desired equilibrium between value and costs is that we have cut the connection between the two.

❖ What Must We Do to Fix It?

No matter what direction our health system takes in the next few years—whether it remains decentralized, turns to a national health care system, or does something in between—resolution of the cost problem will require connecting value to costs. While guidelines can by no means achieve this goal by themselves, they can make major contributions to it. First, depending on how they are designed, guidelines can provide essential information on the value of a medical activity (health outcomes). Until we systematically provide this information, we will never be able to compare value with costs. Second, guidelines can provide information on the costs of an activity for the same reason. Both of these emphasize the importance of explicitly estimating the health and economic outcomes of practices.[16-17]

This brings us to the central question of whether the designers of guidelines (eg, specialty societies, third-party payers, and quality assurance programs) should go on to actually connect value with costs, recommending only practices for which the value is judged to be worth the costs, or whether guidelines should only compare health outcomes (benefits vs harms) and leave it to someone else to connect value and costs. The easiest way to decide whether guidelines should incorporate costs is to examine what happens if costs are not incorporated and leave that job to someone else. Who will do it instead? There are three main candidates: society, practitioners, or no one.

The option of leaving it to society is tempting (largely because it appears to get rid of the problem), but it is also problematic. The biggest question is, who is society? The government? A task force? Practitioners? Patients? In fact, society is all of us, as we express ourselves through the political and economic marketplace. (This chapter is one tiny piece of society's attempt to solve the cost problem.) Thus, one problem with assigning to society the task of connecting value with cost is that there is no single entity that can be identified and given the decision. An additional problem is that, to the extent that society can be considered an entity capable of making decisions, it has shown itself to be severely in conflict with itself about this question. Finally, even if society could determine how to incorporate costs, the main vehicle society would use to express its will on this question would be through guidelines. We would then face the problem that guidelines developed by society would tell practitioners to do one thing based on an incorporation of costs, whereas guidelines from other sources such as third-party payers and specialty societies would tell them to do something else based on an exclusion of costs. This would put practitioners in an intolerable position.

Even worse problems arise if we ask practitioners and patients to incorporate costs on their own. This approach would hand them guidelines derived without considering costs, and then require them to incorporate costs at the time of actual decisions, when patients are not paying the full bill, but are suffering the full emotional burden of their illness. This is not only intolerable, it is quite unrealistic.

The last option is to leave the responsibility to no one. That is, leave the marketplace as it is and do not attempt to connect value to cost. This is the most tempting because it requires no action. The drawback is that it does not achieve what we want to achieve—a connection between value and cost. Costs will continue to rise, inefficiencies and distortions will spread, friction between patients, providers, and payers will grow, and nobody will be happy except those for whom high costs represent high incomes. Another drawback of this approach is that it is unlikely to continue for long. Government and industry are near the breaking point.[18] If the cost problem is not addressed soon through the existing system, they will be forced to move to other solutions such as stricter controls over decisions, greater sharing of financial risk by providers, or a national health care system.

Now consider the merits of making the connection between value and cost through guidelines. This approach has the potential to be a scalpel, not a meat axe; guidelines can address specific health problems, interventions, patient indications, providers, and settings. This approach is natural; practitioners have used guidelines for centuries to guide their decisions.[19] There is a weak precedent; guidelines have implicitly incorporated costs in the past (no one recommends putting every postoperative patient in an intensive care unit); they have just not done it well. Incorporating costs in guidelines provides safety in numbers. Individual practitioners are not only spared the emotional burden of making decisions about costs, but can also take comfort that other practitioners are following the same guidelines. This approach is the only approach in which guidelines serve their intended purpose of being an aid to decision making. Instead of giving practitioners recommendations that ignore economic reality, guidelines that incorporate costs would make those agonizing decisions for them. Incorporating costs in guidelines should ease fears of malpractice. To the extent that lawsuits are determined by "standard practice," the guidelines that define standard practice will be the same ones being used by practitioners. A final virtue is that incorporating costs in guidelines is the only hope for avoiding the other options.

Citing these virtues does not mean that incorporating costs in guidelines will solve the cost problem. There are several limitations to what this strategy can accomplish. First, a problem that plagues medical decision making in general will also plague any attempt to incorporate costs in decisions through guidelines; we lack good information on economic outcomes, as well as the health outcomes, of most medical activities. While this should not stop the effort, it will certainly slow it down. Second, guidelines are only one of several factors that affect costs. Other factors, such as medical education, manpower, facilities planning, efficiency of operations, and financial and professional incentives, have a large effect on costs and will continue to do so no matter how costs are incorporated into guidelines. Third, practitioners and patients can choose to ignore guidelines that incorporate costs and continue to overconsume just for themselves. Although this is unfair, it will happen.

The argument for incorporating costs in guidelines is not that it will solve the cost problem by itself, but that it is an essential part of any solution. No matter what other steps are taken, the conflict surrounding costs cannot be resolved until guidelines connect costs to value.

❖ References

1. Fuchs VR. The health sector's share of the gross national product. *Science*. 1990; 247:534-538.
2. *Health Care Benefit Survey 1988*. New York, NY: Higgins AF & Co; 1989.
3. Freudenheim M. Employers resist accounting rule. *New York Times*. June 19, 1990: C2.
4. Freudenheim M. Volleyball in health care costs. *New York Times*. December 7, 1989: C1, C6.
5. Medical costs become primary issue in labor-management negotiations. *Washington Post*. July 19, 1988:C1, C7.
6. High court rules hospitals can sue on Medicaid rates. *New York Times*. June 15, 1990: A1, A12.
7. Department of Public Policy. *Labor and Management: On a Collision Course Over Health Care*. Washington, DC: Service Employees International Union, AFL-CIO, CLC; 1990.
8. Chassin M, Kosecoff J, Park R, et al. *The Appropriateness of Selected Medical and Surgical Procedures: Relationship to Geographical Variations*. Ann Arbor, Mich: Association for Health Services Research and Health Administration Press; 1989.
9. Newhouse JP, Manning WG, Morris CN, et al. Some interim results from a controlled trial of cost sharing in health insurance. *N Engl J Med*. 1981;305:1501-1507.
10. Valdez R, Brook RH, Rogers WH, et al. Consequences of cost-sharing for children's health. *Pediatrics*. 1985;75:952-961.
11. O'Grady KF, Manning WG, Newhouse JP, Brook RH. The impact of cost sharing on emergency department use. *N Engl J Med*. 1985;313:484-490.
12. Manning WG Jr, Wells KB, Duan N, Newhouse JP, Ware JE Jr. How cost sharing affects the use of ambulatory mental health services. *JAMA*. 1986;256:1930-1934.
13. Manning WG, Bailit HL, Benjamin B, Newhouse JP. The demand for dental care: evidence from a randomized trial in health insurance. *J Am Dent Assoc*. 1985;110: 895-902.
14. Foxman B, Valdez RB, Lohr KN, et al. The effect of cost sharing on the use of antibiotics in ambulatory care: results from a population-based randomized controlled trial. *J Chronic Dis*. 1987;40:429-437.
15. Eddy DM. The challenge. *JAMA*. 1990;263:287-290 (Chapter 1).
16. Eddy DM. Comparing benefits and harms: the balance sheet. *JAMA*. 1990;263: 2493, 2498, 2501, 2505 (Chapter 7).
17. Eddy DM. Guidelines for policy statements: the explicit approach. *JAMA*. 1990; 263:2239-2240, 2243 (Chapter 6).
18. Relman AS. Is rationing inevitable? *N Engl J Med*. 1990;322:1908-1910.
19. Eddy DM. Practice policies—what are they? *JAMA*. 1990;263:877, 878, 880 (Chapter 3).

❖ Source

Originally published in *JAMA*. 1990;264:1161, 1165, 1169-1170.

❖ CHAPTER 11

Connecting Value and Costs

Whom Do We Ask, and What Do We Ask Them?

     As a society, we are in conflict with ourselves about the cost of health care.[1] On one hand, we want the best care possible, regardless of cost. On the other hand, we are not willing to pay the cost of the care we want. Our conflict parallels a flaw in the medical marketplace. An essential condition for achieving an equilibrium between cost and value is that the two must be connected through decisions. When people decide what products and services (goods) they want, they must not only see the value they will receive, but they must also be responsible for the costs. Because of a variety of features of the medical marketplace—most notably third-party coverage, third-party advice, and uncertainty about outcomes—the required connection between value and cost is severed. The result is what we see. One side of our collective mind demands more services while the other side cries that costs are too high.

    Resolving our conflict will require connecting value to cost. An essential step in accomplishing this will be to incorporate costs in guidelines.[1] As controversial as that thought might seem (the great majority of guidelines currently do not take costs into account except in the most rudimentary way), arriving at the conclusion is the easy part. A more difficult issue is how to implement the goal of connecting value to cost. Suppose we agree that, in principle, costs should be considered when guidelines are designed, and that an activity should be recommended and covered only if its health outcomes (benefits minus harms) are deemed to be worth its costs. The next questions are, Who should do the deeming? What should the deemers be asked?

❖ Whom Do We Ask?

The determination of whether the value of a health activity is worth its costs should be made by the people who will both actually receive the value (experience the benefits and harms) and pay the costs. These people are not third-party payers, not legislators, and not government administrators. They are not health planners, economists, or statisticians. Neither are they medical experts, clinical researchers, or practitioners. They are people who either already have a health problem (current patients) or people who might get a health problem some time in the future (future patients). For convenience, I will combine both groups under the general label "Patients" (note the capital P), with the understanding that this is really everybody. These people are clearly the ones who will experience the benefits and harms. What is less obvious but equally true is that they are also the people who will ultimately pay the costs. After all the costs have been sliced and diced and spread around, they will all eventually be paid by people[1]—the same people who are now, or eventually will be, Patients.

If current and future Patients should be the ones to compare value and cost, we must now look more closely at how they think. A key to resolving our conflicting positions on costs is to understand that this is not a debate between different groups that hold different philosophic or economic viewpoints; this is a debate within each of us. Every one of us has two minds when we make a decision about whether a health care activity is worth its cost. We have one mind when we are well, sitting in our living rooms, paying taxes, or writing out a check for health insurance. We have another mind when we have a health problem and are sitting in a physician's office. To appreciate the distinction, imagine a hypothetical example.

A new drug is introduced to treat myocardial infarction. The drug increases 1-year survival by an actual 1% (0.01) compared with other drugs. (For comparison, with conventional care the chance of dying of a myocardial infarction within 1 year is on the order of 12%; with streptokinase it is decreased to about 9%. Assume that this new drug will decrease the probability of death by 1% further, down to 8%.) The drug has no risks, but costs about $10 000. Imagine that a third party has decided to handle coverage for the drug through a rider—each subscriber can decide whether to pay an increase in the premium in order to have the drug covered, should the need arise.

Suppose I am trying to decide whether to add the rider to my policy. To make an intelligent decision I must estimate the benefits and costs to me of covering the drug. The main benefit is a decrease in the probability that I will die of a heart attack. Given my age and risk factors, I have about a five in 1000 (0.005) chance of having a myocardial infarction in the coming year. After taking into account the chance that I will have a heart attack and the effect of the drug on my chance of dying if I should have one (0.01), access to this drug will decrease my chance of dying of a heart attack in the next year by about 0.00005 (0.005 × 0.01), or one in 20 000. The cost of the insurance rider is calculated as the chance I will have a heart attack and need the drug (0.005) multiplied by the cost of the drug ($10 000), or about $50. (For this example, ignore the administrative costs.)

Now, when I am trying to decide whether to pay the $50 premium in order to have access to this drug in case I should have a heart attack, I can weigh the probabilities, compare the expected benefit to the cost, and decide if, to me, the benefit is worth the cost. This is a personal value judgment.[2] Suppose I decide the expected benefit is not worth the cost. That is, suppose I am not willing to pay $50 to decrease my chance of dying of a heart attack in the coming year by one in 20 000. (Perhaps I'd rather buy some compact disks.) I will not buy the insurance rider.

That was one of my minds. Now consider my other mind. Imagine that I am unlucky and have a heart attack. I am now on a stretcher in an emergency department. A physician is leaning over me and asking if I want the new drug. Of course I do. There is no longer any uncertainty about whether I will have a myocardial infarction; I just had it. The benefit is still fairly small (the drug will decrease my chance of dying by 1%), but it is a lot (200 times) larger now than it was before I had my heart attack (0.005%). The benefits are definitely worth $50 and I want the drug to be covered. Give me my drug!

As this example illustrates, our conflicting views on costs correspond to two positions that we can be in with respect to our knowledge about which health problems we might contract, which health interventions we might want, and how much we have to pay. In the first position we do not know which, if any, health problems we will contract, or which interventions we will want, and we know we have to pay for whatever we choose. When we weigh the expected benefits against the costs, we might decide not to pay for some interventions, even some that are effective and for which there is a positive net benefit (the benefits outweigh the harms). In the second position our perspective is quite different; we know precisely which disease we will get and which interventions we will want, and the insurance check has already been sent. The magnitude of the expected benefit has changed, the costs are out of the picture, and an intervention that used to look bad now looks good.

❖ What Do We Ask Them?

A crucial step in connecting value to cost is to agree on which of our minds we should be talking to. In fact, both minds are real and have a legitimate say in whether the value of a health activity is worth its cost. However, it is essential to keep straight which mind should be asked which questions. The person in the first position (the person sitting in his or her living room) can be asked either of two questions.

1. There is a probability of 0.005 that you will have a heart attack in the coming year. *If* you do have a heart attack, the drug we are discussing

will decrease your chance of dying by 1%. Thus, having access to the drug will decrease your chance of dying by 0.005%, or one in 20 000. The additional premium to cover this drug is $50. Are you willing to pay $50 to have this drug covered?

2. *Imagine* that you have just had a heart attack. The drug we are discussing will decrease your chance of dying by 1%. The cost of the drug is $10 000. Would you be willing to pay $10 000 to receive the drug?

The essential element of these questions is that the probability of having a heart attack (0.005) enters both sides of the questions equally. For the first question, the probability that the person will have a heart attack affects *both* the benefits and the costs: the expected benefit is calculated as the probability of having a heart attack (0.005) multiplied by the effect of the drug for people who actually have had heart attacks (1%); the premium is the proportion of people who get heart attacks (0.005) multiplied by the cost of the drug ($10 000). For the second question, the probability of having a heart attack enters *neither* side of the comparison: the heart attack has occurred (the probability is 1), and the cost to be considered is the full cost of the drug ($10 000).

For the person in the physician's office who actually has the disease, the appropriate question is equivalent to the last one, with the only difference being that the circumstances are real.

3. You have in fact just had a heart attack. The drug will decrease your chance of dying by 1%. The drug costs $10 000. Are you willing to pay $10 000 to receive it?

Any of these questions can lead to a proper conclusion about whether the benefits and harms of the intervention are worth the costs to the individual. We might get different answers to the three questions, but they are all fair in the sense that they accurately represent the expected benefits and costs that apply to the respective positions. The third is the best in the sense that the Patient in the physician's office does not have to imagine how he or she would feel if a health problem were to develop; the health problem *has* developed and the Patient knows how he or she feels. However, if the cost of the intervention is beyond reach, an individual in that position might not be able to contemplate this question, as well as the second question (which is why people buy health insurance). For very expensive interventions, the first question must be used. The first question is real in the sense that it corresponds exactly to that faced by anyone making a decision about insurance. The only drawback to this question is that it requires the person to *imagine* what he or she would want if a health problem were to develop.

While it might be difficult for an individual to put himself or herself in those shoes, it is an inevitable part of life that arises whenever a decision is made about anything that has important but uncertain consequences for the future, such as purchasing other types of insurance, choosing a career, or getting married.

While each of these questions poses some theoretical and practical problems, those problems are trivial compared with the problems that are raised by a fourth question. It is *not* appropriate to ask the person who has the health problem (ie, the individual in the second position) the following:

4. You have in fact had a heart attack. The drug will decrease your chance of dying by 1%. The drug will cost you nothing (or some small copayment far below the full cost, or a slight increase in next year's premium). Do you want to receive the drug?

The inappropriateness of this question is that it applies the probability of having a heart attack to only one side of the comparison—the costs. The person has the heart attack, but was asked whether he or she was willing to pay only a small fraction of its full cost (eg, $50 vs $10 000). To ask this question should be just as absurd as asking the following:

5. You have a probability (0.005) of having a heart attack that would make you a candidate for a drug that will decrease your chance of dying by 1%. The cost of the drug is $10 000. Are you willing to pay $10 000 up front to have the drug covered *in case* you should have a heart attack?

Ironically, the least desirable question (question 4) is the one that currently forms the basis for most guidelines, including coverage policies. Any guideline that is based solely on the effectiveness of an intervention or its benefits and harms, without considering cost, is, in essence, asking question 4. Any policy that is based on a "community standard" or "common and accepted practice" is, in essence, determined by decisions made in physicians' offices, where Patients do not see the costs of interventions.

This illustration has been simplified on purpose to isolate the important concepts. For example, most people have group policies in which the majority of an insurance premium is paid by employers; thus, most people do not even face the full premium, much less the full cost of an intervention. Also, relatively few interventions are covered by specific riders, and most policies are for groups, not individuals. Thus, it is rare that an individual has an opportunity to make an insurance decision about a particular intervention. In addition, for most health activities, both the health and economic outcomes are uncertain. Finally, most Patients' decisions in the second position are strongly influenced by practitioners (third-party advice). However, none of these complicating factors changes the three-point moral of the story: first, we have two minds depending on whether we have a disease, and whether we have to back up our choices with our checkbooks; second, a main reason costs are out of control is that decisions and policies are determined by answers to the wrong questions; and third, to connect value and cost, it will be necessary to ask the right questions, and hold ourselves to our answers.

❖ Implementing the Connection

If a commitment is made to resolving the problem of cost by connecting value to cost, implementing the connection will require the following steps: (1) Estimate the health outcomes (benefits and harms) of the intervention.[3] (2) Ask Patients if the benefits outweigh the harms. (3) If the answer is no, stop. The intervention should not be used, recommended, or covered. (4) If the answer is yes, proceed to estimate the cost of the intervention. (5) Ask Patients if the value of the intervention (benefits minus harms) is worth its cost (using questions like questions 1, 2, or 3). That is, are they willing to pay the cost to receive the benefits and harms of the intervention? (6) If the answer is yes, the intervention should be used, recommended, and covered. (7) If the answer is no, the intervention should not be used, recommended, or covered. (8) Finally, adhere to the decision.

This list is simplistic in that it sets aside (for a later chapter) very important issues such as what constitutes a representative group of Patients, how to frame the questions and make them realistic, what to include in costs and how to estimate them, what proportion of Patients must agree in order to conclude whether the benefits are worth the harms and cost, and the very important fact that the Patients' answers will depend on how wealthy they are. These issues are not merely methodological; many of them imply social value judgments. However, given these simplifications, this list identifies the essential steps that must be taken to connect value to cost.

❖ Observations

First, the process described by these steps is not an alternative to administrative approaches to bringing cost into alignment with value. Rather, this process represents what must occur for the successful implementation of *any* rational approach to this problem. Most of the administrative mechanisms employed so far do not attack the problem of cost directly; instead they put pressure on someone else to solve it. Limits on Medicaid budgets, prospective payment, performance targets, physician profiling, and other mechanisms only create incentives; they do not specify what actually should be done. Ultimately they push the difficult choices about costs vs quality to individual decision makers. In the end, practitioners and Patients will have to resolve the conflict at the level of their decisions. This is the point at which the steps for connecting value and cost described in this chapter must be applied. If the resolution of the problem of cost is truly to reflect the interests of Patients (addressing simultaneously their concern for both value and cost), the resolution must follow the steps just outlined.

Second, it is worthwhile to review the essential ingredients of this process. There are three. Connecting cost to value requires (1) information about health and economic outcomes, (2) actual comparisons of health and economic outcomes by Patients, and (3) a conviction on the part of practitioners and Patients to live with their decisions. On the first point, it should be obvious that, if value is to be connected to cost, it is essential to explicitly estimate the health and economic outcomes of alternative interventions. The only reason to belabor this point is that currently few programs that design guidelines explicitly estimate even health outcomes, much less economic outcomes. There is a strong tradition in medicine not to do either. On the second point, there is also a strong tradition in medicine for practitioners to determine what is best for their Patients, rather than turning to Patients for those decisions (third-party advice). While it is neither feasible nor desirable to have every Patient compare benefits, harms, and cost at the time of every decision, it will be necessary to systematically survey representatives of Patients to learn their preferences.

These first two ingredients will be difficult to achieve for methodological reasons. The third ingredient will present an additional challenge. Implementing these steps will mean that there will be some health activities that Patients will determine have benefit, but are not worth their cost. This in turn will mean that some beneficial activities will not be used, recommended, or covered, solely because of their cost. Adhering to a Patient's decision not to pay to have a beneficial activity will require a sharp transformation in our collective and personal instincts to always provide the maximum care possible. If the Patient is in the first position (sitting in his or her living room) when the decision is made, adhering to the decision will mean that *if* he or she should eventually get a health problem for which the intervention might be used, the intervention will not be covered. The Patient will always be able to receive the intervention, but he or she will have to pay for it in full. If the Patient does not have the money, he or she will not get the intervention. If the Patient is in the second position (the individual in the physician's office) when the decision is made, adhering to the decision will mean the Patient does not get the intervention.

What? Not cover an intervention that has benefit, just because of its cost? That's heresy! No, it's not heresy; it is the connection of value and cost. When value and cost are connected, this is the form the connection takes—a conscious comparison of whether some real value offered by an intervention is worth its costs, and a determination to live with the decision. But isn't that rationing? Yes, it is. Isn't that bad? Not necessarily.

❖ References

1. Eddy DM. What do we do about costs? *JAMA*. 1990;264:1161-1165, 1169-1170 (Chapter 10).
2. Eddy DM. Anatomy of a decision. *JAMA*. 1990;263:441-443 (Chapter 2).
3. Eddy DM. Comparing benefits and harms: the balance sheet. *JAMA*. 1990;263:2493, 2498, 2501, 2505 (Chapter 7).

❖ Source

Originally published in *JAMA*. 1990;264:1737-1739.

CHAPTER 12

Rationing by Patient Choice

Resolving our conflict about health care costs will require connecting value to cost.[1,2] Ideally, the connection should be made through individual decisions in the marketplace—each individual would be responsible for paying the financial cost of the health care services he or she chooses to receive. This would force each of us to weigh the value of those services (their benefits and harms) against the cost we would have to pay and would ensure that, both for the individual and for society as a whole, the value of health care would be worth its cost.

Unfortunately, in medicine the connection between value and cost has been cut by some basic flaws in the medical marketplace, most notably third-party coverage, third-party advice, and uncertainty. Individuals do make decisions, but they are based on imperfect perceptions of the benefits, without appreciation of the true costs. The inevitable result is what we see today—an unchecked demand for health care services has driven up costs beyond the point that, when we eventually do see the bill, we are willing and able to pay.

To bring cost into alignment with value, someone must weigh the two. Specifically, someone must decide which health services are "worth" their cost, and which cost "too much." These decisions should not be made by administrators, legislators, economists, ethicists, medical experts, or practitioners, but by the people who will actually receive the value (experience the benefits and harms) and pay the costs, that is, present and future Patients. (The capital "P" denotes that this group includes well people who do not yet have and might never get a health problem—people in the living room as well as people in the physician's office.) Patients are clearly the ones who receive the benefits and harms of health care. As consumers, premium payers, and taxpayers, they also, eventually, pay the costs.[1]

Thus, for each intervention and patient indication in question, the procedure for connecting value and cost involves the following four steps: (1) make available to a representative group of Patients information on benefits, harms, and costs; (2) ask them what they want and are willing to pay for, using questions of the type described elsewhere[2]; (3) consistently implement the choices in guidelines; and (4) adhere to the policies.

The first three steps obviously raise important and difficult methodological issues. Before addressing them, however, we should examine the broader implications. In fact, the last step will be the most difficult. It will inevitably mean that some services that are beneficial will not be recommended, and these services will be denied coverage because they were found (by Patients) to cost too much. Let me paint the grimmest picture: Imagine that a new treatment is found for a disease that strikes one of every 1000 (0.001) men a year and has a poor prognosis. The treatment, which is accompanied by 10% mortality and considerable morbidity, has been shown to increase median survival from 13 months to 16 months and to increase 3-year survival from 15% to 18%. Its effect on long-term survival is not known, but it does offer some hope. Unfortunately, the treatment costs $150 000.

Suppose an insurance company offers to cover this treatment as a rider; for an increase in premiums of $150 ($150 000 × 0.001) per man per year, this treatment will be covered should the man have the misfortune of developing the disease. Suppose further that virtually nobody chooses to buy the rider. That is, suppose every man who is asked says that he would rather have the money than have coverage for this treatment. Perhaps they think that the probability that they will get the disease and the magnitude of the benefit of the treatment are too small. By declining the rider, those men have made the required connection between the value and cost and have stated their personal judgment that the value of the treatment was not worth its cost. Those men's decisions can then be implemented in guidelines; the treatment will not be recommended or covered.

When presented in the abstract, this seems acceptable. However, now picture what happens when a particular man gets this disease and "needs" the treatment. It will not be covered. If he wants to pay $150 000 on his own to receive the treatment, he can do so. But if he chooses not to or cannot afford to, the result will be no coverage for a treatment that increases survival and offers the only hope of cure for a dreaded disease. That's rationing. Because the rationing was based on the decisions of Patients, I will call it "rationing by patient choice."

❖ Rationing

Few words in medicine evoke stronger emotions than *rationing*. Images are conjured up of children dying of liver disease while administrators give lectures on economic theories to grieving parents and angry reporters. When seen in this light, rationing seems medically and ethically abhorrent.

On the other hand, the forces that motivate rationing are real: The cost of medical care already exceeds what many are willing and able to pay, and it is increasing at a rate that is out of control. From this perspective, rationing might be seen as a necessary evil; it might be the only way to keep the cost of health care affordable. The discussion, then, moves between descriptions of British[3] and Canadian-style rationing; pleas that we hold rationing off as long as possible[4]; observations that health care has always been rationed and the question is not *whether* but *how*[5]; and calls that we reexamine our values and goals.[6]

Part of the discussion about rationing is due to the use of different definitions. The dictionary definition is actually quite broad: to ration is to "allocate" or "distribute." The notion is that the supply of a resource is limited, and it is not possible for everyone to receive all of the resource that he or she would ideally like to have. The resource must therefore be divided up and allocated in some way. Classic examples are rationing water among survivors of a shipwreck or rationing gasoline during wartime.

The concept of limited resources certainly applies to medical services. For example, if I need a roentgenogram or laboratory test, I want it performed by the best technicians with the best equipment, I want the roentgenograms read by three experts, and I want the results in an hour. If I need surgery, I want to have it done by the world's most experienced surgeon. I want any test or treatment that might help—even if it costs (someone else) $1 million. Some people actually receive this level of care—President George Bush is an example—but it cannot be provided to all of us. A wide variety of factors already affect which people will receive which medical services. The most obvious is the sheer ability to pay. Some people fly to the Mayo Clinic for routine check-ups, while one in seven Americans has no health insurance. Other factors that limit who gets what include geography, availability of experts or special equipment, queues, and the ability to negotiate the medical system. All these factors affect the distribution of health care services. If *rationing* is defined broadly as the use of various mechanisms to allocate health care services, it is true that we have been rationing medical care for centuries, and the question is indeed not whether but how.

❖ Explicit Rationing

Why then is *rationing* such an emotionally charged word? The current controversy is due to a shift in how we think about rationing. In the past, rationing has been implicit. No one consciously planned it, implemented it, or defended it—it just happened. Most important, it was determined by forces beyond the control of practitioners. They did not have to actively deny their patients effective treatments; rather, the rationing occurred passively by determining which patients got in to see them. While these features did not undo the potential harm of rationing, they certainly made it easier to accept.

In the last few years, we have begun to think about extending rationing beyond its traditional domain to new ground. This new ground, which I will call "explicit rationing," is characterized by six main elements. The first is that, as the word implies, it is explicit. Someone will consciously and publicly define what activities should be rationed and how. The second concerns who will be performing the rationing. The new type of rationing would be implemented by practitioners face to face with patients. The third element addresses who is subject to rationing. Currently, about one in seven Americans has no insurance at all; coverage of their care is already rationed by ability to pay. Today's debate is whether to extend rationing to limit coverage for people who do have insurance. The fourth element is the target of rationing. Explicit rationing is not aimed at peripheral services that have been traditionally excluded by some insurance policies, such as dental, cosmetic, or eye care. Nor is it aimed at unproven, risky, or outmoded services. Explicit rationing is aimed at the heart of medical practice—at "standard and accepted" services that in the past would have been covered without question. The fifth element is the cause of rationing. In the classic examples, the cause of rationing is scarcity of some physical resource, such as water or gasoline. While there are examples of this type of scarcity in medicine (such as donor organs for transplantation), the real cause of explicit rationing is financial cost. The last element addresses what is to be rationed. Explicit rationing does not call for limiting health care services themselves, but rather limiting coverage for health care services from shared resources (ie, private insurance, private plans, and government programs). People would not be forbidden from receiving a rationed service; they would just have to pay for it themselves, in full.

Thus, the subject of real debate is defined by six elements: (1) explicitly, as a matter of policy, (2) having payers (3) withhold payment (4) from people who otherwise have coverage (5) for standard services that have demonstrated benefit (6) because of their cost.

Although medicine has a long history of rationing, several elements of explicit rationing are threatening. First, the explicitness forces us to make and defend decisions we would much rather ignore. Second, explicit rationing puts practitioners in an uncomfortable position. They might have to stand before patients, knowing that it is physically possible to offer them a treatment, and yet withhold the treatment if its coverage has been rationed and the patients cannot or will not pay. This is in clear conflict with providers' emotional, medical, and sometimes financial instincts to provide the maximum care possible. Third, extending rationing to people who already have coverage involves a much larger number of people than the current one in seven who are uninsured. Specifically, explicit rationing affects the other six of seven; it strikes much closer to home. Fourth, targeting core, effective services will undoubtedly remove some existing coverage, and, to the extent that people choose not to pay for the service on their own and that the service is truly effective, will actually reduce the quality of care. While we have come to accept that some services were never covered, we recoil at the idea of losing a service that was formerly covered or denying a new service that would ordinarily have been covered. Fifth, rationing because of financial cost abruptly wakes us from our dream that health care should be free and that cost should play no role in health care decisions.

❖ Meat Axe and Top-Down Rationing

The strengths and weaknesses of rationing by patient choice are best seen in comparison with other methods currently used to ration coverage. The best examples are from government entitlement programs. Current criteria used by various programs to determine who and what will be covered include age, employment status, gender and family status, income, type of disease, category of service, where the service is provided, and how long the service is needed. Because this type of rationing is based on broad categories of populations, diseases, and services, I will call it "rationing by meat axe."

Rationing by meat axe controls the costs of particular programs (eg, Medicaid) by limiting the size or boundaries of the program. However, because it does not address specific patient indications or interventions, it does not control costs within the program. That is, it does not directly ration the content or ingredients of a program. To accomplish the latter, many programs use additional mechanisms that attempt to ration services indirectly by forcing others to determine precisely which services should be curtailed for which indications. This type of rationing, which I will call "top-down rationing," does not specifically designate what activities should be eliminated, but rather puts pressure on others, usually practitioners, to make those decisions. Examples are prospective payment for Medicare payments to hospitals, limits on Medicaid payments to hospitals, and volume performance standards for physician services.

❖ Rationing by Patient Choice

Rationing by patient choice is distinguished from these other mechanisms by several characteristics. First, it is based on a direct comparison of value and cost, not geography, age, gender, family status, point of service, or other broad factors. Nor does it attempt to hide rationing behind queues or administrative hassle. This directness might make us uncomfortable, but at least it is honest. Second, the comparisons are performed at the level of individual interventions and patient indications (eg, signs, symptoms, and risk factors), not broad disease groups or classes of interventions. This means that, in theory at least, rationing by patient choice can be as finely tuned as desired. A third characteristic of rationing by patient choice is that the comparisons are performed by the people who will actually receive the benefits and harms, and eventually pay the costs. This feature of rationing by patient choice has an elegant simplicity. Is it worth $900 to perform magnetic resonance imaging for a patient with a headache if there is a 1% chance of finding a treatable tumor? Ask patients with headaches. Is $10 000 too much for a treatment that reduces 1-year mortality after a heart attack by 1%?[2] Ask people at risk for heart attacks. Do the benefits of colorectal cancer screening in high-risk men outweigh their harms and costs?[7] Ask men at high risk for colorectal cancer. These questions might appear to be purely economic, but in fact they address our basic values and goals.

The principal logic for rationing by patient choice is that it simulates, albeit imperfectly, what would have occurred had the medical marketplace functioned properly. A corollary is that it relieves administrators and legislators from trying to imagine what Patients want and are willing to pay for. The administrator's role shifts from struggling with impossible value judgments to understanding and implementing the judgments expressed by Patients.

The most important consequence of all these characteristics is that rationing by patient choice, if applied properly, should align value and cost in a way that is acceptable to Patients. When Patients make their choices, they would be speaking simultaneously about value and cost. If they want more value, they would simultaneously be expressing a willingness to pay for it through increased premiums or taxes. If they want to spend less money, they would simultaneously be expressing a willingness to settle for less value.

Rationing by patient choice has several drawbacks. Three are technical. First, because it is finely tuned to specific interventions and patient indications, rationing by patient choice requires much more work than, for example, rationing by age, gender, or broad classes of interventions and diseases. This ability for fine tuning is a strong medical virtue, but a methodological liability. Second, actually eliciting Patient preferences for costs will require great care. Issues such as selecting representative Patients, educating Patients, framing questions, adjusting for differences in incomes, and synthesizing divergent preferences are not only methodological but ethical and political. It can be done, but we have had extremely little experience doing it in medicine. Third, rationing by patient choice requires some kind of evidence regarding benefits, harms, and costs, which is often lacking.

However, none of these invalidate the approach. To be done correctly, rationing should be as finely tuned as possible, ideally down to the level of individual interventions and patient indications. With respect to the difficulty of eliciting Patients' thoughts about costs, these thoughts are clearly of fundamental importance in any strategy used to connect value to costs. Our lack of experience is not a reason to delay, but a prod to action; our methodological naiveté should be corrected, not pampered. Finally, the lack of good evidence on outcomes plagues every aspect of medicine. Whether the task is to weigh the benefits and harms of alternative treatments for individual patients, to provide informed consent, or to balance value with costs, there is no option but to proceed with whatever information is available. It can also be argued that attempting rationing by patient choice will be a powerful stimulus to getting better information.

As difficult as these methodological issues will be, there is another drawback that is much more disturbing. Implementing this type of rationing will require accepting the consequences of Patients' choices. If a man declines to pay $150 to have a treatment covered if he should need it, the consequence will be that, if he should need it, it will not be covered. If the man cannot or will not come up with the money on his own, physicians will have to stand by while he goes untreated. This will require a massive change in the way we think about what constitutes acceptable medical care. There are many models to help us—we stand by while people suffer the consequences of failing to buy other types of insurance or making a bad business decision—but it will still hurt.

❖ Questions

"Isn't health inherently different from other aspects of life in that costs truly should not be a part of medical decisions?" or "Isn't it immoral to consider costs when making decisions about health?" If the answer to these questions is yes, it would mean that people are willing to pay any amount of money, no matter how large, to receive any amount of benefit, no matter how small. Rather than debate these questions on a theoretical level, we can let Patients tell us the answer. There is nothing inherent in rationing by patient choice that forces any particular position or philosophy about what role cost should play in health decisions.

"Won't this approach limit access?" First, the process of rationing by patient choice (as distinguished from the actual choices Patients make when they apply the process) will not necessarily limit anything. It is up to Patients to define the limits. If they choose, they can spend $10 000 to buy access to an intervention that will reduce their chance of death by one in 10 million. However, suppose Patients decide not to buy coverage for such an intervention. That still does not technically limit their access to the intervention. The only thing limited by this approach is what is covered from shared resources. Anyone can go on to receive the intervention, at his or her own expense.

"How much money will rationing by patient choice save?" The actual effect on costs cannot be known until the choices are actually made. However, it is likely that rationing by patient choice will decrease costs substantially. Current policies are based on a gross underappreciation of costs. Many activities that look attractive when thought to be free will look unattractive when attached to a real price tag. This said, it is important to understand that the purpose of rationing by patient choice is not to reduce costs; it is to align cost and value. If Patients want to spend more money on health care, so be it. Rationing by patient choice will then tell us how much more they want and that they are willing to pay for it.

"How does rationing by patient choice fit in with other types of rationing?" Aligning value and cost through patient choice should decrease the need for more blunt cost control measures, such as prospective payment and volume performance standards. Those measures are imposed from the top down because cost is currently out of control from the bottom up (at the level of decisions about individual interventions and patient indications). Rationing by patient choice works from the bottom up.

"Given the specialized knowledge required, can Patients ever know enough to make truly informed comparisons of value and cost?" No. This is inherent in any complex decision involving outcomes that are not only uncertain, but that by their nature cannot be truly understood until they actually occur. (One cannot "test drive" an abdominal perineal resection.) However, this does not mean that the decisions cannot be made, or that they should be made by someone other than Patients. First, uncertainty about outcomes is an unavoidable part of medical decision making, no matter who is making the decision. Second, if Patients do not make the choices, who should? Everyone else—third-party payers, administrators, legislators, experts, and practitioners—all suffer from the same uncertainty about outcomes. Most of them also have financial or professional conflicts of interest, and none of them can really know how Patients feel (unless they ask the Patients, which is what rationing by patient choice is all about). To be sure, these decisions will be difficult for Patients, and there will be some bad choices, but that is a fact of life.

"Shouldn't rationing be postponed until all sources of waste and ineffective practices have been eliminated?" First, remember that rationing is already happening; all that is being discussed now is how rationing will be instituted. The real question is whether rationing by patient choice is worse than rationing by other methods, such as rationing by meat axe or top-down rationing. Second, while waste and inefficiency are clearly bad, and while efforts to eliminate waste and inefficiency should definitely be continued,[4,8] there are compelling reasons to proceed with rationing by patient choice. One is that if we wait until all waste and inefficiency have been removed, we will wait forever. A second is that there are relatively few practices that have absolutely no value; most have some value, or at least have proponents who will argue that point. Thus, for the great majority of practices that are candidates for improving efficiency, the question will be whether the small value is worth the cost. That is the question addressed by rationing by patient choice. A third reason to proceed is that making direct comparisons between value and cost, and implementing the decisions, is probably the best way to identify wasteful and inefficient practices and to stimulate reform. A final reason is that even if we eliminated all waste and inefficiency, we would still want to balance the value and cost of the services that remain.

"Won't this approach limit innovation?" No. Innovation does not require that a product be considered free. On the contrary, feedback on the value of a product compared with its cost is a crucial guide to innovation and is the most powerful stimulant possible for innovations that provide true value and that decrease waste and inefficiency.

"Even if people decline to buy coverage for a treatment, when they are actually faced with the disease and need the treatment, won't they change their minds and demand it?" Yes, they probably will, and they can receive it, provided they pay for it themselves and not out of shared resources. As harsh as it might seem, if they cannot or will not pay, the treatment must be withheld. The applicable maxim is, "You can't change your bet after the wheel is spun." Of course, we would all like to receive things without paying for them, but that is not a real option. To yield to demands for things Patients previously said they weren't willing to pay for would not only disconnect value and cost, but would disconnect them in a way that is unfair to others.

Compassion is one of the most noble of human emotions, but it has a price tag. We can choose to pay the price and place no financial barriers in the way of health care. But if we do, we must understand that an inevitable consequence of no financial barriers is uncontrolled costs. The crucial question is whether Patients want to pay the increases in prices, premiums, and taxes (and tolerate the waste and inefficiency) that inevitably follow from pretending that health care is free. If so, we should stop worrying about the cost of health care. If not, we must be prepared to accept the consequences. The main virtue of rationing by patient choice is that it puts the balance in the hands of the people who will live and die by, and pay for the results. In return for the freedom to set the balance anywhere they want, patients, and practitioners, must accept the consequences of patient choices.

❖ Methodological Issues

This discussion has skipped over several important methodological issues. They include the following: What constitutes a representative group of Patients? What do we do if Patient choices are not unanimous (eg, 60% find an intervention worth its cost and 40% do not)? How do we adjust for the fact that the amounts people are willing to pay are dependent on their incomes? Perhaps most important, what do we do about people who are poor who do not have enough money to buy coverage for anything? Each of these issues has not only methodological implications but conceptual, ethical, and political implications as well. They come to a head in the development of an operational definition of "essential care" or "basic health services."

❖ References

1. Eddy DM. What do we do about costs? *JAMA*. 1990;264:1161, 1165, 1169-1170 (Chapter 10).
2. Eddy DM. Connecting value to cost: whom do we ask and what do we ask them? *JAMA*. 1990;264:1737-1739 (Chapter 11).
3. Schwartz WB, Aaron NJ. Rationing hospital care: lessons from Britain. *N Engl J Med*. 1984;310:52-56.
4. Relman AS. The trouble with rationing. *N Engl J Med*. 1990;323:911-913.
5. Fuchs V. The 'rationing' of medical care. *N Engl J Med*. 1984;311:1572-1573.
6. Callahan D. *What Kind of Life: The Limits of Medical Progress*. New York, NY: Simon & Schuster Inc Publishers; 1990.

7. Eddy DM. Comparing benefits and harms: the balance sheet. *JAMA*. 1990;263:2493, 2498, 2501, 2505 (Chapter 7).

8. Relman AS. Reforming the health care system. *N Engl J Med*. 1990;323:991-992.

❖ Source

Originally published in *JAMA*. 1991;265:105-108.

❖ CHAPTER 13

What Care Is 'Essential'? What Services Are 'Basic'?

The concept is very appealing. It postulates that there is a minimum set of services to which everyone should have access, regardless of ability to pay. This set of services would form a floor for insurance policies, health plans, and government programs. People who want to receive more services could purchase them, either by buying more comprehensive (and expensive) insurance policies or plans, or by paying out-of-pocket. But everyone would at least receive the basic level of care. In the concept of essential care we find a compromise between the idealistic view that Society should provide everyone with everything free of charge, and the practical fact that, as a society, we cannot pay the price of doing that. It strikes an ethical balance between Society's obligation to the individual and the individual's obligation to Society.

The concept is indeed appealing. Unfortunately, putting the concept into practice is far more difficult. Despite the fact that terms such as essential care and basic services come up in virtually every discussion of rationing, the uninsured poor, care for the aged, mandated benefits, and national health insurance, they have never been defined in truly operational terms.

The general principles have been well described. For example, Callahan[1] has written:

A "minimal level of adequate care" consists, first, of full support for caring . . .; second, of full support for those public health measures that promote general societal health as well as access to primary and emergency care; and, third, of access to more individualized forms of cure compatible with a sensible allocation of resources to the health sector in relationship to other societal requirements.

94

General definitions of this type serve as useful guides, directing our attention, for example, to a balance between caring and prevention vs curing. But they leave unanswered the specific questions about just which interventions provide "full support" or are a "sensible allocation of resources."

Other definitions that do attempt to be operational usually end up defining broad categories of services. For example, the recent report of the Pepper Commission[2] defines the "recommended minimum benefit package" as:

> hospital care, surgical care and other inpatient physician services, physician office visits, diagnostic tests, and limited mental health services (45 inpatient days and 25 outpatient visits), and preventive services including prenatal care, well-child care, mammograms, Pap smears, colorectal and prostate cancer screening procedures, and other preventive services that evidence shows are effective relative to costs.

This type of definition *is* operational in the sense that a physician or administrator could determine whether an intervention was essential. But with the possible exception of the four cancer screening tests, which for unstated reasons are singled out for special mention, this definition is so broad that it is very unlikely to accurately sort out services that are truly essential in the usual sense of the word. Whether a service is essential appears to depend more on where it is provided, by whom and when, than on its actual value to patients. For example, an extremely expensive, very low-yield diagnostic test provided in a hospital would apparently be considered essential by this definition (because it is provided in a hospital), whereas a lifesaving antibiotic that could be taken at home would not. The definition does include a guiding principle for selecting preventive services ("that evidence shows are effective relative to costs"), but it leaves to others the task of determining what amount of effectiveness is worth what cost.

❖ Defining Essential Care

Suppose we wanted to actually define a set of interventions that would be considered essential. Or let us make the problem even simpler. Suppose we have a particular intervention in mind—how would we actually go about determining if that intervention is essential?

An operational definition of essential care must begin with a clear understanding of the issue that is to be resolved. The central problem that underlies the concept of essential care is that different interventions have different worths, determined by their benefits, harms, and costs. While few would debate the importance of benefits and harms, some might object to including costs. But cost is the very problem that drives the concept of essential care. If costs were of no concern, there would be no problem; everyone could get everything that has benefit, and the distinction between essential and "luxury" care would never arise. To remove costs from the definition of essential care would not only be unrealistic, it would separate the concept of essential care from the problem it is designed to solve.

Whether an intervention is essential will depend on how the benefits, harms, and costs are weighed. Interventions that have great benefits, no harms, and low costs are essential. Interventions that have no benefits, or for which the benefits only slightly outweigh the harms, and that have high costs, are not. The central issue is where and how to draw the line.

This formulation of the problem has several implications. First, in order to determine if a service is essential, it is necessary to have some idea of its benefits, harms, and costs. An operational definition of essential care that is not based on its benefits, harms, and costs is like an automobile without a steering wheel. This might seem obvious, but it is pertinent that we do not yet systematically estimate the benefits, harms, and costs of an intervention.

The second implication is that the need for information about benefits, harms, and costs means that essential care must be defined at the level of particular interventions. "Hospital care," "surgical care," "diagnostic tests," and even "prenatal care" are far too broad to enable any useful estimates of benefits, harms, and costs. Furthermore, for many interventions it will be necessary to narrow the target to specific indications. Carotid endarterectomy might well be considered essential for a 65-year-old man with transient ischemic attacks, 80% stenosis, and history of stroke, but not for a 50-year-old asymptomatic man with 20% stenosis. For some interventions, it might even be necessary to identify a particular protocol. A Papanicolaou smear every 5 years is almost certainly essential; a Papanicolaou smear every 2 months is almost certainly not.

A third implication is that defining essential care will inevitably involve making value judgments. Sometime and somewhere, some group of people will have to compare benefits vs harms, and compare health outcomes vs costs. These three implications add up to the following: to determine what constitutes essential care, it is necessary to (1) identify specific interventions, patient indications, and protocols; (2) estimate their benefits, harms, and costs (compared with specified alternatives); and (3) weigh the benefits vs harms and costs.

Now let us assume that we have identified an intervention and have estimated its benefits, harms, and costs. (This might not be a good assumption for some interventions, but a strong case can be made that if it is not possible to estimate the benefits and harms of an intervention, that intervention cannot be considered essential.) Suppose, for example, we are interested in a hypothetical drug that decreases the probability of dying of a myocardial infarction from 9% to 8% (an actual decrease of 1 percentage point, or 0.01), and that costs $10 000.[3] The decision to cover the drug can also be viewed from the perspective of an insurance rider. A man or woman who has a five in 1000 chance (0.005) of having a heart attack in the coming year would pay $50 (0.005 × $10 000) to buy coverage for the drug that would decrease his or her chance of dying of a heart attack by one in 20 000 (0.005 × 0.01). We now face the third step. Who should decide if this treatment is essential?

❖ Who Should Decide?

In previous chapters[3-5] I have argued that decisions about benefits, harms, and costs should be made by the people who will actually receive the benefits and harms and eventually bear the costs—that is, Patients. It is their lives and their money. The easiest way to appreciate that the choices should be made by Patients is to ask—who is in a better position to weigh the benefits, harms, and costs than the people who will have to live with the benefits and harms, and who will eventually have to pay the cost? Thus the general strategy is to identify some representative Patients (let us call them judges); present them with information on the benefits and harms of the intervention (using questions like those described in a previous chapter[4]); tell them what it will cost them to receive those outcomes (being careful to construct settings in which the options, outcomes, and costs are realistic); and observe their choices.

This approach is clearly a good way to learn how people weigh benefits and harms. However, it faces a major problem in the evaluation of costs. Since costs are at the heart of any definition of essential care, this problem deserves careful thought. The problem is that the amounts of money that people are willing to pay to receive the outcomes of a health intervention depend critically on their financial status (eg, income and net worth). A poor person who makes, say, $5000 a year might well find $50 to be far too high a price to pay for a drug that reduces the probability he or she will die of a heart attack by one in 20 000. In contrast, a person making $300 000 a year might consider it a best buy to pay $50 a year to reduce the chance of a heart attack by one in 20 000. If we use the value judgments of the wealthiest people to define essential care, nearly everything will be essential—which is clearly not helpful (nobody except the wealthiest people will be able to afford it). If we use the judgment of the poorest people, very few interventions will be called essential—which fails to achieve our goal of providing an ethical floor for health services. What financial status should be used as a reference point?

To begin the discussion, let us suppose that we use the median financial status in the United States as the reference for defining essential services. To simplify the description of the main concepts, I will use income as a measure of financial status, with the understanding that if the concept is acceptable, we can return to define a better measure of financial status that incorporates, for example, net worth as well as income. Thus, to be more specific, let us say that an intervention will be considered essential if Patients with median incomes find the health outcomes (benefits and harms) of the intervention to be worth its costs. Other cutoff points could obviously be chosen. For example, if a public debate reveals that we are inclined to be more generous, we can increase the level to say, 125% of the median income. Or if we are feeling less generous, we can make the reference 85% of the median income. But the median has a nice symmetry. It not only corresponds to the criterion we use for most other public decisions—majority vote—but it roughly defines the "average American."

If, for the time being, we accept the median income as an appropriate reference or benchmark, the next task is to build this reference into the process for defining essential care. One strategy is to select at random a group of Patients who have median incomes and let them make their choices. However, this would greatly limit the number of available judges, and might restrict the judges to too narrow a set of personal beliefs, education, occupations, and values.

An alternative strategy is to index the perceived costs of the interventions to the income levels of the individual judges, using the median US income as the reference point. For example, costs could be presented in terms of daily wages. To keep the numbers round, suppose the median daily wage is $100. To a median-income person, coverage for the heart attack drug ($50) would cost a half-day's wage. This could be used to standardize the costs for people with different incomes. For example, a person who earned only $40 a day could be asked if he or she was willing to pay half a day's wage (which to him or her is $20). A person whose average daily income was $1000 would also be asked to pay a half a day's wage (which to him or her is $500). This strategy does not discriminate against gender, race, age, or any other factor that might be connected with income. In fact, it is designed to eliminate income discrimination. It is also important to understand that this strategy does *not* call for actually charging everyone a cost that is indexed to his or her income. Rather, this maneuver would be used only to learn the choices judges would make after adjustment for their incomes to make them "average."

To summarize, the steps for defining essential care that adjust for differences in income now become (1) estimate the benefits and harms of the intervention, (2) estimate the costs in real dollars, (3) convert the costs into an equivalent wage, using the median wage as the reference point, (4) ask each judge if he or she is willing to pay that equivalent wage to receive the intervention, and (5) define as essential anything that the average Patient would want for himself or herself. Others can no doubt improve on the details of this strategy; it is the principle I want to emphasize. The spirit of this proposal is much like the Golden Rule: Do unto others as you would have them do unto you. If the average person would choose the intervention for himself or herself, it should be considered essential for others. But if the average person would not choose an intervention for himself or herself, it need not be considered essential for others.

❖ Design Issues

Implementing a system like this would require careful attention to many methodological issues. In addition to the usual problems that arise in the estimation of outcomes and costs, some obvious examples are the following: How many judges should there be? To what extent should the Patient judges be advised by physicians? What mechanism or forum should be used to elicit the judges' choices (eg, polls, focus groups, face-to-face interviews, a "science court," actual experiments)? How should the questions be framed? Particular interventions will often determine particular genders and age groups, but within those groups, should judges be selected at random, or should a conscious attempt be made to achieve a spectrum across other variables (eg, geography, education, religious background)? If Patients themselves cannot serve as judges (eg, because of age or mental incompetence), who should serve as their proxies? How should judges be calibrated for variables other than income (eg, net worth, family status)? How frequently should the judges' opinions be updated to consider new technologies or possible changes in social values? There is already a rich literature on many of these topics, but this research would require translation to this problem, and no doubt some additional work.

Most of these issues can be addressed using established principles from statistics, psychology, economics, and ethics. Two issues, however, deserve special mention: (1) What if the judges are not unanimous? and (2) How do we deal with interventions whose outcomes affect different parties in conflicting ways? First, we can expect that the decisions of judges will rarely be unanimous. Suppose 37% of men at risk of heart attacks choose to buy coverage for the heart attack drug, while 63% decide that the coverage is not worth the cost. Clearly the degree of unanimity provides very useful information about the degree of "essentialness," as perceived by Patients. But some rule will still be needed to place this treatment on one side of the line or the other. The first step is to see if there are any identifiable factors that separate those who choose the intervention from those who do not. Perhaps there is some subgroup of people who have a different value system that must be respected. If that is the case, it might be possible and desirable to include those factors in the list of patient indications, and develop separate policies for the different groups of people. But assuming that no such factors can be identified or that it is not practical or ethical to separate people by that factor, an obvious strategy for resolving split decisions is to consider an intervention essential if it is chosen by a majority of judges. This not only is consistent with other public decisions, but maximizes the number of people who will be pleased with the results.

The other issue deals with judgments that affect different interest groups. Up to this point, I have tacitly assumed that the outcomes of interventions affect only the people who actually receive the intervention. In fact, many interventions affect several parties, in conflicting ways. A policy to isolate a person who has a highly infectious disease is an obvious example. From a purely selfish point of view, the patient who has the infection would say the harms and costs of isolation outweigh its benefits. But people who might be exposed to the infection would argue the other way. In problems of these types, both sides have reasonable and legitimate interests.

There are several ways to reconcile the interests of the different parties. One is to select a set of judges who are neutral in the sense that they do not represent either party. Preferably, they should be vulnerable to the possibility of eventually ending up in either party. These neutral judges would then be presented with information on the outcomes that affect each party *and* the probabilities that they (the neutral judges) might eventually end up in either party. Because the judges must face the possibility that they will be in either party, their interests will span both parties, and they will be forced to weigh the interests of both parties. This approach is a variation of the "original position" described by Rawls.[6]

When dealing with these or any other of the methodological issues, it is important to keep them in perspective. First, the definition of essential care is in its infancy. Our initial steps must be tentative, open to review, and eager for improvement. Second, it is quite likely that there is no single set of methods, much less a perfect set of methods, that will be applicable to all problems.

Like experimental designs for clinical research, the appropriate methods will undoubtedly be different for different interventions, and will have to be tailored to fit particular problems. Also, like experimental designs, each method will undoubtedly have its strengths, weaknesses, and biases, and will require interpretation. Our immediate goal is not to be perfect, but to improve on what we are doing now. Given that, at present, there is no systematic approach at all to learning how Patients weigh benefits and harms, or how much they are willing to pay for health interventions, that goal should be easy to achieve.

❖ Observations

First, this approach, which for convenience I will call "majority choice by average Patients," does not depend on or promote any particular mechanism for *financing* essential care. This approach could be applied in our current heterogeneous financing system to define a basic insurance policy, a basic managed care plan, or essential services for Medicaid and Medicare. Alternatively, it could be used to define a basic benefit package for a mandated employer-based program for the uninsured poor, or for a national health plan. This approach addresses the *content* of essential care, not its financing.

A second observation is that inherent in this approach, indeed inherent in the very idea of essential care, is that it is acceptable for different people to end up receiving different levels of care. The ethics of having multiple levels of care depends critically on where the levels are set. There is good agreement that it is unacceptable to have some people receive a very high level of care while other people receive virtually no care at all. However, there is also good agreement that it is acceptable to have some people receive a very high level of care while others receive less care, *provided* that the lower level of care covers everything that is essential. The majority choice of average Patients defines that lowest acceptable level of care to be that which an average American would want for himself or herself if he or she were paying the bill. By definition, if people with median financial status were offered a more comprehensive package (at a higher cost), they would turn it down. This is the basis for saying that this level satisfies essential needs. However, we *can* expect wealthier people to buy more comprehensive packages. No doubt several different levels of insurance and health plans would eventually be offered, and bought. It is even easy to imagine insurance companies and health plans competing by offering different levels of care, for different prices.

The third observation is at first thought startling. If this approach were to be used to define essential care, policies that will affect millions of people and billions of dollars would be based on the value judgments of a small group of judges, perhaps 50 to 2000 people. That seems like a very fragile basis for such a huge impact. Ironically, as fragile as that might seem, it is considerably more stable than what we do now. Currently, the great majority of policies are set with no explicit estimation at all of the benefits, harms, or costs of interventions, and no systematic exploration of how Patients weight benefits, harms, and costs. Whatever the methodological flaws of defining essential care by the majority vote of average Patients, they are trivial compared with the methodological flaws of current methods used to set these policies.

Finally, this approach can be applied piecemeal—one intervention at a time—with very little investment, and without any major commitment to legislative change, financing, or even implementation. Whenever a new technology raises questions about benefits, harms, or costs, its outcomes could be estimated, a representative group of Patients could be identified, the questions could be asked, and Patient choices could be learned. Let's pick a few controversial interventions, try it out, and see what happens.

❖ References

1. Callahan D. *What Kind of Life: The Limits of Medical Progress.* New York, NY: Simon & Schuster Inc Publishers; 1990:191.
2. *A Call for Action.* Washington, DC: The Pepper Commission; 1990:61.
3. Eddy D. What do we do about costs? *JAMA.* 1990;264:1161, 1165, 1169, 1170 (Chapter 10).
4. Eddy D. Connecting value and costs: whom do we ask, and what do we ask them? *JAMA.* 1990;264:1737-1739 (Chapter 11).
5. Eddy D. Rationing by patient choice. *JAMA.* 1990;264:105-108 (Chapter 12).
6. Rawls J. *Theory of Justice.* Cambridge, Mass: Harvard University Press; 1971.

❖ Source

Originally published in *JAMA.* 1991;265:782, 786-788.

CHAPTER 14

The Individual vs Society

Is There a Conflict?

Your Hospital Cafeteria: 7:40 AM

DR WILLIAMS: I need to fill you in on Mrs Smith.

DR HART: Oh, yes, I remember her. Breast cancer, about 2 years ago. I saw her family in the hall yesterday. How is she?

W: Unfortunately, she's gotten worse. She now has metastases to the liver and bone.

H: Oh, dear, she's such a lovely woman. What's next?

W: Well, I want to try high-dose chemotherapy with autologous bone marrow transplantation. I've told her about the 10% treatment mortality, about the high complication rates and side effects, and that there are no controlled trials showing benefit, but it's her only hope.

H: Will her insurance company cover it?

W: We're lucky there. Her employer is self-insured. They've agreed to cover the costs from an employee-funded health promotion fund. Apparently they don't want the bad publicity some of the other insurers have gotten when they've exercised their contract exclusions for investigational procedures.

H: What did you think about the talk by Dr Horner at the Grand Rounds last month?

W: The cost does bother me; $150 000 is a lot of money. In Mrs Smith's case, she won't have to pay anything. But Dr Horner's point was that the amount of benefit from this treatment is small compared with its cost. She estimated that if the same resources were put into breast cancer screening, they would deliver about 10 times the benefit compared with high-dose chemotherapy.

H: But what good does that do Mrs Smith? It's too late to screen her now. Given her current condition, your only choices are the chemotherapy or nothing.

W: True. I didn't really understand the point Dr Horner was trying to make. She seemed to be saying that, from a social or public health perspective, it's better to spend the money screening women for breast cancer. She even went so far as to imply that doing high-dose chemotherapy instead of screening was harmful, because it might deprive others of the screening. But what can I do about that? I agree that the chance of success is low, but it's Mrs Smith's only option.

H: What are you going to do?

W: What do you think? I'm going to do the chemotherapy. If somebody else wants to screen women, they should do that. It's not as though I control that money and can spend it on something else if I don't treat Mrs Smith. God knows, I don't want to see any more cases of metastatic breast cancer, but we've got to treat the patients we've already got. The way I see it, the best way to fight this disease, even from a social perspective, is for each of us to do everything we possibly can for the people we're responsible for.

❖ What Is the Conflict?

First, let's amplify the point being made by Dr Horner, who is hypothetical. Although there are no controlled trials showing any benefit of high-dose chemotherapy with autologous bone marrow transplantation (HDC-ABMT), and although many oncologists consider the treatment investigational,[1] the treatment does offer hope. To try to capture the value of this hope to Mrs Smith, let us *suppose* that this treatment provides a 5% chance of completely curing women who have what is otherwise considered "terminal" metastatic breast cancer. Let us further suppose that the treatment is 5% effective and is indicated regardless of a woman's age, type of breast cancer, sites of metastases, or other factors. It is important to stress that this effectiveness is, at present, hypothetical.

Now consider a 50-year-old woman with metastatic breast cancer. If this treatment has a 5% cure rate, and if she might live, say, 30 more years if she is cured, then this treatment would increase her life expectancy by about 1.5 years (0.05×30 years). Suppose that instead the $150 000 was used to provide screening for breast cancer. At approximately $100 per screening examination, $150 000 would buy 10 years of mammograms (from age 50 to 60 years) for about 150 women. Assuming that mammography can reduce breast cancer mortality by about 40% in this age group, in a group of 150 women this implies a gain of approximately 12 person-years of life. That is about eight times the impact of HDC-ABMT.

Furthermore, mammography screening by itself is not very cost-effective. Consider what would happen if the $150 000 was spent on antitobacco education. Imagine giving $10 000 to each of 15 high schools, and suppose that each school was successful in getting just *one* child to switch from becoming a smoker to becoming a nonsmoker. Smoking decreases a person's life expectancy by about 7 years. Thus, converting 15 children to nonsmokers would gain approximately 105 person-years of life, about 70 times the effect of HDC-ABMT.

All of these are rough estimates, but there is considerable room for error and room to still make two points. First, there can be vast differences in the yields of different activities (in the amount of benefit that can be achieved with a specified amount of resources). The differences can exist not just between heroic treatments and preventive activities, as in this example, but between any types of activity. Second, if the $150 000 had been spent on other activities, more health care could have been provided to more people.

These differences are the seeds of a potential conflict between individuals and society. The conflict can arise whenever an individual receives a disproportionate amount of resources (eg, services) without replenishing them (eg, paying for them). Failure to replenish a resource can occur directly (eg, the individual is billed for a service but does not pay the bill) or indirectly (eg, an insurance premium does not anticipate the cost of the service). When either occurs, other people can be harmed in two main ways, depending on whether and how the resources eventually are replenished. If the funds are not replenished, the harm is to health; other people do not get the benefits of the lost services. If the funds eventually are replenished, the harm is financial; other people must pay to replenish the funds. In both cases, the "other people" are what we call "society."

If the care that is received by the individual is considered "essential" and if the individual is incapable of paying, then this use of "social" funds is considered acceptable. It is viewed as part of society's responsibility to individuals in need. However, as the cost of the service increases, as the value of the service becomes more questionable, and as the individual's ability to pay increases, the conflict grows.

The story at the beginning of this chapter is one example of such a conflict simplified to expose the main elements. In this case, society consists of Mrs Smith's coworkers. If the employees' health promotion fund is not replenished, they lose the health benefits they might have derived from the fund (eg, breast cancer screening). If Mrs Smith's coworkers have to replenish the fund, they suffer financial harms. Dr Williams might not have direct control over how money from the fund is spent, but by drawing $150 000 from the fund, Dr Williams has affected either the health care or wallets of other people.

In short, many activities in medicine that make great sense from the point of view of an individual patient might not make sense when the perspective is widened to encompass other activities for other people—what we call society. To the extent that maximizing the care of individual patients either restricts resources available for other activities for other people or drives up costs that other people will have to pay, there is indeed a conflict between the individual and society.

❖ Who Are the Conflicting Parties?

But how can that be? Society is nothing more than a collection of individuals. How can it be that what is best for one is not also best for the other? If we maximize the care for every individual in the society, as Dr Williams suggests, why doesn't that maximize the care for society as a whole? Conversely, if a guideline is designed to be the best for society, why isn't that guideline also the best for all the individuals who make up society?

The most obvious explanation of this paradox is that, in fact, we do *not* maximize care for every individual in society. We pour resources into some individuals with low expectations of benefit, while other individuals get few or no resources, even though the benefit would have been great. In this context, the conflict between the individual and society is really a conflict between different groups of individuals. The different groups can be rich vs poor, old vs young, urban vs rural, patients with highly funded diseases vs patients with poorly funded diseases, aggressive patients (or patients with aggressive physicians) vs passive patients, and so forth. Society is the entire collection of individuals. When one group receives a disproportionate amount of resources compared with another group, society suffers in the sense that the aggregate health of all its individuals—measured by such indexes as mortality rates, morbidity rates, and life expectancy—is lower than would occur with a more even distribution.

But suppose we corrected that. Suppose we took steps to ensure that every woman in Mrs Smith's corporation who developed metastatic breast cancer would receive HDC-ABMT. Even if resources from the corporation's fund were made available evenly to every individual who needed it, there would still be a conflict between the individual and society. It is important to understand this deeper conflict because it affects everyone, even those who appear to be the winners of the first type of conflict. This conflict goes straight to the paradox that individuals can both *be* society and be in conflict with society. This conflict is not *between* individuals, but *within* each individual.

❖ Two Positions

As I have described previously,[2] each of us can be in two positions when we make judgments about the value of different health care activities. We are in one position when we are healthy, contemplating diseases we might get, and writing out checks for taxes and insurance premiums. Call this the "first position." We are in a different position when we actually have a disease, are sitting in a physician's office, and have already paid our taxes and premiums (the "second position"). The deeper conflict is between the different positions that each of us can be in as we progress through life.

The conflict between the two positions can be illustrated with a simplified example. Imagine that you are a 50-year-old woman employed by Mrs Smith's corporation. The corporate medical director has called all the female employees to a meeting where she explains that, currently, neither breast cancer screening nor HDC-ABMT is covered by the company's health program. However, the company plans to expand the program and is considering two options: (1) cover screening for breast cancer for all women between the age of 50 and 65 years; or (2) cover HDC-ABMT for any woman younger than 65 years (retirement age) who develops metastatic breast cancer. Because this fund can benefit only middle-aged women, the cost will be paid by each female employee as a one-time payment at age 50 years (with appropriate refunds and prorated costs for women who leave or enter the corporation after age 50 years).

Now imagine that you are in the first position. You do not have breast cancer, at least not yet. From your perspective, the health and economic outcomes of the two possible programs are as shown in Table 14.1. Which do you prefer?

No matter what your risk of developing or dying of breast cancer, as long as you do not yet have the disease (the first position), option 1 will always deliver greater benefit at lower cost than option 2. This is true even if you somehow knew that you were destined to get breast cancer or, even worse, that you were destined to get terminal breast cancer (the outcomes for these two scenarios can be calculated by dividing each of the entries in Table 14.1 by 8.22% and 3.57%, respectively).

Now, let us switch you to the second position. Imagine that you already have breast cancer and have just been told that it has metastasized and is terminal. The outcomes of the two programs from this perspective are shown in Table 14.2. The value to you of the screening option has plummeted because you already have breast cancer and can no longer benefit from screening. The

TABLE **14.1**   Health and Economic Outcomes of Two Health Plans From the Perspective of a 50-Year-Old Asymptomatic Average-Risk Woman*

	Baseline	Option 1, Screen	Option 2, HDC-ABMT
Probability of getting breast cancer, %	8.22	8.22	8.22
Probability of dying of breast cancer, %	3.57	2.88	3.54
Increase in life expectancy, d	0	44	2.5
Cost, $†	0	1195	1506

*Calculations performed on CAN*TROL.[3] Screen indicates screening of women between the ages of 50 and 65 years for breast cancer, and HDC-ABMT, high-dose chemotherapy with autologous bone marrow transplantation to age 65 years.
†Present value of costs, discounted to age 50 years at 5%.

TABLE **14.2**   Health and Economic Outcomes of Two Health Plans
From the Perspective of a 50-Year-Old Woman with
Terminal Metastatic Breast Cancer*

	Baseline	Option 1, Screen	Option 2, HDC-ABMT
Probability of getting breast cancer, %	100	100	100
Probability of dying of breast cancer, %	100	100	95
Increase in life expectancy, y	0	0	1.5
Cost, $†	0	1195	1506

*Calculations performed on CAN*TROL.[3] Screen indicates screening of
women between the ages of 50 and 65 years for breast cancer, and HDC-
ABMT, high-dose chemotherapy with autologous bone marrow transplantation
to age 65 years.
†Present value of costs, discounted to age 50 years at 5%.

screening option would benefit your fellow employees, as shown in Table 14.1,
but not you. Which program do you prefer now?

Maximizing care for individual patients attempts to maximize care for
individuals when they are in the second position. Maximizing care for society
expands the scope of concern to include individuals when they are in the first
position. As this example illustrates, the program that delivers the most benefit at the least cost for society (option 1) is not necessarily best for the individual patient (option 2), and vice versa. But as this example also illustrates,
individual patients and society are not distinct entities. Rather, they represent
the different positions that each of us will be in at various times in our lives.
When we serve ourselves in the second position, we can harm ourselves in
the first. Given that, at present, most decisions and guidelines are made from
the second position, it is important to understand this potential for harm.

❖ What Harm Is Done?

The amount of harm that is done by defining guidelines from
the second position depends on the specific features of the problem. To continue the example of breast cancer, suppose there are 1000 women in the corporation who would be affected by the new program. If the first position is
used to define the program and if option 1 is chosen, the number of breast
cancer deaths will be reduced from 36 to 29, a reduction of seven deaths at a
cost of about $1.2 million (1000 × 3.57% = 36 deaths; 1000 × 2.88% = 29 deaths;
and 1000 × $1195 = $1 195 000). If the second position is used and option 2 is
chosen, the number of deaths will be reduced by one at best (from 36 to 35),
and the cost will exceed $1.5 million. More money will be spent and less ben-
efit will be achieved.

Choices made from the second position have one main virtue: they give
the appearance that everything that can possibly be done for an individual

patient is being done. I use the word *appearance* because, in fact, while everything will have been done for a patient *after* he or she gets a disease, everything will *not* have been done for that *person* if you consider the person's entire lifetime. Nonetheless, if the women choose option 2 rather than option 1, neither patients nor physicians will have to face the emotional anguish of knowing that some potentially beneficial treatment was available but not covered.

Unfortunately, this virtue has a very high price—in this example, $300 000 and six deaths. What is worse is that this price is largely invisible, which means it is very likely to be ignored and allowed to continue. Dr Williams sees Mrs Smith face to face. Dr Williams does not see her coworkers. When six more of them die over the next several years, their deaths will not be connected to the heroic attempt to save Mrs Smith with HDC-ABMT. Chances are, those women themselves will receive whatever heroic treatment is currently available at the time, perpetuating the cycle. The harm done is seen only in statistics like morbidity and mortality rates, which are removed in space and time from the events that caused them. But behind every statistic is a real person, just as real as Mrs Smith. We do not know who they are yet, but Mother Nature does. One is Mrs Swenberg, sitting in the third row, fourth seat from the left, one is Mrs Williams, in the first row. Even if we do not see these people at the time we maximize health care for individual patients, they exist and they are harmed.

❖ Observations

Two observations are important. First, while this example has contrasted an investigational treatment with a preventive activity, the problems it identifies can occur with any types of activities. Whether the services involve life support at $500 000 a year for a Medicaid patient who is brain dead from a drug overdose, a patient with vague knee pain insisting on a magnetic resonance imaging test, or a visit to the emergency department for an uncomplicated sore throat, the potential for conflict between the individual and society exists.

Second, in order to expose the main concepts, this example has been simplified to the extreme. In reality, society is millions of people, not a thousand 50-year-old women. There are thousands of diseases and tens of thousands of services, not just screening and high-dose chemotherapy for breast cancer. Explicit choices between two types of services for a population are rare; most decisions involve the treatment of a particular patient. When choices are made, they are rarely made by patients, and the costs of services are usually laundered to the point of invisibility.[4]

But these simplifications do not change the basic conclusions. After Mother Nature completes all the bookkeeping, the result is that well-intentioned attempts to maximize the care of individual patients can harm other people. The sense of harm is lessened by depersonalizing these other people as society and seeing them only through statistics. But in reality, they are just as real as the individual patients we see face to face; what is society or a statistic to one physician is another's patient. The conflict between the individual and society not only exists, it affects all of us.

❖ What Is the Solution?

Resolving the conflict between the individual and society requires answering several additional questions, including the following: What is the source of the conflict? What constitutes a "disproportionate" use of resources? Why not fund both options? Which position is "correct"? And, most important, what are we trying to achieve?

❖ References

1. Canellos G. Who should pay for clinical research? *J Clin Oncol.* 1990;8:1775-1776.
2. Eddy DM. Connecting value and costs: whom do we ask, and what do we ask them? *JAMA.* 1990;264:1737-1739 (Chapter 11).
3. Eddy DM. A computer-based model for designing cancer control strategies. *NCI Monogr.* 1986;2:75-82.
4. Eddy DM. What do we do about costs? *JAMA.* 1990;264:1161, 1165, 1169, 1170 (Chapter 10).

❖ Source

Originally published in *JAMA.* 1991;265:1446, 1449-1450.

decision maker faces a limited resource and must determine which of two options yields the greatest benefit from the resource, either the choice will be obvious or it will not make much difference. However, most medical decisions do not take this form. Instead of facing a limited resource and being asked to pick which patient would benefit the most from the resource, most decision makers, especially practitioners, face a patient and must decide which services to provide to that patient. For this type of decision, the connection between individuals is less obvious, and it is more difficult to appreciate that trying to maximize care for a particular patient will affect the financial or health outcomes of other people.

To understand the conflict between the individual and society, it is helpful to distinguish the two perspectives. In one, which is often called the public health or societal perspective, the decision maker sees a resource and wants to allocate it as efficiently as possible across patients. In the other, which might be called the patients' perspective, the decision maker sees an individual patient and wants to choose resources to optimize that patient's care. Both decision makers have the same goal of providing the best possible health care to the people they serve. However, because they see different people in different settings and make decisions in different directions, the strategies they propose are often in conflict.

❖ Two Positions

The two perspectives roughly correspond to the two positions each of us can be in with respect to a health care service.[3] We are in one position (the "first position") when we do not yet have a health problem that would need the service and are deciding whether to buy coverage for the service. We are in another position (the "second position") when we have a disease, we know much more about what services we want, and this year's bills have already been paid. With admitted simplification, society is people when they are in the first position, whereas patients are people when they are in the second position. The conflict arises because what is best for us when we are in one position is not necessarily best for us when we are in the other position.[1]

❖ The Conflict

Unfortunately, when decisions are made from the patient's perspective, it is more difficult for the decision maker to determine when an individual is getting a disproportionate share of resources. First, from the patient's perspective, with its narrow focus on one person, it is not obvious that the level of care given to one person will affect the health and economic outcomes of other people. But even when this is appreciated, practitioners and patients can easily depersonalize the other people as "society," an insurance company, or the government, forgetting that these entities are really other patients, premium payers, and taxpayers. Some practitioners even see it as their duty to try to capture a disproportionate share of services for their patients. They perceive themselves as having an ethical responsibility to place the needs of their individual patients above the ill-defined needs of society, to serve as their patients' advocates in a battle with society. Any concern that their patients might receive an unfair share can be rationalized by assuming that if all practitioners look out for other patients with equal vigor, everything will work out fine.

There are several problems with this reasoning. One is that, in fact, we do not maximize the care of all individuals evenly. Some receive large amounts of resources, with little expectation of benefit, while others get far fewer resources even though the yield would have been much greater. The discrepancies affect not only the uninsured who draw from the pool only for urgent care, but also people who ostensibly have full insurance coverage. The discrepancies can occur because of such factors as geography, place of treatment (eg, a research center vs a community hospital), availability of resources, variations in providers' opinions about the outcomes of particular interventions, aggressiveness of the patient, aggressiveness of the physician, recent court cases or news articles, and the strength of a lobby for a particular disease. A second problem is that attempts to maximize every patient's care are likely to drive costs beyond the point that the people who will eventually pay the bill are willing to pay. But an even more impressive problem is that decisions from the perspective of the patients, where the attention is directed toward individuals after they seek care, do not maximize the health of even those individuals.

❖ An Illustration

In Chapter 14, I illustrated these problems with a purposely simplified example of a hypothetical corporation that offered to 1000 of its 50-year-old female employees two options. One option would cover breast cancer screening from age 50 to 65 years; the other would cover high-dose chemotherapy with autologous bone marrow transplantation (HDC-ABMT) for women who develop metastatic breast cancer. To a woman in the first position (and from the public health perspective), breast cancer screening would reduce her chance of dying of breast cancer by about 0.7 percentage points (from 3.57% to 2.88%), increase her life expectancy by about 44 days, and cost her about $1200. To the same woman, coverage of HDC-ABMT would decrease her chance of dying of breast cancer by about 0.03 percentage points (from 3.57% to 3.54%), increase her life expectancy by about 2.5 days, and cost her about $1500. (The estimates for HDC-ABMT assume that the treatment has a 5% cure rate, which has not actually been demonstrated. The implications of other assumptions can be calculated proportionately. For example, a cure rate of 15% would imply a decrease in probability of dying of 0.09 percentage points and an increase in life expectancy of 7.5 days.) When applied to the 1000 women in the corporation, the first option would prevent about seven breast cancer deaths, add about 120 person-years of life, and cost about $1.2 million. The second option would prevent, at best, one death, would add about 7 person-years of life, and would cost about $1.5 million. Thus, from the first position, the public health perspective, or society's point of view, option 1 provides considerably greater benefit at lower cost and is the preferred program. However, from the perspective of an individual patient who has terminal breast cancer (the second position), a program that covers HDC-ABMT is preferable.

❖ Why Not Do Both?

How can the conflict be resolved? In addition to highlighting the conflict, this example illustrates several approaches that might be used to try to resolve it. The most obvious question is, "Why not cover both screening and high-dose chemotherapy?"

That is a possibility. Its merits depend on whether women find the additional benefits to be worth the costs. To appreciate the issues, imagine that you are a 50-year-old average-risk woman employed by the corporation. From your point of view, the options appear as shown in Table 15.1.

Compared with option 1, are you willing to pay about $1100 more to buy option 3 ($2303 − $1195 = $1108), which will reduce your chance of dying of breast cancer by an additional 0.02 percentage points (from 2.88% to 2.86%) and add 2 days of life expectancy? Think hard and understand that if you choose option 3 you will actually have to pay the money; you will not be allowed to pass the cost off to someone else. If you and your coworkers truly prefer option 3, then indeed the solution to the conflict is to cover both screening and HDC-ABMT. This resolves the conflict because although you will be covered for HDC-ABMT, which draws a resource from the pool, you will be paying enough money into the pool to replace the expected cost. Thus, one

TABLE 15.1   Health and Economic Outcomes of Three Health Plans From the Perspective of a 50-Year-Old Asymptomatic Average-Risk Woman*

	Baseline	Option 1, Screen	Option 2, HDC-ABMT	Option 3, Both
Probability of getting breast cancer, %	8.22	8.22	8.22	8.22
Probability of dying of breast cancer, %	3.57	2.88	3.54	2.86
Increase in life expectancy, d	0	44	2.5	46
Cost, $†	0	1195	1506	2303

*Calculations performed on CAN*TROL.[4] Screen indicates screening of women between the ages of 50 and 65 years for breast cancer, and HDC-ABMT, high-dose chemotherapy with autologous bone marrow transplantation to age 65 years.

†Present value of costs, discounted to age 50 years at 5%.

way to resolve the conflict is to ask people if they are willing to pay for the additional services, and if they are, respect their wishes.

Now suppose you and your coworkers do not think that the benefits of adding HDC-ABMT to screening are worth the cost. Three remaining approaches might be tried to resolve the conflict. One is for the company to give you no choice—it might unilaterally create and bill you for a program that provides coverage for both screening and HDC-ABMT, even though you would rather keep the money than have coverage for HDC-ABMT. This approach, which might be called the "do-it-anyway" approach, does eliminate the health side of the conflict because it covers the service and replenishes the fund. However, this approach does not address the financial side of the conflict; you and your colleagues will be forced to pay for something you did not consider to be worth its costs. The do-it-anyway approach only converts the effect of the conflict from a health harm to a financial harm.

A second approach is to make option 3 an employee benefit and pass the costs on to consumers of the corporation's products. Call this the "pass-the-buck" approach. If you are an employee of the corporation, you should like this approach; it gives you a benefit at no cost. The fact that the benefit is not worth the cost is moot as far as you are concerned because you do not have to pay the cost. However, this approach is obviously unfair to the consumers of the product. Not only will they have to pay for a benefit they will never get—the benefit will go to you and your coworkers—but they will be paying for a benefit that the recipients themselves (you) determined was not worth its cost. Consumers might tolerate this for one company and one coverage policy because the costs would be highly diluted. But if this were to become the general method for resolving the conflict between the individual and society, everyone would use it, the costs of all products (and Social Security taxes and income taxes) would be affected, and the total burden on consumers would be huge. Furthermore, this approach boomerangs; you will end up paying for other peoples' health benefits. For example, when you buy a car, about $700 of your money goes to pay for other peoples' health benefits (Walter B. Maher, Chrysler Corporation, written communication, March 4, 1991). Every year, one way or another, every household in the country pays about $7000 for somebody's health care (calculated by dividing the total expenditures for health care by the number of households). Like the previous approach, this one does not solve the conflict between the individual and society; it only hides it better by spreading the financial burden to a larger number of people.

The third approach is to respect your wishes when you say you are not willing to pay for option 3. If you decide that the health benefits of covering HDC-ABMT are not as important to you as the money required to buy that coverage, this approach would take you at your word, not bill you for the cost of HDC-ABMT, and not cover the cost of HDC-ABMT if you should get metastatic breast cancer. This approach, which might be called the "patient-choice" approach, is consistent with rationing by patient choice.[5] It resolves the conflict because it does not ask anyone else to pay the cost of a service you yourself were unwilling to pay for. The drawback to this approach is that if you should develop metastatic breast cancer, HDC-ABMT would not be covered. You could change your mind in the sense that you would not be forbidden from getting HDC-ABMT, but you would have to pay for it yourself, in full. You might end up regretting this decision, but that is not a conflict between you and society; it is a choice you made for yourself. You would be in conflict with society only if you tried to demand coverage for the HDC-ABMT, even though you declined to buy it when you had the chance.

An important conclusion of this exercise is that all the approaches that resolved the conflict are based on the same principle—let people decide what they are willing to pay for, respect those decisions, and adhere to those decisions. Notice that this principle would also allow you to choose none of the options. That is, if you look at Table 15.1 and decide that not even the benefits of option 1 are worth its cost, this principle would say that neither screening nor HDC-ABMT should be covered. This principle is difficult to apply for a variety of practical reasons, such as incomplete information about the relative merits of interventions, variations in peoples' preferences, and the interposition of third-party payment. Nonetheless, the principle must be understood if practical methods are to be developed to implement it.

The only remaining question is, when should people be asked to make their decisions—when they are in the first position or the second? To determine the guideline for treating breast cancer, should we show Table 15.1 to women before they get breast cancer, or should we show women who have metastatic breast cancer a modified table that indicates no benefit for screening (see Table 14.2 of Chapter 14)?

❖ Which Position Is 'Correct'?

Both positions are real and have important things to say about the use of health care resources. When resolving the conflict between the individual and society, however, there are several reasons to give precedence to decisions made in the first position. One is that a person in the first position can look into the future to anticipate what he or she would want when he or she reaches the second position. In contrast, once a person reaches the second position, it is too late to fulfill the desires of the first position, at least with respect to that disease. Thus, the first position includes the second, but not vice versa.

But a more impressive reason is that by any aggregate measure of health care quality, such as morbidity rates, mortality rates, life expectancy, measures of health status, or quality-adjusted life-years, and for any specified level of resources, choices made from the first position can always provide as high a quality of care as choices made from the second position and can often provide a higher quality of care. This means that if guidelines are systematically defined from the first position (the public health perspective) more people will live longer, with higher quality, at lower cost than if guidelines are defined from the second position (the patient's perspective). Policies designed from the first position provide greater good for the greater number.

These statements are true because people in the first position always have more options from which to choose. Any option available to the second position is also available to the first position, but there are often options available to the first position that are not available to the second position. To the extent that the additional options available to the first position offer greater benefit and/or lower cost than the options available to the second position, decisions made from the first position will result in a higher quality of care and/or lower cost. In the example, individuals in the first position could choose from any of the options in Table 15.1. But by the time a person reaches the second position, the only viable option is option 2. Option 1, which would have provided more benefit at lower cost, is no longer available.

One might wonder if guidelines defined from the first position can always provide benefits and costs that are at least as good as guidelines from the second position, are there any advantages to making guidelines from the second position? Choices made from the second position have two main virtues. First, they give the appearance that everything that possibly can be done for an individual patient is being done. I use the word *appearance* because, in fact, while everything will have been done for a patient after he or she gets a disease, everything will not have been done for that person if the person's entire lifetime is considered. Nonetheless, if option 2 or 3 is chosen rather than option 1, neither patients nor physicians will have to face the emotional anguish of knowing that some potentially beneficial treatment was available but not covered.

The second virtue is closely related to the first. Patients in the second position tend to be much more visible than people in the first position. To the extent that other people who are unrelated to the patient (call them onlookers) place value on attempts to maximize care for an identified individual as opposed to unidentified people, setting policies from the second position can provide the onlookers with vicarious benefit. Memorable examples are a little girl who falls in a well or even whales trapped in Alaskan ice. The vicarious benefit onlookers derive from attempts to save identified individuals offsets at least some of the harm caused by spending large amounts of money that could have yielded greater benefit if used in other ways.

However, both of these virtues can be incorporated in decisions made from the first position. To address the first, add a line to the balance sheet to register the fact that if a woman chooses option 1 but ends up developing breast cancer, she will suffer the anguish of not having HDC-ABMT covered (Table 15.2). People should think hard about this additional outcome when making their choices because, under the patient-choice approach, they must live with the decision.

To address the second benefit, the pertinent question is whether the amount of vicarious benefit received by the onlookers is sufficient to outweigh the harm that results from the inefficient use of resources. The amount of such benefit will depend on the nature and visibility of the particular case. Whether

TABLE 15.2   Health and Economic Outcomes of Three Health
Plans From the Perspective of a 50-Year-Old
Asymptomatic Average-Risk Woman*

	Baseline	Option 1, Screen	Option 2, HDC-ABMT	Option 3, Both
Probability of getting breast cancer, %	8.22	8.22	8.22	8.22
Probability of dying of breast cancer, %	3.57	2.88	3.54	2.86
Increase in life expectancy, d	0	44	2.5	46
Probability of suffering the anguish of not having HDC-ABMT covered, %	. . .	3.57	0	0
Cost, $†	0	1195	1506	2303

*Calculations performed on CAN*TROL.[4] Screen indicates screening of
women between the ages of 50 and 65 years for breast cancer, and HDC-
ABMT, high-dose chemotherapy with autologous bone marrow transplantation
to age 65 years.
†Present value of costs, discounted to age 50 years at 5%.

right or wrong, live television coverage of attempts to rescue a 5-year-old girl
from a well will provide more vicarious benefit than newspaper coverage of a
50-year-old woman fighting with an insurance company for an investigational
breast cancer treatment, which in turn will provide more vicarious benefit
than hearing about a homeless person who needs better nutrition. To incorporate this feature of a guideline, each option should be studied for the potential
of vicarious benefit; a helpful measure is its "newsworthiness."

❖ What Happens Now?

Our current practices tend to accentuate rather than resolve the
conflict. We have little idea of the level of services for which people are willing to pay, we make most decisions from the second position, and we use the
pass-the-buck approach to pay for those decisions. The lack of systematic
information about the relative benefits and harms of many interventions,
and about peoples' preferences for benefits, harms, and costs, deprives us of
the anchor we need to determine the total size of the pool, or to determine
what constitutes a fair share of services. Most decisions that reflect the second position are not the result of any careful analysis or public debate but
simply a consequence of the fact that the great majority of the encounters
between individuals and the health care system occur when patients are in
the second position. As for paying for services, we have raised the pass-the-
buck approach to a fine art. For example, not only do employees get health
benefits covered by their employers, who pass them on to consumers, but
employees do not have to pay taxes on the benefits as income, the employers

can deduct the costs as a business expense, and the government can pass all the lost tax revenues on to future generations through budget deficits. The fact that most decisions are made from the second position and reflect the patient's perspective produces just what we would expect: most patients want everything possible and expect somebody else to pay for it. Practitioners undoubtedly sense that many of the services they provide are excessive, but their responses vary widely, with some discouraging their use, some staying neutral, and some encouraging them.

Thus, to a great extent the current "solution" to the conflict between the individual and society today is for individuals to try to extract as much from society as possible. We are in a tailspin: individual patients drive up costs, which are passed on to other people, who try to recover their "fair share" by overusing services when their turn comes around.

❖ What Is the Solution?

Because of the magnitude and complexity of the problem, resolving the conflict will be extremely difficult. To begin, it is helpful to describe what we want to achieve and then try to get closer to that goal than we are now. Ideally, we would have good information about the benefits, harms, and costs of services, about the level of health care for which people are willing to pay, and, correspondingly, about the level of resources that should be made available for health care. Ideally there would be some agreed-on measure of benefit per resource that would serve as a threshold for deciding when coverage of a particular service is fair. When the yield of a service is below the threshold, physicians and patients would voluntarily restrain themselves from seeking coverage for that service from the pool. Conversely, if a particular service has a high yield but is underused, steps would be taken to stimulate that service.

Many problems will prevent us from reaching this ideal. They include lack of good information about the health and economic outcomes of many activities; the fact that the outcomes of a service depend on the specific indications for which it is used (which means there will be few simple guidelines); the lack of a tradition of asking patients their preferences; the fact that preferences are highly personal and variable (which means there will be few single correct answers); and the fact that physicians and patients have strong incentives to maximize services after patients seek care.

Despite these problems, it is certainly possible to improve on our current approach. The first step is to recognize the problem. Physicians and patients must understand that when they attempt to maximize care from the patient's perspective, they might not only be in conflict with society, but they might well be fostering guidelines that are not even in their own long-term interest. Everyone must also understand that behind the abstract label of society are real people; when individuals receive a disproportionate amount of services at the expense of society, they harm the health and finances of other people just like themselves.

The second step is to learn more about the benefits, harms, and costs of the most important interventions and about what people want from the health care system. We should pick two to three dozen representative health problems that span the most important diseases and types of activities, estimate their benefits, harms, and costs, and ask people whether the benefits and harms are worth the costs, using the type of questions described elsewhere.[3] This exercise would provide essential information about whether we are currently spending too much or too little on health care and would provide the threshold that determines the fair share to be covered from pooled resources. The recent programs of the Agency for Health Care Policy and Research are an important step in this direction. The third step is to identify some services that, on the basis of clinical judgment and common sense are suspected to be overused or underused, estimate their health and economic outcomes, and ask people if they are worth their costs. While uncertainty and variability will limit our progress, we can achieve some success by analyzing the extremes. The last steps are to incorporate what we learn into practice policies and then to adhere to those guidelines.

Because it involves human behavior and self-control, the last step will be the most difficult and will require great leadership from practitioners. Medicine has a long tradition of trying to maximize care for individual patients, a tradition not only based on compassion, but strongly reinforced by medical education, pressure from patients, families, the press, the courts, and professional and financial incentives. But the act of pooling resources across individuals requires that that tradition be modified. In return for gaining the benefits derived from sharing costs, individuals must also accept some responsibilities and limitations. A responsibility is to respect others who contribute to the pool. A limitation is to not withdraw from it an unfair share.

❖ References

1. Eddy DM. The individual vs society: is there a conflict? *JAMA*. 1991;265:1446, 1449-1450 (Chapter 14).
2. Eddy DM. What care is essential? what services are basic? *JAMA*. 1991;265:782, 786-788 (Chapter 13).
3. Eddy DM. Connecting value and costs: whom do we ask, and what do we ask them? *JAMA*. 1990;264:1737-1739 (Chapter 11).
4. Eddy DM. A computer-based model for designing cancer control strategies. *NCI Monogr*. 1986;2:75-82.
5. Eddy DM. Rationing by patient choice. *JAMA*. 1991;265:105-108 (Chapter 12).

❖ Source

Originally published in *JAMA*. 1991;265:2399-2401, 2405-2406.

❖ CHAPTER 16

What's Going On in Oregon?

Few programs have attracted more attention than Oregon's recent Medicaid legislation.[1-3] Whatever the ultimate verdict, there is no doubt that this program has become a focal point of debate on virtually every aspect of national health policy: access, cost, effectiveness, rationing, and basic care.

Oregon's interest in modifying its state Medicaid program first attracted national attention in 1987 when the legislature decided to stop paying for transplants. The decision was forced when the state faced $48 million in immediate social program needs but had only $21 million in the budget. Given a choice between expensive transplants for approximately 30 individuals and basic health care for 5700 women and children, the legislature chose the latter.

One individual whose transplant would not be covered was Coby Howard, a 7-year-old boy with acute lymphocytic leukemia. His plight and his family's efforts to raise money from public contributions received intense press coverage. When Coby died, the family was within $20 000 of the $100 000 needed for his treatment. The case was a classic example of the conflict between an individual and society.[4,5]

The debate over Coby Howard's transplant, however, only brought into national view work that had been in progress in Oregon for several years. In the early 1980s, a grass-roots effort led by Oregon Health Decisions began holding community-based meetings to discuss the state's health care priorities. A variety of other organizations—such as the Center for Ethics in Health Care at the Oregon Health Sciences University and the Oregon Health Action Campaign—added to the public debate. In September 1988, a Citizens' Healthcare Parliament met to define the state's needs and values. At approximately the same time, John Kitzhaber, MD, president of the Oregon State Senate, began to work with the various political constituencies (eg, professional, consumer, and business groups) to develop a consensus on principles that should guide the state's health care programs.

This work culminated in July 1989 when the Oregon legislature passed the Oregon Basic Health Services Act, a three-part program designed to ensure that every person in Oregon would be covered for at least basic health care. The three components are to expand Medicaid to include all citizens with a family income below the federal poverty level, to require that employers offer workplace-based coverage for employees and their dependents through a small-business insurance pool, and to establish an all-payers' high-risk pool. Thus, the public sector would be responsible for everyone below the federal poverty level, while the private sector would be responsible for those above it. The act also stipulates that providers should be fully reimbursed for the cost of their services.

A central feature of the program is to set priorities for health services. The act created the Oregon Health Services Commission and charged it with producing a ranked list of services that could be used to define a basic care package for coverage by Medicaid. The same package would also define the minimum set of services to be covered by the private sector insurance pools. The commission defined *services* as pairs of conditions (defined by the *International Classification of Diseases, Ninth Revision* [ICD-9] codes) and treatments (defined by *Current Procedural Terminology, Fourth Edition* [CPT-4] codes) and proceeded to analyze more than 1600 condition-treatment pairs. The initial method used a benefit-cost formula that incorporated the health outcomes that could be expected from the condition with and without the treatment, the duration of benefit, the values Oregon residents place on the outcomes, and the cost of the treatment.

When the initial draft of the priority list was released in May 1990, several problems were apparent. The major ones were that (1) some condition-treatment pairs were defined too broadly (eg, minor esophageal strictures that require only medical treatment were grouped with extreme strictures that require resection); (2) there was inadequate differentiation of the durations of the benefit of different treatments (eg, the same "lifetime benefit" was assigned to treatments for self-limited measles, chronic diabetes mellitus, and life-threatening appendicitis); (3) the cost data were incomplete or inaccurate; and (4) there were questions about whether the cost-benefit calculations captured social values accurately, especially values relating to lifesaving treatments. In response to these problems, the commission regrouped and narrowed the definitions of condition-treatment pairs, refined the calculations of duration of benefit, and reviewed the cost assumptions. The commission also loosened the method for ranking the services to incorporate subjective judgments about the types of services and outcomes, along with the objective estimates of benefits and cost.

A revised priority list was published February 20, 1991, and received wider acceptance. Actuaries then estimated the cost of each service and the budget necessary to cover different packages of services. A final priority list and actuary report were submitted to the governor and legislature May 1, 1991. In June, the legislature voted on the reports and a specific funding level. This funding level defines the basic health care package—services covered in order of their ranking in the priority list until the allocated funds are exhausted. Services that rank below the cutoff point are not covered from public funds.

Implementation of the program will require a waiver of the federal law, which can be granted administratively by the Health Care Financing Administration (HCFA) or statutorily by the US Congress. Two components in particular require a waiver: Oregon needs permission to modify the types, amounts, and scopes of services and to add new groups who have incomes below the federal poverty level but who do not currently qualify. Oregon will apply to both the HCFA and Congress for the waiver. If the waiver is approved by either the HCFA or Congress, Oregon will implement the Basic Health Services Program in the summer of 1992.

❖ The Current Program

Evaluating the impact and merits of the proposed program requires an understanding of Oregon's current Medicaid program. Oregon's program today is the result of a collection of laws, built up over the years by both federal and state governments, that define who is eligible and what they are eligible for. Six main building blocks define who is eligible: the presence of children in a family, the ages of the children, whether a woman is pregnant, whether someone is aged, the presence of a major disability, and income. Using criteria based on these building blocks, federal law defines certain groups of people who must be covered, other groups of people for whom coverage is optional, and still other groups of people for whom coverage is forbidden. The result truly justifies the adjective *patchwork*. The next few paragraphs give a sense of the variety of combinations possible.

The largest group for whom federal law requires coverage consists of families who qualify for cash assistance through the Aid to Families with Dependent Children (AFDC) program. The eligibility requirements are that a family must have a child younger than 18 years with a single parent (or two parents if the chief wage earner is unemployed or disabled) and have an income less than the threshold defined by the state, provided it is not more than 100% of the federal poverty level ($880 per month for a family of three in 1990). Oregon has set the threshold at 50%. Another federal program is the Poverty Level Medical Program, which requires coverage for pregnant women and children younger than 6 years old if the family income is less than 133% of the federal poverty level. The state cannot modify that threshold. Additional requirements extend coverage to such groups as children born after September 30, 1983, if their families earn less than 100% of the federal poverty level; children in foster care; children in subsidized adoptions; the aged, blind, and disabled if they qualify for Supplemental Security Income (SSI)—which in Oregon requires an income less than 74% of the federal poverty level (Oregon can set this threshold anywhere between its threshold for AFDC and 133% of the AFDC threshold); and Medicare beneficiaries with incomes less than 100% of the federal poverty level.

Examples of optional groups are "medically needy" people (families and SSI-qualified adults and children whose family incomes are between 50% and 67% of the federal poverty level), individuals in nursing facilities who would be eligible for SSI if they lived at home, children between 18 and 21 years old in families that qualify for AFDC, and pregnant women as well as children younger than 1 year old in families with incomes between 133% and 185% of the federal poverty level. Oregon currently covers some but not all of these groups.

If a person qualifies for Medicaid coverage, the coverage itself is generous. Federally mandated services are defined by broad categories, depending mainly on where the service is provided and who provides it, with relatively little attention given to what the service actually is. Examples of coverage defined by where a service is provided are inpatient hospital services, outpatient hospital services, home health services, nursing facility services, services provided in federally qualified health centers, and rural health services. Examples of covered services defined by who provides them are nurse-midwife services and physician services. Only three categories are defined by the type of service: family planning services and supplies, medical transportation, and laboratory and roentgenographic services. Within these broad categories are extremely few restrictions, and those restrictions themselves are based on broad categories. The tightest restriction affects inpatient hospital services, where federal law limits coverage to 18 days per year, except for people younger than 21 years. Oregon also covers a wide variety of optional services for adults, such as eyeglasses; chiropractors' services; private duty nursing; and speech, hearing, and language disorder services. All these optional services and many more are required by federal law for people under age 21. The only services not currently covered in Oregon are dentures, nonemergency dental services for adults, hospice, and adult screening services.

The net result of all this is a program that covers virtually every medical service for a subset of poor people but covers nothing for a far larger number of people who are poor or nearly poor. Approximately 200 000 people fit the criteria for Medicaid eligibility in Oregon. However, more than twice that number—approximately 450 000 people, or 18% of the state's population—do not have any health insurance. Approximately 120 000 of the 450 000 have incomes below the federal poverty level, but they are not poor enough (eg, incomes below 50% of the federal poverty level) or they do not have the right family status (eg, no children, not pregnant, or children too old) to qualify for Medicaid. A family of four with an income of $541 a month is "too rich" to qualify, even though private insurance would cost them about $204 a month.

The financial cost of the program is high, approximately $230 million in 1990. This cost is shared between the federal government (63%) and the state (37%). But more alarming and frustrating is that, under current laws, the costs grow without control. The budget for physical medical services alone (excluding mental health and chemical dependence services and long-term care) has risen at an annual rate exceeding 18% since 1984, more than twice the rate for other goods and services in the economy. The next biennial budget for medical services will be up 30% over the previous budget. Part of this increase reflects the inexorable inflation of medical care that affects both private and public sectors. But another cause is the propensity of the federal government to add patches to the Medicaid quilt. For example, the Omnibus Budget Reconciliation Act of 1990 added coverage for children born after September 30, 1983 (currently 8 years old) whose families have incomes below 100% of the federal poverty level. This will gradually expand the age limit for children until the year 2004, when the limit will be capped at 21 years.

As the cost of the current program climbs, states have relatively few choices under current federal law. They can raise taxes, reduce payments to providers, pull money from other social programs, or tighten the criteria for coverage. The last option can be accomplished by lowering the income threshold that qualifies a family for coverage (eg, lower the income limit for AFDC from the current 50% of the federal poverty level to 40%), by dropping some of the optional groups (eg, pregnant women and children under 1 year old with family incomes between 133% and 185% of the federal poverty level), or by dropping some of the optional categories of services (eg, respirator care services for ventilator-dependent adults).

All of these have obvious drawbacks. Raising taxes is often blocked by the public's view that current taxes are already too high. Reducing payments to providers such as physicians and hospitals selects them out to absorb the costs, forces them to shift the costs to others, or prompts them to refuse to treat Medicaid patients at all. Pulling funds from other social programs such as education, housing, transportation, and nutrition not only deprives the recipients of those programs but has an indirect effect on health that can cause more harm than good. The last option of restricting the criteria for coverage is the most cynical; it "corrects" the imbalance between people and resources by dropping people. Unfortunately this is often the easiest solution politically, and the effects can be extreme. For example, Alabama has set the income threshold for AFDC at 14% of the federal poverty level.

The available options are especially frustrating because, even when they are implemented, they leave the majority of the poor and near poor with no coverage. At best, they prop up for one more budget cycle a program that is inadequate to begin with.

❖ Effect of the Proposed Program

Faced with the system just described, it is not only reasonable but laudable for states to search for better approaches. Oregon has identified another option—one that is not permitted under current federal law. In essence, it attempts to achieve a better balance between who receives coverage and what services are covered. Instead of covering virtually all services for a fraction of the poor while leaving the remainder uncovered, Oregon proposes to expand *who* is covered to ensure the availability of coverage for everyone but to contract *what* is covered by eliminating coverage of low-priority services.

The current program covers approximately 60% of the poor (those below the federal poverty line) for virtually every service, including services of relatively low or even unknown value, but leaves approximately 40% of the poor with no coverage, even for services that are well documented to have high value. It also leaves uncovered approximately 330 000 other people whose incomes exceed the federal poverty level. The proposed program would offer coverage for all 450 000 Oregon residents who currently have no coverage, but only for services that pass a priority threshold. The shift in balance between who and what is well symbolized by the two main components of the program that require waivers—one would permit Oregon to be more selective in determining what services are covered, allowing the state to cut coverage for low-priority services, and the other would give Oregon more freedom to define who is covered, allowing it to expand the criteria to everyone below the federal poverty level.

The objective of the Oregon plan is not to save money, nor will it have that effect. The proposed program is estimated to cost at least 25% more than the current program. Rather, the objectives of the Oregon plan are to provide better coverage, better incentives, a better balance between health services and other social services, and, most important, better health.

❖ Contributions

In taking these steps, Oregon has made major contributions to the national debate on the cost, access, and quality of health care.

First, Oregon has focused national attention on important problems with the current Medicaid system.[6] One problem is that the current Medicaid system rations people (or for those who dislike the word *ration*, the current system "prioritizes" people). A 6-year-old child is in, a 7-year-old child is out; a woman who is pregnant is in, but if she is not pregnant, she is out; a single adult with a child is in, but single adults without children and two-parent families and childless couples are out. The current system is an excellent example of rationing by meat axe.[7] A second problem is that the current system does not recognize that different medical services have different degrees of effectiveness. It is willing to place different values on different people but not on different services. A third problem is that the current system does not curb Medicaid's appetite for resources that belong to other social programs, even programs that are important to health. Keeping a child healthy requires more than periodic physical examinations and vaccinations; it requires good playgrounds, schools, parents with jobs, crime-free neighborhoods, and counseling about drugs, tobacco, and reproduction. A fourth problem is that the current system fails to address the conflict between the individual and society.[4,5] It has no mechanism for shifting hundreds of thousands of dollars from supportive care for one brain-dead accident victim to basic prevention or medical care for thousands of people.

A second contribution from Oregon is that the state and its leaders have demonstrated the political courage to take action. It is easy to talk about how problems of cost, quality, and access should be addressed (the way I do). It is far more difficult to actually address the problems. Solving these problems will require that someone step out front, take the initial heat, and welcome others to improve on the initial steps. Oregon has done that.

Third, Oregon has created an open and explicit social process for addressing the state's health care needs. The importance of this contribution extends far beyond the immediate goals of the Basic Health Services Act. It provides a framework and an orderly process for review, debate, and resolution. If you disagree with the rank given your favorite service, there is a phone number to call (503 378 6575) to review the reasoning, methods, and assumptions. If there was a mistake in the numbers (eg, about expected effectiveness or cost of a service), you can examine the assumptions and find the mistake, and the commission will correct it. If you disagree with the values assigned to a particular outcome, you can review the results of telephone surveys and town hall meetings.

A fourth contribution is the initial focus on principles and the subsequent derivation of methods from principles and results from methods. This strategy directs attention to the desired goals of the program, not to the political acceptability of particular results. The principles provide an anchor for debates that could otherwise be driven by extraneous factors or churn aimlessly.

Fifth, Oregon has used explicit outcomes-based and preference-based methods to set its priorities.[8] Oregon practitioners used the literature and their subjective judgments to estimate the probabilities of outcomes with and without treatment, and the duration of the treatment effect. Rather than waffle with words like *rarely*, *many*, and *probably*, they described their beliefs precisely, with numbers. This explicitness improves communication and allows others to review their reasoning. With respect to eliciting preferences, Oregon has implemented the most comprehensive process in existence, conducting dozens of town-hall and statewide meetings, a telephone poll of 1001 randomly selected citizens, formal interviews of representatives of special groups, and legislative votes.

Finally, Oregon included costs and cost-effectiveness as important factors in setting priorities for services. This is political dynamite but is the only way to achieve the desired balance between value and cost.[9]

❖ Controversies

As can be expected with any plan that addresses an extremely difficult and entrenched social problem, the Oregon plan has been controversial. The controversies range from academic details to broad concepts. The motivations range from philosophical disagreements, to displeasure that a favorite service was not ranked high, to frank misunderstandings of what Oregon actually did.

The criticisms are of two basic types: one objects to *what* Oregon is doing, the other objects to *how* the state is doing it. There are two main complaints in the first category. One is that before the state cuts any people or services from coverage, it should eliminate waste and inefficiency in the current system. Although, no doubt, considerable waste exists in the current system, states have no direct way to control it. The most direct way to reduce waste is to identify ineffective services and cut their payments. But that is precisely the type of selective coverage not allowed under current law, and permission to do that is one of the main objectives of Oregon's request for a federal waiver. Another approach is to create an incentive system that seeks out services with low effectiveness and high costs. The proposed approach, with its rankings based on benefits and costs, will do just that. In general, the most a state can do today to decrease waste is to reduce reimbursement to physicians and hospitals and hope that this "top down" rationing will stimulate efficiency.[7] Unfortunately, a far more likely response is that providers treated this way will shift costs or even refuse to treat Medicaid patients. States have tried to reduce waste for at least a decade and will continue to do so. The need for a new approach is indicated by the fact that both costs and the size of the uninsured population continue to grow.

A second complaint about what Oregon is doing—as voiced by Henry Waxman (D, Calif)—is that the state is "drawing an arbitrary line and denying access to medically necessary services" for the most vulnerable population.[10] Three observations are appropriate. First, the complaint about an arbitrary line is weak; the current system has dozens of lines. The proposed process will reduce the number of lines to two. One will be the federal poverty level of income, which is no more arbitrary than the federal process that defined it. The other will be the line drawn on the priority list. This line was not arbitrary either; it was the result of an explicit, 2-year publicly accountable process. A second observation is that the proposed program will add many more people to the Medicaid rolls. For example, it will add families with children between 8 and 21 years of age and incomes between 50% and 100% of the federal poverty level, and all childless adults with incomes below 100% of the federal poverty level. Oregon Medicaid will continue to cover pregnant women as well as children under 6 years of age with family incomes between 100% and 133% of the federal poverty level. However, the new plan will ensure that those who do not qualify for the expanded Medicaid program will have access to coverage through the private sector. A third observation addresses the part of the complaint that *medically necessary* services will be denied. If the priority-setting process functions correctly, it should rank services by their degree of medical necessity and drop coverage only for services that are thought to have low necessity.

This brings up the other type of criticism. Even if Oregon's goals are accepted, the success of the plan depends critically on the methods used to implement those goals. Several critics have claimed that the methods are so inherently flawed that the process itself is doomed.

❖ References

1. Hadorn D. Setting health care priorities in Oregon: cost-effectiveness meets the rule of rescue. *JAMA*. 1991;265:2218-2225.
2. Dixon J, Welch H. Priority setting: lessons from Oregon. *Lancet*. 1991;1:891-894.
3. Daniels N. Is the Oregon rationing plan fair? *JAMA*. 1991;265:2232-2235.
4. Eddy DM. The individual vs society: is there a conflict? *JAMA*. 1991;265:1446, 1449-1450 (Chapter 14).
5. Eddy DM. The individual vs society: resolving the conflict. *JAMA*. 1991;265:2399-2401, 2405-2406 (Chapter 15).
6. Kitzhaber J. A healthier approach to health care. *Issues Sci Tech*. 1991;7.
7. Eddy DM. Rationing by patient choice. *JAMA*. 1991;265:105-108 (Chapter 12).
8. Eddy DM. Practice policies: guidelines for methods. *JAMA*. 1990;263:1839-1841 (Chapter 5).
9. Eddy DM. Connecting values and costs: whom do we ask, and what do we ask them? *JAMA*. 1990;264:1737-1739 (Chapter 11).
10. Mjosbeth J. Oregon plan. *Health Legislation Regul*. 1991;17:1.

❖ Source

Originally published in *JAMA*. 1991;266:417-420.

CHAPTER 17

Oregon's Methods

Did Cost-effectiveness Analysis Fail?

The Oregon approach, although well intentioned, will inevitably lead to gross misallocations of resources. . . . Those who take rationing seriously should back away from the Oregon Plan before it gives a promising approach an irretrievably bad name.

New York Times
July 9, 1990

The methodological basis for this is insane. Patients are not bundles of isolated procedures. You have patients in care who have multiple needs depending on a whole series of factors.

Sarah Rosenbaum
quoted in the *Oregonian*
August 29, 1990

This counterintuitive preference order [of the first draft of the priority list] did not occur as a result of faulty data, as was suggested by the Oregon Health Services Commission, or by chance, but as an inevitable consequence of the application of cost-effectiveness analysis.[1(p2219)]

Oregon's plan to revise its Medicaid program is performing an important national service.[2] It is providing a focus for a national debate, a target to shoot at, a starting point for improvement. The current Medicaid program is a patchwork program that covers virtually all services for certain groups of people defined by family status and income but leaves uncovered more than one third of all those under the federal poverty level and fails to address an even larger number of people who are near the poverty line but have no insurance. A primary objective of Oregon's Basic Health Services Act is to ensure that everyone has access to coverage for health services—through the state if their incomes are below the federal poverty line and through the private sector if they earn more. However, the Oregon plan goes beyond a concern for coverage to address the content of medical care. In addition to examining *who* should be covered, the Oregon plan examines *what services* they should be covered for. Specifically, the Oregon Basic Health Services Act created the Oregon Health Services Commission and charged it with developing a list that ranks services by priority. On June 30, 1991, the state's legislature determined the total Medicaid budget, which had the effect of drawing a line on the list; specific services will be covered in order of their appearance on the priority list until the budget is exhausted. An important consequence of this is that some services that are currently covered fall below the budget line and will be dropped from coverage. To proceed with its plan—both to expand the categories of people to be covered by Medicaid and to restrict the services for which they will be covered—Oregon must obtain a waiver from either the Health Care Financing Administration or Congress.

The success of Oregon's program depends on the methods it used to develop the priority list. Methods are the bridge between goals and results. If Oregon's methods are seriously flawed, more harm than good might be done, and the state's plan should be stopped in its tracks. On the other hand, if the state's methods are sound, its priority list could be considered a model for the nation. The methods used in Oregon to rank medical services are important to analyze not only because of their effect on Oregon's citizens, but also because of their implications for national policies.

❖ Oregon's Initial Method Failed

The most visible fact about Oregon's methods is that they were changed in midstream. In the initial phase of the project, the commission conducted a cost-effectiveness analysis. It estimated measures of the benefits and costs of each service, calculated the ratio of costs per benefit, and ranked services in order of their ratios. A draft of the priority list derived by this approach was released on May 2, 1990. That list was widely criticized by both commission members and outside reviewers. The immediate reaction was that many of the rankings were clinically counterintuitive, assigning higher priorities to some services that were clearly less important than other, lower-ranked services. Hadorn[1] cites two examples: dental caps for pulp exposure were assigned a higher priority than surgery for ectopic pregnancy, and splints for temporomandibular joints were ranked higher than appendectomies for appendicitis.

In response to apparent inconsistencies like these, the commission identified several technical problems: (1) Some condition and treatment pairs were defined too broadly. (2) The duration of the benefits of treatment were inaccurately estimated. (3) Some cost data were incomplete or inaccurate. In response to these problems, the commission regrouped and narrowed the definitions of condition and treatment pairs, refined estimates of duration of benefit, and reviewed the cost assumptions. In addition to these technical problems, the commission also questioned whether the cost-benefit calculations captured social values accurately, especially values relating to lifesaving treatments. In response to this problem, the commission undertook a major revision of the cost-benefit approach. First, it created 17 major categories of services based on the types of conditions and/or outcomes of treatment. Examples are "preventive care for children" and "treatment of acute life-threatening conditions where treatment prevents death, with a full recovery and return to previous health state." The commission then ranked these categories according to three criteria: value to society, value to an individual, and whether they are essential to health care.

Next, the commission sorted all the services into appropriate categories and within each category ranked the services by their revised estimates of net benefits. A final step was then added. The commissioners examined each service one by one to identify any remaining counterintuitive rankings and rearranged services by hand until, in the commissioners' judgment, the list seemed reasonable. Factors considered in the final hand-tuning were the seriousness of the condition, the effectiveness of the treatment, the relative cost of the treatment, the prevalence of the condition, the importance of the service to the public, and the commissioners' own values. A final list derived by this revised approach was released on May 1, 1991.

The change in methods was major. The initial method was an attempt at a formal, objective, "numbers-based" approach that ranked services by their cost-benefit ratios. It clearly failed, to be replaced by a more subjective approach in which costs and cost-benefit ratios were considered much less formally, if at all. This change frames two questions that must be answered before the appropriateness of Oregon's final list can be judged. First, why did the initial method fail? Second, did the revised method correct the failings sufficiently to justify proceeding with Oregon's plan? The answer to the second question should affect any decision to actually implement Oregon's priority list, such as the federal government's decision to grant Oregon the waivers it requests. The answer to the first question, however, has even broader implications and is the focus of this chapter. The initial method used in Oregon was the first large-scale public attempt to apply cost-effectiveness analysis to set priorities for medical services. Everyone agrees it failed. If that failure documents an inherent flaw in cost-effectiveness analysis, the implications are enormous. An entire school of thought would have to be reevaluated. Other attempts to apply cost-effectiveness analysis to public programs should be halted, such as the Health Care Financing Administration's new regulations that would apply cost-effectiveness analysis to coverage decisions. The meaning of individual cost-effectiveness analyses, such as those on cholesterol treatment[3,4] would be thrown into limbo. The failure of Oregon's initial method is an important case study that deserves careful scrutiny.

❖ What Did Oregon Do?

To make judgments about why the initial method failed, we have to examine exactly what it did. The first step was to define the services to be ranked. The commission defined a "service" as a particular treatment or procedure applied to a particular diagnosis or condition. Thus, each service is really a condition and treatment pair. Examples are "medical therapy for hypoglycemic coma," "septoplasty/repair/control of hemorrhage for life-threatening epistaxis," and "stabilization for open fracture of the ribs and sternum." For obvious reasons, the commission used codes from the *International Statistical Classification of Diseases, Injuries, and Causes of Death, Ninth Revision* (*ICD-9*) to define conditions, and codes from *Current Procedural Terminology, Fourth Edition* (*CPT-4*) to define treatments. While the use of *ICD-9* and *CPT-4* codes has definite administrative benefits, it does limit the commission to the degree of specificity described by those codes. For example, *ICD-9* and *CPT-4* codes cannot distinguish between a carotid artery bypass procedure done for a man with 90% occlusion and symptoms vs an asymptomatic man with 40% occlusion. Furthermore, to limit to a reasonable number the services that required analysis, several *ICD-9* and *CPT-4* codes had to be combined. For example, "office visit, magnetic resonance imaging for pituitary neoplasm" was defined by *ICD-9* codes 237, 253.0, 253.1, 253.6, 253.9, 226, and 227 and *CPT-4* codes 90000 through 90080, 70551, and 80084. The initial list of services condensed all the possible condition and treatment pairs to approximately 1600 services.

Once the services were defined, the crux of the priority-setting process was to calculate a cost-benefit ratio for each service. For the cost of a service, the commission used the charges for the treatment, including all medications and ancillary services. To estimate the "net benefit" of a service, the commission developed a formula based on a set of health and functional states described by Kaplan and Anderson—the Quality of Well-Being (QWB) Scale.[5] The scale defines 24 health or functional states, or "QWB states," ranging from perfect health to death. Examples are "loss of consciousness, such as seizure, fainting, or coma"; "burn over large areas of face, body, arms, or legs"; "general tiredness, weakness, or weight loss"; and "spells of feeling upset, being depressed, or of crying." Each QWB state was assigned a "weight" (W) to reflect the quality of life associated with any symptoms or limitations related to that category. Weights for QWB states were anchored by 0 (death) and 1 (no significant decrement in quality of life), although there was no restriction against assigning a negative number to a QWB state thought to be worse than death.

These QWB states were then used to calculate a measure of benefit (the "net benefit") for each service. The net benefit is the difference in QWB with treatment (QWB_{Rx}) vs QWB without treatment (QWB_{No}) multiplied by the duration of the effect of treatment. In turn, QWB with or without treatment was calculated by multiplying the QWB weight (W_i) of each QWB state (indexed by i) by the probability (P_i) that symptoms in that QWB state would occur, and then adding across QWB states. Thus, the steps for calculating QWB with treatment are to identify the potential outcomes of the treatment, associate each outcome with a particular QWB state, estimate the probability of the outcome with treatment, multiply that probability by the weight for the associated QWB state, and add across all the QWB states. This method can be summarized in the following formulas:

$$\text{Cost-Benefit Ratio} = \frac{\text{Cost of Service}}{\text{Net Benefit of Service} \times \text{Duration}}$$

$$\text{Net Benefit of Service} = QWB_{Rx} - QWB_{No}$$

$$QWB_{Rx} = \sum_i P_{i,Rx} \cdot W_i$$

$$QWB_{No} = \sum_i P_{i,No} \cdot W_i$$

where i indexes the different potential QWB states affected by a service, $P_{i, Rx}$ is the probability of the ith outcome with treatment, $P_{i, No}$ is the probability of the ith outcome without treatment, and W_i is the weight of the ith outcome.

To implement the formulas just described, the commission asked panels of physician specialists to estimate the patient age at which the condition occurred, estimate the duration of the benefit, and estimate the probabilities of various types of outcomes both with and without the treatment. To the greatest extent possible the panels based their estimates on the literature, but they used clinical judgments when necessary to fill the gaps. Estimates of costs were based on Medicaid and health insurance records as well as on subjective judgments. The weights for various QWB states were obtained from a random telephone survey of 1001 Oregon citizens, supplemented by surveys of people in special categories, such as people who were economically and educationally disadvantaged, bedridden, and chronically depressed.

❖ An Example

The main ideas behind the method can be clarified by walking through an example: calculation of the cost-benefit ratio for "acute appendicitis/appendectomy" (*ICD-9* code 540.9 and *CPT-4* codes 44950, 44900, and 44960). Begin with the calculation of the patient's QWB_{Rx} and QWB_{No}. The main potential outcomes of appendicitis and appendectomies were determined to be (1) complete cure of the condition with no residual symptoms; (2) survival with abdominal pain; (3) survival with symptoms such as vomiting, fever, and chills; and (4) death. Abdominal pain is in the sixth QWB state: "pain, stiffness, weakness, numbness or other discomfort in chest, stomach (including hernia or rupture), side, neck, back, hips or any joints in hands, feet, arms or legs." Vomiting, fever, and chills are in the eighth QWB state: "sick or upset stomach, vomiting or loose bowel movement, with or without fever, chills or aching all over." The weights assigned to the four QWB states to reflect a patient's quality of life were (1) complete cure, 1; (2) survival with symptoms in category six, 0.747; (3) survival with symptoms in category eight, 0.63; and (4) death, 0. The probability that appendicitis would cause death if untreated was judged to be 99%. With treatment, the probability of death was judged to be only 1%. Of the 99% of patients who survive with treatment, 97% were expected to be asymptomatic, 1% were expected to have symptoms in the sixth category, and 1% were expected to have symptoms in the eighth category. The median age for appendicitis was judged to be young adulthood (age 19 through 35 years), and the benefit of treatment was expected to last for the remainder of a person's life (expected to be 48 years).

The QWB_{No} of a patient with appendicitis can be calculated from these numbers to be 0.01 (Table 17.1). Similarly, the QWB_{Rx} is 0.984 (Table 17.2). The net benefit resulting from treatment is then calculated as the QWB_{Rx} minus the QWB_{No}, or 0.974 (0.984 − 0.01 = 0.974). The denominator of the cost-benefit ratio is the net improvement in health status (0.974) multiplied by the duration of the benefit (48 years), or about 47. The cost of an appendectomy and related services was estimated from Oregon Medicaid records to be $5744.

TABLE 17.1   Quality of Well-being Without Treatment

Outcome	Probability × Weight	Score
Death	0.99×0	0
No adverse outcome	0.01×1	0.01
Sum across all outcomes	. . .	0.01

TABLE 17.2   Quality of Well-being With Treatment

Outcome*	Probability × Weight	Score
Death	0.01×0	0
QWB state 6	0.01×0.747	0.00747
QWB state 8	0.01×0.63	0.0063
No adverse outcome	0.97×1	0.97
Sum across all outcomes	. . .	0.98377

*QWB indicates quality of well-being.

Thus, the cost-benefit ratio is the cost of the treatment ($5744) divided by the net benefit times the duration (47), or about $122. This is the priority score for the service "appendicitis/appendectomy."

Priority scores were calculated in this fashion for approximately 1600 services. The resulting scores ranged from a high priority of about 1.5 (the lowest cost per unit benefit) to a low priority of 2 782 350 (the highest cost per unit benefit). A score of 122 for appendicitis/appendectomy gave this service a priority of 397 out of about 1600.

❖ Why Did Oregon's Initial Method Fail?

As has already been described, application of this process led to many rankings that did not make sense clinically, and it is widely agreed that the approach failed. The crucial question is why. The possible reasons can be divided into two basic types—conceptual and technical. Conceptual reasons would argue that the objective of the initial method—to rank services by the amount of benefit they provide per unit of cost—was inherently the wrong thing to do. Technical reasons would argue that the intention to perform a cost-effectiveness analysis was sound, but the execution was flawed. The distinction is very important. If the reasons for failure are conceptual, an entirely new approach to setting priorities must be used, and many technical questions become moot. For example, if the attempt to incorporate costs was fundamentally incorrect, the commission need not waste time improving the accuracy of cost estimates. Even more extreme, if the flaw was the very attempt to set priorities, the commission does not even need to estimate the benefits of different services. On the other hand, if the basic approach of ranking services by the amount of benefit they deliver per unit of cost was conceptually correct, we would want to ensure that it was transferred properly to the revised method and that any technical problems were corrected.

The argument that the use of cost-effectiveness analysis in Oregon's initial method was conceptually and fundamentally flawed has been made most forcefully by Hadorn.[1] He argues that cost-effectiveness analysis is inherently incapable of capturing the value people place on lifesaving technologies and rescuing individual, identifiable lives. "This counterintuitive preference order did not occur as a result of faulty data, as was suggested by the Oregon Health Services Commission, or by chance, but as an inevitable consequence of the application of cost-effectiveness analysis."[1 (p2219)] The fact that the list "seemed to favor minor treatments over lifesaving ones . . . reflects a fundamental and a irreconcilable conflict between cost-effectiveness analysis and the powerful human proclivity to rescue endangered life: the 'rule of rescue.' "[1 (p2218)] "There is a fact about the human psyche that will inevitably trump the utilitarian rationality that is implicit in cost-effectiveness analysis: people cannot stand idly by when an identified person's life is visibly threatened if effective rescue measures are available."[1 (p2219)] He went on to propose a priority-setting approach based on "necessary care guidelines," in which "cost is not considered in determining the importance of treatment."[1 (p2223)]

To evaluate this argument, we must first determine whether the apparently counterintuitive results can be explained by any other reasons or can only be explained as a failure of cost-effectiveness analysis. Suppose everyone agrees that surgery for ectopic pregnancy is more important than dental caps for pulp exposure. How can the initial ranking, which assigned them similar priority scores, be explained? (Actually, *surgery* for ectopic pregnancy was assigned a slightly better priority score [116.04] than dental caps [117.3]; Hadorn[1] mistakenly substituted the numbers for salpingectomy/salpingoophorectomy for ectopic pregnancy in his example. Nonetheless, the point he intended to make stands.)

First, it is important to understand that a priority-setting process based on cost-benefit ratios should not be expected to rank services according to our intuitive sense of their "importance" or degree of benefit. Indeed, the entire purpose of the exercise is *not* to rank services by their benefit but rather to rank them according to the amount of benefit they deliver per unit of cost. If you want to check the results against your intuition, you should compare the *volumes* of different services that can be offered with a particular amount of resources. In this example, the appropriate comparison is not between treating a patient with dental caps for pulp exposure vs treating a patient with surgery for ectopic pregnancy but between treating 105 patients with dental caps at $38 each vs treating one patient with surgery for ectopic pregnancy at $4015 (4015 ÷ 38 = 105). The priority list says that these two choices are approximately equivalent. The intuition to compare adjacent services directly (one to one) is not only inappropriate, it is misleading. When this is kept in mind, many of the apparent inconsistencies disappear.

However, suppose some rankings still appear counterintuitive. That is, suppose it still appears that the amount of benefit provided by 105 dental caps is not nearly as great as the amount of benefit provided by one surgery for ectopic pregnancy. There are several other explanations that do not impugn the use of cost-benefit ratios. Specifically, an attempt to rank services by their cost-benefit ratios can fail if there are problems either with the numerator (the estimated costs) or the denominator (the estimated benefits). To test for possible errors, let us begin with some of the technical problems identified by the commission itself. With respect to the numerator, even a cursory examination of the costs assigned to different services confirms the commission's claim that there were inaccuracies in the cost data. For example, scores of treatments ranging from medical treatment of tinea pedis to magnetic resonance imaging for pituitary hypofunction to percutaneous transluminal coronary angioplasty for heart attacks were all assigned the same cost, $98.51. There is obviously something wrong with the cost estimates; this by itself could explain inconsistencies in rankings.

However, there are more important and interesting problems with the denominator—the estimation of benefit (net benefit times duration of benefit). The commission identified two problems: errors in estimating the duration of benefits and overly broad definitions of the QWB states. As an example of the former, in the initial calculations, the same "lifetime benefits" were assigned to treatment for a self-limited childhood disease (measles), a chronic adult disease (diabetes), and a life-threatening disease of young adults (appendicitis). The problem with the breadth of the QWB states is that they do a poor job of registering differences in the severity of symptoms. For example, the category "trouble speaking" ranges all the way from a mild lisp to mutism. With so much room in each category, it is easy to generate inconsistent rankings. When a person is assigning a weight to "trouble speaking," he or she might be visualizing a mild lisp but the weight might end up being used to rank a treatment for mutism.

Beyond these two problems, there are many more signs of technical problems with the denominator that could explain counterintuitive results. One of the most obvious is that 55 services involving biopsies were assigned the same net benefit, even though they involved very different medical conditions. For example, biopsies for psychosis, dyspnea, leukoplakia, and aseptic meningitis with human immunodeficiency virus infection were all assigned the same benefit—an improvement in QWB of 0.269 for a duration of 10 years. In summary, even a superficial review of the priority list reveals a large number of technical problems that could explain counterintuitive rankings. There is no need to look to the use of cost-effectiveness analysis for the explanation.

What about Hadorn's point that cost-effectiveness analysis is inherently incapable of addressing the "rule of rescue"? There is no question that society places a high value on heroic attempts to save certain types of identifiable, highly visible lives, such as little girls who fall down wells (although not homeless people dying of pneumonia on park benches), and the commission itself observed that the initial method did not adequately take into account the value people place on lifesaving technologies. Why did Oregon's initial methodology fail to capture this? Specifically, was the failure due to an inherent problem with cost-effectiveness analysis or another technical problem?

The failure to capture the rule of rescue was due not to any inherent features of cost-effectiveness analysis but to problems with the denominator of the cost-benefit ratio. Specifically, the measure of benefit used by the commission was probably inappropriate for its intended use. There are two main problems: The method focused attention on outcomes, not services, and the questions were asked from the viewpoint of an individual, not society. On the first point, the application of cost-effectiveness analysis requires a measure of the benefit of each *service*. The method used by the commission, however, did not ask that question directly. Rather, it used the potential *outcomes* of a service, as described by the QWB states, as stepping stones from which to calculate the desirability of the service itself. By focusing on the outcomes of services instead of the services themselves, some important information was lost about the *nature* of the services that might affect their desirability. For example, reducing carcinogens in drinking water and surgery for breast cancer both affect the same outcome—death from cancer, but they have very different social connotations; the first affects outcomes in anonymous people in the future, while the second affects the survival of an identifiable person right now. Thus, one problem was that the use of QWB states filtered out important information about features of particular services that could affect their desirability.

That problem was compounded by the fact that the question people were asked about the QWB states did not correspond to the use to which the answers were put. To derive weights for the QWB states, Oregon citizens were asked to describe how different types of symptoms and health states would affect their quality of life as individuals. The form of the question was, "If you had [some collection of symptoms or limitations], how much would that decrease the quality of your life, on a scale of 0 (death) to 1 (perfect health)?" To say that living with symptoms in QWB state 8 (vomiting, fever, and chills) has a weight of 0.63 means that having these symptoms was judged to decrease the quality of an individual's life by about 0.37 ($1 - 0.63 = 0.37$), or about one third as much as death itself (which moves the QWB from 1 to 0). Assuming that the responders truly understood the implications of the question, an appropriate use of such a weight would be to help individual patients and their physicians choose between treatments that affect those outcomes.

In Oregon, however, the weights were used in a different way. They were used to determine how to *allocate* different types of treatments *across* people. That is, the purpose of the Oregon exercise was not to compare the desirability to an individual of vomiting vs death but rather to determine how many people treated for vomiting are equivalent to one person treated to prevent death. Thus, the score of 0.63 for category 8 would imply that, if the costs and durations of two treatments were the same, treating three people to prevent vomiting would be equivalent to treating one person to prevent death ($3 \times 0.37 \cong 1$). Even if responders answered the original question accurately, they might not agree that the answer should be interpreted or used this way. For Oregon's purposes, a more appropriate approach would be to address the allocation question directly. To return to the comparison of surgery for ectopic pregnancy and dental caps, the commission could have asked, "If you had a choice of performing surgery on one person with ectopic pregnancy or providing dental caps to x number of people with pulp exposure, how large would x have to be to make you indifferent between those two alternatives?" To summarize, the failure of Oregon's initial method to incorporate the rule of rescue can be explained by flaws in the method for measuring benefit.

Can cost-effectiveness analysis incorporate the rule of rescue? Yes. The rule of rescue represents the fact that people other than the patient can derive benefit or utility from an attempt to save the patient. In a previous chapter[6] I described this benefit obtained by others as *vicarious utility*. This benefit can be incorporated in a cost-effectiveness analysis by using a measure of benefit that includes the vicarious utility that accrues to the bystanders along with the benefit to the individual patient. One way to do this is to ask "allocation" questions of the type I just described. The allocation question addresses not only the desirability of outcomes to an individual, but also the desirability of a service and its outcomes to people other than the patient. When people decide how many dental caps are equivalent to one treatment for ectopic pregnancy, they can incorporate in their conclusions the vicarious utility that they as bystanders would obtain from the two treatments, as well as the direct effects of the treatments on the patients. If policymakers still want to use QWB states, another way to incorporate vicarious utility in a cost-effectiveness analysis would be to structure the QWB states to include information that might affect the desirability of the outcome to people other than the patient. For example, a QWB state "death from cancer" could be split into several states to reflect differences in the propensity for vicarious utility: "anonymous death from cancer," "identifiable death from cancer," and "identifiable death from a cancer that the media has publicized." To the extent that people place a higher value on preventing the last type of death over preventing the first type of death, they can assign those QWB states different values.

This discussion of different measures of benefit emphasizes two general facts about cost-effectiveness analysis that are important to understand when evaluating its success or failure. One is that cost-effectiveness analysis is not a particular method, any more than mathematics is a particular formula or chemotherapy is a particular drug regimen. Rather, cost-effectiveness analysis is a collection of methods bound together by a set of principles. It is applicable to any problem in which there are multiple activities, the activities produce different amounts of "goodness" and require different amounts of resources, the total amount of resources is limited, and the objective is to maximize the total amount of goodness that can be produced with the available resources. To achieve this objective, however, cost-effectiveness analysis must be tailored to particular applications in the same way that chemotherapy must be tailored to particular diseases and patients. A corollary of this is that, if a particular application of a cost-effectiveness analysis fails, the proper response is to examine the specific methods, not to discard the entire discipline. Of specific interest in this example is that the measures of "goodness" must be chosen carefully to reflect the true preferences of the parties to whom the analysis will be applied. For some problems, an appropriate measure of benefit will be a score based on QWB states such as those used in Oregon; for others, it might be person-years of life saved; and so forth.

A virtue of cost-effectiveness analysis is that it is very flexible in accommodating different measures of both goodness and resources. For example, if society places an extremely high value on saving little girls from wells, it can assign an extremely high benefit score to the service "girl in well/extraction." Thus, no matter how expensive such rescues might be, the analysis will preferentially allocate resources to that service, even if it means that 50 people will die from carcinogens in drinking water or 10 000 women will go without prenatal care. There is nothing inherent in cost-effectiveness analysis that prohibits it from assigning different values to different modes of death or even different values to different individual people (eg, a higher value to President Bush than to me). To give another example, in his article Hadorn[1] proposes giving priority to services according to how "necessary" they are. Assuming the term "necessary" can be defined (if it cannot, it is of little value in any priority-setting method), "necessity" can be used as the measure of benefit in a cost-effectiveness analysis, and the analysis will maximize the amount of "necessity" that can be obtained with the available resources.

The second general fact about cost-effectiveness analysis is that it does not assume or promote any particular philosophy about how resources should be allocated. Much of what Hadorn describes as a failure of cost-effectiveness analysis is really a consequence of a particular philosophy—what we might call "medical egalitarianism." According to medical egalitarianism, it is just as important to prevent an invisible or statistical death by a public health measure as it is to prevent a highly visible death by a heroic, high-technology, media-pleasing treatment. Put in more personal terms, medical egalitarianism would say that it is as important to prevent your son from dying of cancer by removing carcinogens from your water as it is to prevent Coby Howard from dying of leukemia under intense media coverage.[1,2] The initial method used in Oregon was egalitarian in this sense. In contrast, the rule of rescue is not egalitarian, because it assigns a higher value to preventing visible deaths than statistical deaths. Whether Oregon *should* use an egalitarian or nonegalitarian approach to priority-setting is worthy of deep debate (and a future article), but the point for now is that cost-effectiveness analysis is philosophically neutral. It does not take one side or the other and could be used to serve either objective. It is up to the people who assign the values to different services to decide whether they want to assign a higher value to preventing visible deaths than statistical deaths. Similarly, cost-effectiveness analysis is not synonymous with utilitarianism, nor is utilitarianism incompatible with the rule of rescue. The principle of utility, which is the basis of utilitarianism, is that the highest ethical good provides the greatest happiness to the greatest number of people. This can easily incorporate the vicarious utility (happiness) that gives rise to the rule of rescue. In summary, there is nothing inherent in cost-effectiveness analysis that prohibits it from incorporating the rule of rescue. The key is to define the measure of benefit correctly.

A final point is that, even if, for some reason, cost-effectiveness analysis could not incorporate the rule of rescue in a particular application—that is, even if policymakers were unable to assign values to services or outcomes to register the high value they place on lifesaving technologies for visible deaths—that is no reason to completely discard costs and reject cost-effectiveness altogether, as Hadorn appears to recommend. If worst came to worst, cost-effectiveness analysis could still be applied to set priorities for all the remaining services that are not subject to the rule of rescue.

❖ Conclusions

In conclusion, as the Oregon Health Services Commission itself determined, the initial method it used to set priorities was crude. There were many technical problems that caused it to generate counterintuitive results, and its failure can easily be explained without impugning the use of cost-effectiveness analysis. Furthermore, there is nothing inherent in cost-effectiveness analysis that renders it incapable of being used in a priority-setting exercise such as that undertaken in Oregon.

When the Oregon commission identified the problem with its initial methodology, it took the appropriate step of revising its methods to try to correct the problems. This chapter has focused on the lessons that can be learned from the failure of the initial method. However, whatever the methodological and philosophical issues raised by the initial priority list, the ultimate question for Oregon is whether the revised method used to develop the final priority list corrected the problems sufficiently to justify approving Oregon's plan.

❖ References

1. Hadorn DC. Setting health care priorities in Oregon: cost-effectiveness meets the rule of rescue. *JAMA*. 1991;265:2218-2225.
2. Eddy DM. What's going on in Oregon? *JAMA*. 1991;266:417-420 (Chapter 16).
3. Goldman L, Weinstein MC, Goldman PA, Williams LW. Cost-effectiveness of HMG-CoA reductase inhibition for primary and secondary prevention of coronary heart disease. *JAMA*. 1991;265:1145-1151.
4. Schulman KA, Kinosian B, Jacobson TA, et al. Reducing high blood cholesterol level with drugs: cost-effectiveness of pharmacologic management. *JAMA*. 1990;264:3025-3033.
5. Kaplan R, Anderson J. A general health policy model: update and applications. *Health Serv Res*. 1988;23:203-235.
6. Eddy DM. The individual vs society: resolving the conflict. *JAMA*. 1991;265:2399-2401, 2405-2406 (Chapter 15).

❖ Source

Originally published in *JAMA*. 1991;266:2135-2141.

❖ CHAPTER 18

Oregon's Plan

Should It Be Approved?

On August 19, 1991, the Oregon Department of Human Resources submitted to the Health Care Financing Administration (HCFA) a proposal to conduct its new Medicaid program as a 5-year demonstration project. If approved, the most visible and controversial plan to reform health care coverage for the poor and uninsured will be set in motion. If denied, the results of 2 years of hard planning and negotiations will disappear, and 2 years of debate will become moot.

Frustrated by uncontrollable increases in Medicaid costs, a large population of uninsured, and a nagging sense that resources were being misallocated, the Oregon state legislature passed the Oregon Basic Health Services Act in July 1989.[1] The act had three parts designed to ensure that every citizen was covered for at least basic health care. One part would expand Medicaid to cover all people with incomes less than the federal poverty level; the second would require employers to cover workers and their dependents; and the third would reform the small insurance market by creating an all-payers' high-risk pool.

A central feature of the act was to set priorities for health services. Recognizing that not all services have the same value, the act created the Oregon Health Services Commission and charged it with defining a set of "basic" services that would be required for coverage by all public and private programs. Using methods that were innovative for public programs and that caused considerable debate, the commission ranked 709 services in order of their priority. After actuaries had estimated the cost of covering each service on the list, the state legislature compared the benefits and costs of the services, and on June 30, 1991, they drew a line on the list. The line identified the top 587 services as "basic" and required for coverage. The remaining 122 services would go uncovered in the basic package. This exercise caused some services that were previously uncovered to be added, such as hospice care and preventive services for adults, and caused some services that were previously covered to be dropped, such as treatments for temporomandibular joint disorder (service 620), bursitis (service 631), diaper rash (service 649), and the common cold (service 695). In essence, when it drew the line, the legislature was saying that services above the line were deemed to be worth their costs to publicly mandated programs, even within the context of competing social needs, whereas services below the line were not.

Before it can implement the program, the state needs to receive several waivers to the Social Security Act under Section 1115(a) and an agreement from the HCFA to provide the federal share of the costs. Although 11 waivers are needed in all, two are especially important. One would permit the state to expand the criteria for coverage to include people whose incomes are less than the federal poverty level but who currently do not meet categorical or financial requirements for Medicaid. The other would permit the state to re-define the services it would cover, ie, to define the basic package.

❖ The Proposal

The state is proposing to conduct a 5-year demonstration during which the program would be implemented and its effects on access, utilization, outcomes, health status, and costs would be monitored. The demonstration would start July 1, 1992, when the newly qualified people would begin to enroll in Medicaid. Beginning in the fourth year of the program (July 1, 1995), the employer-based insurance program mandate would take effect. Throughout the 5 years, an aggressive managed care program would be implemented to ensure high-quality provision of the basic services and to control costs.

The proposal is a package deal. Although the state legally could have created a mandate that employers cover workers and their dependents, and although the state could have defined the basic services to be covered through that program, the Basic Health Services Act of 1989 linked the employer-based insurance program to federal approval of the new Medicaid program. The employer mandate cannot be initiated unless Medicaid is re-formed as well.

❖ Should the Proposal Be Approved?

The proposal will be evaluated on two main levels: technical and conceptual. Technical questions will address such issues as whether the cost of the program has been estimated accurately and whether an effective system will be in place for monitoring access and outcomes. Evaluation of these issues requires a detailed analysis of the proposal, to which I do not have access.

The main conceptual question is whether the proposed program is something that should be demonstrated. That is, if this demonstration is completed as expected, will the results be something the federal government will want to offer as a possible model for other states? The first step in answering these questions is to agree on the criteria that should guide the decision. Reasonable criteria include the following: There should be good reason to believe that the new program will improve on the current program; the program should have the capacity for self-improvement; and there should not be any other programs that are obviously superior and that would be preferable to Oregon's, no matter what the demonstration showed. Notice that these criteria do not ask that the proposed program be perfect or that everyone like it. The problem of financing care for the poor and near-poor in this country is too complex, there are too many constraints caused by current regulations, and there are too many constituents with conflicting objectives to achieve that. Instead, all anyone can ask is that the proposed program take a step in the right direction.

❖ A Balance Sheet

Is the proposed program an improvement over the current program? To answer this, it is helpful to develop a balance sheet (Table 18.1).[2] The balance sheet for this problem has three components: the number of people covered, the services for which they are covered, and financial costs. For the first component, it is convenient to define three groups. Group 1 consists of the individuals who are currently covered by Oregon's Medicaid program. There are approximately 200 000 such individuals. Group 2 consists of the individuals whose incomes are less than the federal poverty level but who currently do not qualify for Medicaid. There are approximately 120 000 in this group. Group 3 consists of people whose incomes exceed the federal poverty level but who currently have no health insurance. Approximately 330 000 of Oregon's citizens are in this group.

Under the new plan, group 1 would continue to be covered by the state Medicaid program (or possibly through the employer mandate, as will be described). Group 2, which is currently not covered by any program, would gain coverage through the employer mandate if they are employed for more than 17.5 hours a week (or if they are dependents of such people) or would gain coverage by Medicaid if they are not.

Approximately one half of the people in group 2 are either employees or dependents of employees and therefore would be eligible for coverage by employer-based insurance rather than by Medicaid. Oregon's planners estimate that about half of them, or one fourth of group 2, would elect coverage through their employers. Group 3, which includes people who are also currently uninsured, would either gain coverage through the employer mandate if they are employed or if they are dependents of employed people, or would be offered the opportunity to buy coverage at their own expense at a reasonable price through the all-payers' high-risk pool.

TABLE **18.1**   Balance Sheet of Expected Effect of Demonstration
Program on Number of People Covered, Services
Covered, and Financial Costs

	Current	Proposed	Change
People covered, No.*			
Group 1	200 000	200 000	0
Group 2	0	120 000	+120 000
Group 3	0	330 000	+330 000
Total	. . .	. . .	**+450 000**
Services covered, code No.			
Group 1	1-709†	1-587	lose 588-709‡
Group 2	0	1-587	gain 1-587
Group 3	0	1-587	gain 1-587
5-year costs, $ (in millions)			
Federal government (Medicaid)	3806	3915.6	+109.6
State government (Medicaid)	2236	2331	+ 95.0
Total	. . .	. . .	**+204.6**
Fifth-year annual cost, $ (in millions)			
Federal government	974	976.9	+ 2.9
State government	572	586.5	+ 14.5
Total	. . .	. . .	**+ 17.4**

*Group 1: current Medicaid recipients would remain qualified; group 2:
persons who are currently under the federal poverty level but who are not
qualified for Medicaid would become qualified; group 3: persons who are
currently over the federal poverty level but who are uninsured would be
covered by business mandate if employed or if a dependent of the employee.

†Some services on the list are not currently covered, eg, hospice care,
preventive and dental care for adults, and transplants for adults. The code
numbers indicate the 709 services in order of their priority.

‡Group 1 will gain some previously uncovered services, such as hospice
care, preventive and dental care for adults, and most transplants for adults.

The net effect of all this is to add approximately 90 000 people to Medicaid, to cover approximately 330 000 people through employer-based plans, and to offer reasonably priced coverage to approximately 30 000 people through the all-payers' insurance pool. Although this plan is intended to be comprehensive and seal all the cracks, inevitably some individuals who qualify for the various programs will decline them. When these dropouts are taken into account, approximately 97% of Oregon's population will have some insurance coverage by the fourth year of the program.

The next issue concerns the services. The changes that will be experienced by an individual depend on which group the individual is in. People in group 1 will lose coverage for services 588 through 709, but will gain some new services that are currently not covered by Medicaid but that were ranked higher than 588. In addition to hospice care and adult preventive services, this includes dental services and most transplant procedures for adults. The new program will also expand coverage for people in group 1 by removing the 18-day limit on coverage of inpatient hospital care. Thus, the new program will cause a net loss to group 1 of approximately 115 services. People in group 2 currently have no coverage at all. They will gain coverage for all the services listed higher than 588. Similarly, people in group 3 have no coverage now and will gain all the services listed higher than 588.

The cost of this program will be borne initially by five parties: (1) the state, (2) the federal government, (3) Oregon's employers, (4) Oregon's employees (through sharing the premiums, copayments, and coinsurance), and (5) unemployed people in group 3 who buy insurance through the pool. Although the first three will eventually pass their costs to people (eg, Oregon state taxpayers, US taxpayers, and the consumers of the services and products of Oregon's businesses), they will be the first to notice the costs in their budgets. During the 5 years of the program, total Medicaid costs will increase about $204.6 million, of which approximately $95 million will be borne by the state and approximately $109.6 million by the federal government. This amounts to an increase in Medicaid costs of approximately 3.4%. The 5-year cost to business has not been estimated as precisely because it does not affect the costs to the federal government, to which the proposal is being made, but it is the same order of magnitude. The actual cost to each employer and individual employee will vary widely, depending on the share of the premium the employer chooses to cover (the mandate requires the employer to pay a minimum of 75% of the premium for employees and 50% of the premium for dependents) and on the use of deductibles and coinsurance.

The increase in cost to Medicaid over the 5 years of the demonstration will be determined by several factors. Just increasing the number of people covered by Medicaid (adding the people in group 2) would cost approximately $680.2 million. To this would be added the cost of administering the demonstration ($61 million over 5 years). However, these costs will be offset by several factors. First, businesses will cover some of the people who would otherwise qualify for Medicaid because they are employed. This should reduce the cost to Medicaid by approximately $108.9 million. Second, redefining the services in the basic care package should save approximately $169.2 million, and implementation of aggressive managed care is expected to save an additional $224.8 million. Finally, the employer mandate should reduce the costs to the Medicare program by about $33.7 million because some people who are older than 65 years are employed. Taking all the factors into account yields the expected increase in 5-year Medicaid costs of approximately $204.6 million, which is to be split between the federal government ($109.6 million) and the state government ($95 million).

These costs will not be distributed equally over the 5 years. The greatest cost to both federal and state governments will occur in the first 3 years when new enrollees enter Medicaid but before the employer mandate begins. For example, the cost in the third year of the program will be $48.8 million for the federal government and $31.2 million for the state. The costs to both governments will then dramatically decrease in the fourth and fifth years. In the fifth year of the demonstration, the additional cost to the federal government is expected to drop to $2.9 million.

An actuarial model predicts that within 2 years after the termination of the demonstration, both the federal and state governments will save money. This is an important point: although the cost of the 5-year demonstration to the federal government will be on the order of $100 million, the actual cost to the government of maintaining the program after the demonstration has ended should be very low or possibly free. It is Oregon's citizens (eg, employees and consumers) who will eventually absorb the long-term increases in costs.

❖ Is This an Improvement?

The net effect is a trade—a cutback in coverage of approximately 115 services for the 200 000 people in group 1 and an addition of coverage for 587 services for 450 000 people in groups 2 and 3. The desirability of this trade depends on the priorities that you assign to the services and the values that you place on the people in the three groups. These are complex issues involving both technical and ethical judgments.[3] To sort through the issues, it is helpful to make an a fortiori argument. If the trade makes sense under several simplifications that bias against the trade, then the trade will make even more sense when the simplifications are removed.

The first simplification is to ignore the fact that group 1 will gain several services, such as hospice care, adult preventive services, and most transplant procedures. That is, imagine that group 1 loses 122 services (588 through 709) and gains nothing. The second simplification involves the setting of priorities for the services. The intention of the Oregon Health Services Commission was to rank services according to their priority. To the best of the commission's knowledge and judgment, activities ranked 1 through 587 provide much greater health and social value than do services ranked 588 through 709. Even a cursory review of the rankings indicates that services the commission placed above the line (eg, surgery for a ruptured spleen) are more important than services below the line (eg, treatment of chancre sores), but there is debate about the methods and some specific rankings. This debate can be finessed with the second simplification: imagine that the commission completely failed in its attempt to rank the services by their true priorities and, instead, achieved nothing better than a random list. Third, let us completely ignore the benefits of Oregon's plan for people in group 3. Clearly, providing access to insurance for 330 000 people in group 3 is a major benefit for Oregon's plan. However, the incomes of people in group 3 are more than the federal poverty level, which complicates comparisons with the people in group 1, who are the only people who will lose any coverage. By limiting the discussion to compare only the benefits to people in group 2 vs the losses to people in group 1, we restrict the comparison to people below the poverty line and eliminate income as a distinguishing feature.

Finally, let us use a "person-service unit" (PSU) as a rough measure of the benefits of coverage for a group. The PSU is calculated as the number of people covered at any time in a year, multiplied by the number of services for which they are covered. This measure is admittedly rough. For example, individual people come in and out of coverage over the course of a year, whereas this measure is based on the number of people covered at a particular time (eg, July 1). Also, not all services are of equal value, although our assumption that the services are listed randomly makes this a more acceptable simplification that, if anything, biases against the trade.

Under these assumptions and simplifications, adding 587 services for 120 000 people in group 2 (ie, 70 440 000 PSUs) would justify the loss of 122 services by 200 000 people in group 1 (ie, 24 400 000 PSUs) if we consider people in group 2 to be only one third as deserving of coverage as people in group 1 (24 400 000 ÷ 70 440 000 = 0.35). We can frame the question more specifically by noting that the majority of people in group 1 are recipients of Aid to Families with Dependent Children, the distinguishing feature of which is the presence in the family of a child younger than 18 years. Does the federal government believe that a childless adult is only one third as worthy of coverage from public funds as an adult who has a child?

Now reexamine the simplifications. All of them argue that the relative worth of the people who would be added can be much lower than one third the worth of current Medicaid beneficiaries and still make the trade desirable. For example, if we consider the provision of access to insurance for people in group 3 to be a benefit of Oregon's plan, that would mean that if people in groups 2 and 3 (450 000 people) are just one tenth as worthy of coverage as people in group 1, the trade is worthwhile ([122 × 200 000] ÷ [587 × 450 000] = 0.1). If services above the line provide, on average, just twice as much value as services below the line, the factor drops to 0.05, and so forth. Even given the roughness of the PSU as a measure of benefit of coverage, it is reasonable to conclude that the plan is an improvement.

❖ Are the Benefits Worth the Additional Costs?

Oregon's legislature and businesses have already decided that the benefits are worth the costs. (In general, medium and large businesses in Oregon are enthusiastic about the plan; small businesses are not, but everyone has agreed to compromise on the current proposal.) The only remaining question is whether the federal government believes that the benefits of the plan are worth the costs it will bear.

When addressing this question, it is important to keep separate the cost of the 5-year demonstration and the eventual cost of the program to the federal government after the demonstration is complete. After the business mandate and managed care have been fully implemented, the annual increase in cost to the federal government for its portion of Medicaid should be small or possibly negative (ie, a savings). To achieve this, however, the federal government must be willing to pay $109.6 million over 5 years to help support the program before all the savings are realized.

There is a strong clue that the federal government should be willing to do this. First, let us determine what the federal government is currently willing to pay for. If Oregon had never proposed its plan, over the next 5 years the federal government would have paid approximately $3800 million to cover 709 services for 200 000 people in group 1 for 5 years (1 million person-years), for a cost per PSU of about $5 (ie, $3800 million ÷ [709 × 1 million] = $5.36). Now examine what the federal government would get with the proposed program. To simplify the issues, let us again make an a fortiori argument. Ignore the fact that if the proposal is approved, 330 000 people in group 3 will gain access to coverage during the 5-year period at no cost to the government. Also ignore the long-term benefits of the program, including that after 5 years, coverage will be expanded to 450 000 more people at little or no cost to the government. Thus, focus only on the benefits and costs of covering group 2 for 5 years. Finally, assume that the rankings of the services are no better than random. Taking into account the delay in phasing in the newly eligible people in group 2 over 5 years, the proposed demonstration will cover 587 services for 528 000 person-years in group 2 (or 309 million PSUs). However, the program will eliminate coverage for 122 services for 200 000 people in group 1 for 5 years (or 122 million PSUs), for a net gain of 187 million PSUs. The cost to the government of achieving this gain will be $109.6 million, or about 60 cents for a PSU, which compares favorably with what the federal government has already shown it is willing to pay for ($5 per PSU). Even under this simplification, if people in group 2 are just 45% as worthy of coverage as are people in group 1, this program should be desirable to the government ($109 000 000 ÷ [$w$309 000 000 − 122 000 000]) = $5.37 [solve for w]). The case becomes much stronger when the simplifications that were introduced to make the a fortiori argument are dropped and when the benefits to group 3, the long-term benefits, and the fact that the rankings are not random are taken into account.

❖ Is There a Capacity for Self-improvement?

Even though a strong case can be made that Oregon's plan is a step in the right direction, it is far from perfect.[4] The second criterion for approval is intended to ensure that approving this particular plan will not lock in place imperfect methods or undesirable results. There are several reasons to believe that Oregon will continue to improve its program. First, Oregon's leaders have already shown a remarkable commitment to improving their process by reaching out aggressively to citizens, businesses, professional groups, and methodologists. Second, the structure and political process Oregon developed to design the current plan provide excellent mechanisms for evaluating the program's progress and making changes. Third, the basic approach Oregon used to set priorities, while admittedly crude now, is quite capable of refinement. The current method does not lock the state into a flawed process.

❖ Is There a Superior Plan?

Several other states have proposed or implemented programs to increase access and coverage. Notable examples are Hawaii's aggressive use of mandated employer-based insurance, the less aggressive program recently introduced by Massachusetts, and the use of managed care to control costs in Arizona. While each of these programs has merits, none of them trumps Oregon, which not only proposes to use both employer mandates and managed care but is the only state thus far to explicitly set priorities for services. Furthermore, unless there is a massive change in the US health care system, with intense centralization of control, it is highly unlikely that there will be a single solution to the problem of providing access to health care for the poor and uninsured. New ideas are still needed.

❖ Criticisms and Questions

"This is rationing." Many people are repulsed by the fact that Oregon's priority-setting process will remove coverage of some services that are acknowledged to have benefit. If resources were unlimited, this would be a valid argument against Oregon's plan, but as the HCFA, federal legislators, and state legislators can verify, resources are not unlimited. As a consequence, Medicaid programs already ration. Currently, the rationing is extremely blunt, withholding coverage of all services for about 40% of people under the federal poverty level, and allowing 330 000 of the near-poor in Oregon to go without insurance.[1] Oregon is seeking a better balance between who is covered and what they are covered for. Oregon's plan takes advantage of what medical practitioners and researchers have known for years: that within the extremely broad categories of services currently covered by Medicaid (eg, inpatient hospital services, physician services, and laboratory and roentgenographic services), there are broad ranges of specific services that have widely varying benefits and costs. Some are essential, some are worthless, and some are harmful. Oregon's plan attempts to shift resources from low-priority services for currently covered individuals to help provide high-priority services for people who currently have no coverage. That is rationing, but it is a more justifiable type of rationing than what is occurring now.

The acceptability of the type of rationing espoused in Oregon can be appreciated by examining the flip side of rationing, which is basic care. While most people consider it acceptable to talk about basic care, many who espouse the concept become anxious when they first see it in action and realize that basic care is not "all-inclusive" care. If the concept of basic care is to be meaningful, it will necessarily involve not covering some services that have benefit.

"But is the method that the commission used to set priorities sound enough to justify proceeding?" The most daring and controversial aspect of Oregon's plan has been its methods for setting priorities. This visibility and the acknowledged problems with the methodology have tended to distract attention from the fact that the full proposal more than doubles the number of people who will have access to coverage for all but low-priority services. As I have described in this chapter, even if the priority list were completely random, the net effect of the plan would still be positive. Nonetheless, it is reasonable to examine the implications of the flaws in Oregon's methods.

There are two main problems. One is that the categories of services are defined too broadly. Ideally, in a priority-setting exercise, services should be defined narrowly enough so that every person who receives a particular service will have the same expected benefits and costs. This usually requires that the services be defined at the level of detail of particular patient indications, diagnostic tests, drug regimens, screening frequencies, and so forth. Because the definitions of services used in Oregon are based on *Current Procedural Terminology, Fourth Edition (CPT-4)* and *International Classification of Diseases, Ninth Revision (ICD-9)* codes, and because of a need to keep the priority-setting exercise manageable, the definitions of services could not be specified at that level of detail. For example, the services generally do not distinguish patients by age, severity of symptoms, or specific indications for a treatment. The second methodological problem is that because of deficiencies in both methods and data, the commission was not able to estimate either the benefits or costs of services accurately enough to use a pure cost-effectiveness ranking. Recognizing these problems, the commission wisely backed away from its attempt to perform a rigid quantitative analysis and used an alternative method that was more subjective. It classified services into 17 general categories (eg, "prevention care for children" and "acute fatal, prevents death, full recovery"); ranked the categories according to general values described in public meetings by Oregon's citizens; focused on the most appropriate indications for each service; ranked services within categories by their net benefit (de-emphasizing costs); and then hand-tuned the entire list using traditional clinical judgment.

There is no question that the final method was crude. The pertinent questions are whether it is better than the current method, whether the inaccuracies of the new method led to any unacceptable results (fatal flaws), and whether there is anything about the methodology that prohibits gradual correction of the problems. The first question is easy. Currently, Medicaid uses *much broader* categories to determine who should be covered and the services for which they should be covered; does not even determine the *existence* of benefit for covered services, much less the magnitude of benefit; does not consider the costs of services or alternative uses of resources *at all*; and makes *no attempt* to rationalize the use of resources. It is safe to say that if the current Medicaid program were being proposed as a 5-year demonstration, it would be rejected immediately.

On the second question, two types of harms can be caused by the problems in Oregon's methods. One is that some services that are worthy of funding might be put below the line and not covered. The other is that services that are not worthy of funding might be put above the line and covered. By focusing on the best indications for a service and by ranking services by net benefit rather than a cost-effectiveness ratio, the alternative method used by Oregon was biased away from the first type of error and toward the second type of error. That is, the crudeness in the method caused the final list to be not nearly as efficient as it might have been in restricting coverage for low-priority services and saving resources. This inefficiency is almost certainly acceptable to the federal government; the current Medicaid program is far *less* efficient. It covers virtually every service and makes no attempt to determine how much benefit a service provides for the resources it consumes. The danger of not covering an important service is not only much smaller, but it can be assessed directly. Anyone can examine the list of services that will not be covered and determine the harm that might be caused. Keep in mind that the Oregon Health Services Commission and state legislature did just that and determined that the uncovered services were not worth their costs.

On the third question, both the problem of overly broad definitions of services and the limitations caused by poor data can be corrected within the framework of the current method. For example, the *CPT-4* or *ICD-9* codes can be divided into finer categories, a precertification process based on more specific patient indications can be implemented, and assessments of benefits and costs can be revised as better data become available.

"Does the plan put an unfair burden on women and children?" A frequently heard complaint is that the burden of Oregon's plan is being borne by women and children. First, the actual impact on women and children will be small. A simple reading of the priority list reveals that relatively few services that specifically serve these two groups will be dropped from coverage (14 for children and nine for women) and they are relatively simple and inexpensive services (eg, treatments for diaper rash, pharyngitis, and superficial wounds without infection) or have little effectiveness (eg, life support for anencephaly). Second, while it is true that the children and women who are in group 1 will lose coverage for some services, it is not correct to say that they will bear the burden of the plan, as though they were paying for it in some way. Coverage for health care for the poor, both with the current program and with the proposed program, is paid for by federal taxpayers, state taxpayers, and businesses and their customers. People in group 1 used to be the only beneficiaries of this generosity, but with the new program, they will share the generosity with people in group 2, who are also poor but who do not happen to fulfill the current qualifications of Medicaid. It is no more correct to say that women and children in group 1 will bear the burden of the proposed program than to say that people in group 2 are now bearing the burden of the current program.

"Is there a danger that Oregon or other states will use priority lists to cut covered services down to nothing?" This is not a real danger. First, Oregon has agreed that it will not make any substantive changes to the list without returning to the federal government for approval. Second, Oregon's actions show that it is far more interested in expanding coverage than contracting it. Third, if states choose to, they already have the legal ability to reduce coverage substantially. For example, Oregon could lower the income threshold for families who are qualified to receive Aid to Families with Dependent Children to zero.

"Will this program expose the federal government to unacceptable increases in costs?" Recall that after 5 years this program will be very inexpensive or even free to the federal government. But more important is that the federal government is already exposed to far larger potential increases in costs. Without changing any laws or getting any waivers, Oregon can already increase its Medicaid costs far beyond what the state is requesting in this proposal. Just by exercising existing options to raise provider reimbursement amounts to Medicare levels and to cover all the optional groups, the state could increase Medicaid costs to a level that would exceed the cost of this proposal by $600 million.

❖ Conclusions

As with any public proposal that attempts to solve a complex social problem, everyone has something they would like to change about Oregon's plan. I myself am unhappy with the priority-setting method. But however stimulating those debates might be, they should not confuse the real issue raised by Oregon's proposal. That proposal is the result of years of work and political compromise, conducted under severe restrictions imposed by current laws and competing constituencies. The decision today is not how to fine-tune Oregon's plan, but whether the plan, as it is currently configured, deserves a demonstration. The main criterion should not be whether the plan is ideal. As Oregon's leaders are the first to admit, it is not. Indeed, it is highly unlikely that any plan that emerges from a political process will ever be ideal. The criterion should be whether Oregon's plan improves on what is currently happening.

Perhaps the best way to determine if Oregon is moving in the right direction is to examine the flip side of Oregon's proposal. Suppose the current program looked like what Oregon is now proposing. That is, imagine that today Oregon had an employer mandate that covered all employees and their families, a high-risk pool that offered insurance at a reasonable cost to everyone over the federal poverty level, and a Medicaid program that covered everyone with incomes under the federal poverty level for services 1 through 587. Imagine further that all this was established after extensive public hearings, citizen surveys, and legislative debate. Now suppose that Oregon was proposing to change that to the current Medicaid program. That is, imagine that Oregon was proposing to (1) dismantle the employer-based insurance and the high-risk pool by discarding coverage for 330 000 people; (2) eliminate all coverage for 120 000 people under the poverty line; and (3) give 200 000 people who currently qualify for Medicaid an additional 122 services that are at the bottom of a priority list developed by medical specialists and thought by the state's legislators to be not worth their costs. Imagine further that the "new" proposal was developed with no public debate or explicit methodology. Executing the proposal would save the federal and state governments about $200 million over 5 years but would save them little if anything after that. Would the HCFA approve this proposal? Would ethicists argue that it is fair and just? Would academics applaud the methodology? Would specialty societies cheer at the shift in coverage for their favorite procedure? Would advocates for the uninsured and poor congratulate Oregon for correcting an unjust burden on Medicaid recipients? I doubt it.

❖ What Happens Next?

The Office of Acquisitions and Grants of the HCFA has created a panel of outside advisers to review the proposal for both technical and conceptual merit. The panel's recommendations will be submitted to the administrator of the HCFA and to the Secretary of Health and Human Services. If the HCFA and the secretary recommend approval, the proposal would then be sent to the Office of Management and Budget for a budget analysis. To be funded, the proposal must be approved by both the Secretary of Health and Human Services and the Office of Management and Budget. Because this proposal is being submitted to the HCFA in the Executive Branch, formal approval by Congress is not required. However, if congressional leaders have strong feelings, they can no doubt make them known to the HCFA, the Secretary of Health and Human Services, and the Office of Management and Budget.

If the proposal is funded, it will continue to focus attention on methods for setting priorities. Given the failure of the initial cost-effectiveness analysis, an important question is whether Oregon and others should try to resurrect the cost-effectiveness method or abandon it for some other approach.

❖ References

1. Eddy DM. What's going on in Oregon? *JAMA.* 1991;266:417-420 (Chapter 16).
2. Eddy DM. Comparing benefits and harms: the balance sheet. *JAMA.* 1990;263:2493, 2498, 2501, 2505 (Chapter 7).
3. Daniels N. Is the Oregon rationing plan fair? *JAMA.* 1991;265:2232-2235.
4. Eddy DM. Oregon's methods: did cost-effectiveness analysis fail? *JAMA.* 1991;266: 2135-2138, 2140-2141 (Chapter 17).

❖ Source

Originally published in *JAMA.* 1991;266:2439-2445.

❖ CHAPTER 19

Cost-effectiveness Analysis

A Conversation With My Father

MAXON H. EDDY, MD: All right. I've read your chapters about what's going on in Oregon.[1-3] I agree with you that their first attempt to use cost-effectiveness analysis to set priorities failed but that that failure did not necessarily doom the entire method. I also understand that even now Oregon's commission is not totally satisfied with the priority-setting process it eventually used and that it is seeking ways to improve the process. Based on what you've already written, I'll bet you're going to try to convince me that Oregon should use cost-effectiveness analysis to rank its services. I've got to warn you that you're going to have a hard time. In 40 years of practice I never withheld a test or treatment that I thought would help my patients, even when I had to absorb the cost myself. I believe that what we do in medicine should be determined by the value it provides, not by what it costs.

DAVID M. EDDY, MD, PHD: You're right. I am going to try to convince you that Oregon should use cost-effectiveness analysis to rank its services. In fact, I'm going to go further to argue that cost-effectiveness analysis should be used to determine the content of medical care in most settings, not just programs for the poor.

MHE: Fair enough. Give it a try.

DME: First, are we clear about what the term *cost-effectiveness analysis* means?

MHE: Go over it again.

DME: Cost-effectiveness analysis is a collection of methods for solving the following problem: There are multiple activities. Each activity produces different amounts of some desirable outcome, such as health benefits. Each activity requires different amounts of resources, such as money. There are not enough resources to do all the activities. The objective is to allocate the avail-

156

able resources across the activities to maximize the desirable outcome. In the medical context, a typical objective is to allocate a budget to activities in a way that maximizes the health of the population being served.

MHE: Where does the *cost-effectiveness ratio* come in?

DME: The cost-effectiveness ratio is a measure of the amount of benefit provided by an activity for a specified amount of cost. It is the criterion used to rank activities and therefore is the basis for setting priorities.

MHE: Before you go on, I've also heard the term *cost-benefit analysis*. Is there a difference between that and cost-effectiveness analysis?

DME: Yes. The distinction is that they use different types of units to measure the outcomes of a treatment. (For simplicity I will use the word *treatment* in a general sense to describe any kind of a health intervention, including primary prevention, screening, and diagnosis.) I'm sure you can appreciate that, if you are going to set priorities for treatments on the basis of the desirability of their outcomes and costs, you need to have some measures that describe the outcomes and the costs. The measure for costs is easy—it's dollars. The measure for health outcomes causes the problem. In a cost-effectiveness analysis, the units for measuring the benefits and harms of a treatment are either the natural units that we think about in clinical practice—such as the probability that a patient will survive 5 years after a cancer treatment, the weight loss after a treatment for obesity, or the mortality rate of a surgical procedure—or some composite measure based on natural units. An example of such a composite measure is the quality-adjusted life-year, which combines information about the effect of a treatment on both length of life and quality of life.

In cost-benefit analysis, the health outcomes are not left in their natural units but are instead converted into dollars. Thus, a cost-benefit analysis requires placing a dollar value on such outcomes as achieving 5-year survival, losing weight, or preventing an operative death.

MHE: That's confusing. In both cases you're measuring the *benefits* of a treatment. If you measure the benefits in their natural units you call it *effectiveness*, but if you measure the benefits in dollars you call it *benefits*.

DME: You're right; it is confusing. I wish we could go back to redefine the terms. Unfortunately, they've been in use long enough that I'm afraid we're stuck with them.

MHE: Why make the distinction at all? That is, why not just call everything *cost-effectiveness analysis* and leave it up to—what should we call them—the "analysts" to determine whether the appropriate measure is dollars or some natural unit?

DME: I'm not sure why the people who originally coined the separate terms thought the distinction was important. I think the main reason is that the original applications of these techniques were to set priorities for public projects such as highways, parks, and dams. In those applications, the benefits of the projects were estimated in economic terms. When the techniques were applied to medicine, however, many people found it both difficult and obnoxious to place a dollar value on health outcomes such as a human life. I imagine that the term *cost-effectiveness analysis* evolved to distinguish the method from the original applications that focused solely on money—to avoid the bad connotations. The irony is that, in a cost-effectiveness analysis, whenever a judgment is made about whether the health outcomes of a treatment are worth its costs, or whenever priorities are set, a dollar value for the health outcomes has implicitly been specified. Nonetheless, for most people it is easier to accept an implicit valuation than to explicitly place a dollar value on a life.

MHE: Wait. I don't see how a cost-effectiveness analysis that focuses on health outcomes implies a dollar value for those outcomes.

DME: It's a fairly simple idea. Suppose a state is considering several cancer-control programs. To keep it simple, let's say they all cost the same amount of money—about $1 million. Suppose health planners estimate that one would prevent 20 cancer deaths, one would prevent 15 deaths, and one would prevent three deaths. The department of health services requests money for all three programs but the legislature will allocate funds only for the first one. That decision implies that the value of preventing a cancer death is somewhere between $50 000 ($1 million ÷ 20 deaths), which the legislature was willing to pay, and $66 667 ($1 million ÷ 15 deaths), which the legislature was not willing to pay.

MHE: I see. I can also understand that, while it is difficult not to fund a program that will prevent 15 deaths, it is a lot more difficult to state that preventing a cancer death is not worth $67 000.

Where do the harms and risks of a treatment come in?

DME: They are included in the measure of benefit. When we talk about the *effectiveness* or *benefit* of a treatment in a cost-effectiveness or cost-benefit analysis, we really mean the *net effectiveness* or *net benefit*—that is, some measure that combines both the treatment's benefits and harms.

MHE: That's helpful, but I'm still uncomfortable. The word *cost* is prominent in both *cost-effectiveness analysis* and *cost-benefit analysis*. Isn't cost-effectiveness analysis just a smokescreen for cutting costs at the expense of quality?

DME: Not really. Remember that cost-effectiveness analysis is just a tool. Its role is to help people find the most efficient way to allocate whatever amount of money they want to pay. The use of cost-effectiveness analysis does not by itself imply that any particular amount of money is right or wrong; those decisions are made outside of cost-effectiveness analysis.

MHE: Why consider costs at all? I believe that the purpose of health care is to maximize quality at whatever cost that requires.

DME: Costs must be considered because of two facts. First, everything we do in health care costs people money, whether they pay it directly through out-of-pocket expenses or indirectly through insurance premiums, HMO (health maintenance organization) payments, or taxes (eg, Medicare).[4] Second, there is a limit to how much money people have. To put this in perspective, for every man, woman, and child we spend about $2500 each year for health care—that's about $10 000 for a family of four. Compare that with the median family income of about $30 000 (US Department of Housing and Urban Development).

Given these facts, we must ask two questions. First, are the benefits and harms of a treatment worth whatever costs people will have to pay? Second, if there are many treatments to choose from and if there are not enough resources to do them all, which treatments should receive priority? Answering both of these questions requires estimating not only the treatment's benefits (and harms) but also its costs.

MHE: That's pretty abstract. In actual practice we don't stop to ask those questions. It's pretty clear what we must do and we do it.

DME: Oh, but I think you do address those questions. You just do it intuitively. Tell me, do you put all your patients in an intensive care unit (ICU) when they leave the recovery room after surgery?

MHE: All of them? No.

DME: Why not?

MHE: Because it isn't necessary.

DME: What do you mean by "not necessary"? Isn't there some chance that the patient would have a myocardial infarction, an embolism, or some other emergency and that being in the ICU might save his or her life?

MHE: Well, I suppose there is *some* chance. But if you select your patients carefully, it's terribly small.

DME: You agree there would be some benefit. So why not put all your patients in the ICU?

MHE: Well, aside from the fact that it's not a very pleasant place to be, I wouldn't put all my patients there because the amount of benefit would be too small to justify it.

DME: To justify what? The cost? Taking up a bed that might be used by another patient at higher risk who would derive greater benefit?

MHE: I see where you're going.

DME: The fact is that we do not put all our postoperative patients in ICUs because we believe the benefits would be too small to justify the costs. Instead, we reserve the ICU for patients who have a sufficiently high risk of emergencies so that the expected benefits are believed to be worth the costs.

MHE: But what if people were willing to pay the additional costs? Or what if there were empty beds and extra nurses in the ICU? Doesn't it follow from what you've said that if there were no limits on those resources, there would be no need for cost-effectiveness analysis?

DME: You're right. The key question that determines whether cost-effectiveness analysis is needed is whether resources are limited. If indeed people truly were willing to spend any amount of money, no matter how large, to receive any amount of benefit, no matter how small, then there would be no need for cost-effectiveness analysis. We would still need to do a—what should we call it?—an *effectiveness analysis* to determine that the treatment did have some benefit, but we could ignore the costs.

MHE: How does that affect your example about the ICU?

DME: If we filled up the ICU, we would simply build a wing to the hospital and add more beds. To raise the money, we'd hold a hospital fundraising benefit—there's that word again—and raise the money to expand the ICU. While we're at it, let's collect some more money so that we can station paramedics on each neighborhood block. No, wait, let's put a paramedic in each apartment building to minimize the time required to respond to emergencies like heart attacks and strokes.

MHE: Come on. You're pushing this to the extreme.

DME: Yes, I am. Because that's where we can all reach agreement about the principles. You've correctly stated the principle that, if people truly didn't care about the cost of health care and truly wanted to do everything possible to maximize quality or benefit no matter what it costs, then there would be no need to compare the benefits of a treatment with its costs. But another principle is that, if there are limits on resources and if the number of possible treatments exceeds the available resources, then some method must be used to determine which treatments should get priority. That's what cost-effectiveness analysis is designed to do.

MHE: How will cost-effectiveness analysis do that? I still don't see why you don't give priority to treatments according to the amount of benefit they provide. Isn't that more or less what they ended up doing in Oregon?

DME: Cost-effectiveness analysis will do several things. First, it will estimate the health outcomes of each treatment and develop a measure of its benefit—recall that you need that aspect of cost-effectiveness analysis even if you only want to rank treatments by their benefits. Second, cost-effectiveness analysis will estimate the cost of the treatment. Then it will divide the two to calculate the amount of benefit each treatment provides per unit cost—what we loosely call its *cost-effectiveness ratio*. Fourth, it will rank the treatments by their cost-effectiveness ratios. Finally, it will select treatments in order of their cost-effectiveness ratios until the resources are exhausted.

MHE: Wait a minute. Why did you say that the ratio of benefits per unit cost is "loosely" called the cost-effectiveness ratio?

DME: Technically speaking, the ratio of benefits (in the numerator) to costs (in the denominator) is the *effectiveness-cost ratio* or *benefit-cost ratio*, depending on whether the benefits are measured in natural units or dollars, respectively. The cost-effectiveness ratio is the reciprocal of the effectiveness-cost ratio—the cost-effectiveness ratio is the amount of resources consumed by a treatment (in the numerator) per unit of effectiveness it provides (in the denominator). Technically, we want to rank treatments in order of their effectiveness-cost ratios. Because that term sounds so unfamiliar, however, it's easiest to bow to the common usage and refer to the cost-effectiveness ratio. The point is that the highest priority should be given to the treatment that provides the greatest amount of benefit per unit cost.

MHE: Well now, I guess we're at the crux of the issue. Cost-effectiveness analysis ranks treatments by their cost-effectiveness ratios. My instinct would be to rank them by their effectiveness—the amount of benefit they provide. Are you saying that if one treatment provides *greater* benefit than another treatment but its costs are such that it has a worse cost-effectiveness ratio, the more effective treatment should be rejected in favor of the less effective treatment?

DME: Yes.

MHE: Show me.

DME: Okay. So that we don't get confused by a lot of extraneous calculations, let's reduce the problem to its simplest form. Imagine that you are responsible for the health of a group of people, say, 1000 people. Your objective is to maximize their health as measured by some units, which we'll call *health benefit units* (HBUs). Imagine that a lot of thought has gone into defining and measuring the HBU; everyone agrees that this measure of benefit captures all the features of the treatments and their outcomes that people believe are important. Now suppose there are 10 different treatments that might be covered. For the particular patients who are candidates for each treatment, the treatments offer the amounts of benefit (HBUs) shown in Table 19.1 in the second column from the left. For convenience, I've listed the treatments in order of the amount of benefit they provide. The next column of the table shows the cost of each treatment. The columns in the center of the table, under "Population," show the expected number of patients who will need each treatment in the coming year and the total amount of benefit and cost for the population. Ignore the last column for the moment.

Now I tell you that you have a budget of $600 000. You can't provide all the treatments because that would cost almost $1 million. Which treatments are you going to cover?

MHE: Since you've listed the treatments in order of decreasing benefit, I would start at the top with treatment 1 and march down the list until I'd spent $600 000. I guess that would mean covering treatments 1 through 6 at a total cost of . . . let's add it up . . . $593 000. What would you do?

DME: Are you done?

MHE: Well, I've got $7000 left over. I sure would like to include treatment 10, to pick up those 190 HBUs. All I need is an additional $8000 to bring me up to the $15 000 I need for treatment 10. But you say I'm limited to a total of $600 000. Can I spend the $7000 I have left to buy treatment 10 for half the patients?

DME: Yes. But why did you skip over treatments 7, 8, and 9?

MHE: Because they cost much more than treatment 10. Besides, with treatment 10 I get more benefit at lower cost than with treatment 7 or 8. For $7000 I could buy almost half of treatment 10 ($7000 ÷ $15 000 = 47%) to get about 90 HBUs, but $7000 would buy only 3% of treatment 7 ($7000 ÷ $252 000 = 3%) to get 13 HBUS. . . . Oh, I see it. That's the cost-effectiveness ratio.

DME: Bingo. Look at column 7: It's the cost-effectiveness ratio (technically, the effectiveness-cost ratio) for each treatment—the number of HBUs per $1000. For example, for treatment 10, 190 HBUs divided by 15 (thousand

TABLE 19.1　Health Benefit Units (HBUs) and Costs of 10 Treatments

| Treatment | Individual | | Population | | | Cost-effectiveness Ratio |
	HBUs	Cost, $	No. of Patients	Total HBUs	Total Cost, $	
1	9.5	3000	20	190	60 000	3.17
2	9.0	3800	15	135	57 000	2.37
3	8.6	2300	30	258	69 000	3.74
4	8.3	1000	5	42	5000	8.3
5	7.5	5200	70	525	364 000	1.44
6	6.8	950	40	272	38 000	7.16
7	5.4	3000	84	454	252 000	1.8
8	4.3	2200	18	77	39 600	1.95
9	4.0	875	65	260	56 875	4.57
10	3.8	300	50	190	15 000	12.67
Total				2403	956 475	

dollars) is 12.67. Let's list the treatments in order of their ratios. That would be treatments 10, 4, 6, 9, 3, 1, 2, 8, 7, and 5. We could fund all the treatments except the last one, treatment 5, for $592 475. Indeed, we could fund everything but treatment 5 within the $600 000 budget.

MHE:　Let's see what difference it makes. If, as I wanted to, we covered the treatments in order of their benefits (HBUs), we would provide 1422 HBUs to the population. On the other hand, if we covered the treatments in order of their cost-effectiveness ratios, we would provide 1878 HBUs, a difference of 456 HBUs. That's an increase in benefit of about 32% at a slight *decrease* in cost.

DME:　This example illustrates a general principle that can be proven mathematically or that you can demonstrate for yourself by trial and error. For any resource limit, ranking the treatments by their cost-effectiveness ratios will deliver more benefit than any other method of ranking. Similarly, for any quality objective, ranking the treatments by their cost-effectiveness ratios will achieve that objective at the lowest cost. But don't take my word for it, try it out. For example, set any resource limit less than $1 million and see if you can find any other way to rank the treatments that will deliver more effectiveness within that budget than ranking them by their cost-effectiveness ratios.

MHE:　I can't. In retrospect, the point you're making seems obvious, even trivial.

DME:　It is.

MHE:　Then what's all the fuss about? Why are attempts to use cost-effectiveness analysis so controversial? Why did Oregon back off its original cost-effectiveness analysis and instead rank the services by their net benefit?

DME:　Those are crucial questions. Cost-effectiveness analysis clearly has something to offer. To get the most out of it and to use it properly, however, we must understand the sources of controversy, so that we can separate the signal from the noise, so to speak.

One problem is misunderstanding. Many people have never seen a simple presentation of the concepts like the one we just walked through. Most discussions of cost-effectiveness analysis are so embedded in arguments about budgets, politics, mathematical models, and personal interests that it's easy to miss the forest for the trees. Indeed, as you just said, many people see it as a smokescreen for cutting costs.

But even when the principles of cost-effectiveness analysis are clearly understood, there are several issues that can cause controversy. I'll group them into four categories: clinical, methodological, psychological, and philosophical.

The main clinical reason is that the results of a cost-effectiveness analysis are usually counterintuitive. Because it ranks treatments by their cost-effectiveness ratios instead of by their benefits, cost-effectiveness analysis inevitably ranks some less-beneficial treatments ahead of some more-beneficial treatments. In our example (Table 19.1), treatment 10, which offered a benefit of only 3.8 HBUs per patient, was ranked on top, ahead of treatments that offered almost three times as much benefit. In particular, treatment 5, which offered more than twice as much benefit to a patient as treatment 10, was excluded. Indeed, at 525 HBUs, treatment 5 was the most important single treatment available to the population, yet we rejected it. For a real example, remember how critics of Oregon's initial priority-setting process pointed out that tooth caps were ranked ahead of surgery for ectopic pregnancy?[2,5] If you focus only on the benefits of the treatments, the rankings appear to be out of order and run contrary to clinical judgment. To appreciate the results of a cost-effectiveness analysis, you have to understand that the important feature of a treatment is not the benefit it provides to an individual patient or even the total benefit it could provide to a population, but the total benefit it could provide to a population for a specified amount of resources.

MHE: Run that last sentence by me again.

DME: It is confusing. From the practitioners' point of view, the relative importance of a treatment is determined by the amount of benefit it provides to a patient. Surgery for ectopic pregnancy, which can prevent death, is more important than tooth caps, which affect pain and function but not life and death. In our hypothetical example, treatment 5, which provides 7.5 HBUs, is more important to a patient than treatment 10, which provides only 3.8 HBUs. Thus, if a practitioner were asked to rank these two treatments, it would be natural to rank treatment 5 ahead of treatment 10. If you focus on the individual patient and set costs aside, this makes sense. The superiority of a treatment like treatment 10, which appears to a practitioner to be less important, becomes apparent only when you think beyond an individual patient to consider the total amount of benefit that could be provided by offering the treatment to a group of patients within a specified budget. For example, treatment 5 provides 7.5 HBUs to one patient at a cost of $5200. For the same amount of money, 17 patients could be offered treatment 10 ($5200 ÷ $300 = 17.3) for a total of 65 HBUs (17.3 × 3.8 = 65.7). Clearly, we serve the population better if we spend the $5200 to provide 17 people with 3.8 HBUs each for a total of 65 HBUs than if we provide 5.8 HBUs to a single person. But it's difficult to see this unless you do two things: (1) Take a broad perspective that encompasses a large number of patients. (2) Think about the total *volumes* of the different treatments that you could offer with a fixed amount of resources.

MHE: I find those two things difficult to do. As a practitioner, I only know the "population," as you call it, through my individual patients, and they give me an unambiguous message. They say "Give me the best treatment" and "I don't care what it costs." If I asked my patients to rank treatments 5 and 10, they would put treatment 5 above 10. Actually, they'd insist on both.

DME: I agree with you. In fact, that's such an important point that we should come back to it. For now, let's just register the fact that one of the reasons cost-effectiveness analysis causes a fuss is that, while its application is obvious from what we might call the population perspective, it produces results that are counterintuitive from the practitioner's perspective.

MHE: Fascinating. Now you're going to have to convince me that the population perspective is the correct one.

DME: I plan to do that when we talk about the philosophical issues.

MHE: Before we go on, clarify something for me. You calculated the cost-effectiveness ratios from the perspective of the population. Does that create a bias against rare diseases, for which the total benefits of the treatment in the population are small?

DME: No. The cost-effectiveness ratio is the same whether it's calculated from the perspective of the total population or an individual patient—the number of patients cancels out. Try it on one of the treatments in the table. Look at treatment 4. It affects the rarest disease (five patients) and provides the smallest amount of benefit to the population (42 HBUs) yet was ranked second (8.3 HBUs per $1000). The prevalence of a disease in the population doesn't affect the priority of its treatment.

MHE: That's good. Now, what are the methodological issues?

DME: As you can appreciate from the example, the success of a cost-effectiveness analysis depends critically on the accuracy of the measures of benefit and cost. In our example (Table 19.1) I was careful to point out that the HBU accurately captured the features of the treatment and its outcomes that are important to people. The methodological problem is that developing such a measure requires great care.

Several things can go wrong. For example, most treatments have multiple benefits and harms; they all have to be properly weighted and integrated. Another problem is that the measures of benefit must be additive across people. For example, the HBUs had to be defined so that 5 HBUs for two people were equivalent to 10 HBUs for one person. A third problem is that the nature of the treatment itself, independent of its actual effect on outcomes, might be important. For example, two treatments that both prevent a cancer death could have different desirabilities if one treatment uses a highly visible technology to prevent an identifiable death (eg, heroic chemotherapy with bone marrow transplantation for Alice Smith) whereas the other treatment uses a mundane technology to prevent an anonymous death (eg, antitobacco education for the students of Longfield High School). All these factors can be incorporated in a measure of benefit, but it does require care. There can also be problems with the estimation of costs. Simply measuring the direct medical costs is difficult enough. Estimating indirect costs (like the effect of a screening test on treatment costs) and adjusting for the occurrence of costs and savings over time are even more difficult. The bottom line is that, if the measures of benefit or cost used in a particular analysis are inaccurate, the results can discredit the method.

MHE: Is that what happened in Oregon?

DME: Yes. For example, one of their problems was that the outcome of "vomiting, fever, and chills" was assigned a value that made it one third as bad as the outcome "death."[2] This meant that a treatment that prevented death would be considered only three times more desirable than a treatment that prevented chronic vomiting, fever, and chills. Oregon's planners also discovered that their initial measures of benefit did not accurately reflect the public's values regarding lifesaving techniques. To their credit, we should acknowledge that they spotted the problems and revised their methods to minimize the chance of dropping an effective treatment. The final priority list isn't as efficient as it could have been but it is a good starting point.[2,3]

MHE: These problems sound awful. In practice, is the method well enough developed yet to justify its use?

DME: You have a sharp pencil. Let's bring that up again after I've finished listing the other problems. The third set of problems relates to some psychological and territorial issues that cost-effectiveness analysis can raise. One obvious psychological issue is that cost-effectiveness analysis is relatively new to medicine. That newness by itself causes a certain amount of skepticism. Another psychological problem is that understanding cost-effectiveness analysis involves some abstract thinking, which a lot of people aren't used to. Listen to us talking about "HBUs," "treatment 5," and "reciprocals." Many people find it difficult to follow the abstractions, much less trust them enough to apply them to their patients. A third psychological issue is that, while the principles of cost-effectiveness analysis are old and appealing, the explicit application of those principles to health care forces us to think at a conscious, public level about things we would much rather leave at a subconscious, private level. It's one thing to write orders that a postoperative patient should be taken directly to ward 2B. It is quite another thing to publish a list of criteria for transplantations and show a patient that, although he or she would derive some benefit from the transplant, the patient falls just short of the criteria.

MHE: I can tell you another problem you'd probably label *psychological*. Cost-effectiveness analysis uses a language—mathematics—that I don't understand and that is foreign to most practitioners. This can be a bit demoralizing. I sometimes feel as though clinicians are being left out or even put down by the people who conduct the analyses.

DME: I can appreciate that. Actually, analysts are very dependent on practitioners and clinical experts to keep their analyses on target, and analysts don't intend to belittle the contributions of clinicians. But the mere fact that analysts are second-guessing clinical judgment and coming up with results that run counter to conventional wisdom can create that impression.

MHE: Something else that bothers me is that I can't check their results and fear that they might not be doing it right. Some of the problems people address with cost-effectiveness analysis have very high stakes. I get quite uncomfortable when I can't follow their calculations, especially when their results contradict conventional wisdom.

DME: I have to admit that sometimes even I can't check the results, and I have a PhD degree in engineering mathematics. In my case, the reason is usually that the formulas, data, and assumptions are often too cumbersome to publish in the usual format of medical articles, so I don't get the information I need. But occasionally an analyst will use a method I'm not expert in. Your point is well taken.

Let me ask you about something I've worried about. Because cost-effectiveness analyses require quantitative skills, they are usually conducted by people who have different training and interests than the clinical experts and practitioners who traditionally have made the decisions about medical activities. The result for the experts and practitioners is a loss of control. Decisions that used to be their private domain must now be shared. I imagine that this could be threatening. I also wonder whether some of the general criticism of cost-effectiveness analysis doesn't actually represent frustration about control.

MHE: I'm not sure *threatening* is the right word. We're used to sharing decisions—the "team approach" to planning the management of a cancer patient is a good example. I think the problem goes back to the fact that cost-effectiveness analysis uses mathematics, which most physicians don't know. Unless you know the language, it's difficult to participate and difficult to assure yourself that the conclusions are sound.

DME: There's yet another psychological problem, or perhaps *territorial* is a better word. As you can see from our example, when you apply cost-effectiveness analysis there will be winners and losers. The losers will be unhappy. The most obvious result is that patients who need the rejected treatments, and their physicians, will challenge the cost-effectiveness analysis. For example, some pediatricians were unhappy with Oregon's list, and specialists who deliver treatment 5 will be unhappy with the results of our analysis. While some of this displeasure reflects an instinct for self-preservation, it also reflects the justifiable concern of a practitioner for his or her patients. The facts that other patients are being served and that the total population is better off provide little comfort. The displeasure comes out as a criticism of cost-effectiveness analysis. In a sense, they're shooting the messenger.

MHE: You're building up quite a list of problems.

DME: Wait until you hear the last two. I call them *philosophical* because they involve personal and social values and because I can't think of a better word. One involves the conflict between the population perspective and the practitioners' perspective that we talked about earlier. You pointed out that, from your perspective as a clinician, the "population" you serve consists of your individual patients, and their priorities are clear. I'll reinforce your argument with this observation. Considering the instructions that society has given you—through the demands of your individual patients and their families, the press, and the courts—you are doing exactly the right thing. If you define the "population you serve" as your individual patient and if you consider the patient's insurance when you determine the "available resources," you are already practicing good cost-effectiveness analysis. That is, you are effectively using the available resources (which are made virtually limitless by the insurance) to maximize care for the population you serve (your patient). That is, you try to do everything possible for your patient.

MHE: So I'll re-ask the question I asked before. How do you know the population perspective is the correct one?

DME: The answer is in the table. If we followed the practitioner's perspective and gave priority to the treatments according to the amount of benefit they provide, the result would be a quality of care for the population of about 1422 HBUs. On the other hand, if we follow the population perspective and rank treatments by their cost-effectiveness ratios, the quality of care goes up to about 1878 HBUs. You tell me: which is better?

MHE: The latter.

DME: Even though patients who need treatment 5 won't get it? Even though the practitioners who specialize in treatment 5 will attack you?

MHE: Yes, because if I take the first approach and fund treatments 1 through 6, physicians and their patients who need treatments 7, 8, 9, and 10 won't get those treatments, and they will be even angrier. In essence, if resources are limited and it's not possible to do everything, somebody is bound to be unhappy. The mere fact that one constituency or another doesn't like the results cannot be interpreted to mean that the cost-effectiveness analysis was wrong. . . . Wow! Who was that talking, you or me? I've got to watch out. If I talk like that around the hospital, I'll lose all my friends.

. . . Having said all that, why am I still uncomfortable? Here is what bothers me. With rare exceptions, we're not using cost-effectiveness analysis now, yet we don't hear any complaints from the patients and practitioners who want to use treatments like treatments 7 through 10 that wouldn't be covered if the practitioners' perspective were used to set priorities. There's got to be an inconsistency in our reasoning somewhere . . . I see it. When we follow the practitioners' perspective, we don't stop at treatment 6; we give our patients all the treatments. That's why no practitioners are complaining now. Furthermore, the approach of funding all the treatments generates a quality of care of 2400 HBUs, which beats your plan by more than 500 HBUs.

DME: But that plan costs almost $1 million. You had only $600 000 to spend.

MHE: I guess what it comes down to is that I don't believe that. I believe that if people really understood that setting the limit at $600 000 would deprive them of treatment 5 under your plan or deprive them of treatments 7 through 10 if the practitioners' instincts were followed, they'd raise more money.

DME: You've just identified the last reason why cost-effectiveness analysis causes such a fuss. In a very real sense it's an innocent victim caught up in a national debate about how much we are willing to spend for health care. Recall that the justification for a cost-effectiveness analysis depends on whether resources are limited. If resources are not limited, you don't need cost-effectiveness analysis. If they are, you do. If resources are not limited the practitioners' perspective works fine, because everyone gets everything anyway. If resources are limited, however, the population perspective is correct, and the practitioners' perspective will truly harm the health of the population. Most of the controversy that appears to be about cost-effectiveness analysis is really about whether resources are limited. Even in settings like Oregon's, many people still disagree.

MHE: I have to tell you that I side with the people who don't think we've hit the limits yet. One reason is that I believe that there is still a lot of waste out there that, if eliminated, would free up enough resources to fund all the effective treatments. I want to be certain that all the waste has been eliminated before we start cutting services. Another reason is that my patients talk a lot more about the treatments they want than they do about what the treatments cost.

DME: On the matter of waste, I think that we all would agree that we should get rid of waste and that eliminating services should not be used as a substitute for eliminating waste. On the other hand, it's not all that easy to detect and eliminate waste. The health care system has been under pressure for a long time to eliminate waste and inefficiency, and it's not clear how much more can be squeezed out without major changes in structures and incentives. For example, I'm sure you realize that a lot of the waste is at least partially under your control—unnecessary tests, unnecessary hospital admissions, treatments of unknown value, overuse of specialist consultants. Some people would even point to your fees. If waste is that easy to eliminate, why don't you just do it?

The fact is that, while efforts to decrease waste must be continued strenuously, we'll probably not be able to eliminate that problem right away, at least in time for this year's or next year's budget. One more fact to consider is that an important type of waste is the use of tests and treatments that have little or no value. The best way to ferret those out is to do a cost-effectiveness analysis.

MHE: I'll grant all that. I just don't want the waste to be ignored. What about the fact that my patients tell me to spare no cost?

DME: Their demands become less compelling when you realize that they're spending somebody else's money. But a deeper problem is that the "population we serve" is sending out very mixed signals. When people talk to us through their collective voices—as taxpayers, insurance premium payers, businesses, unions, and governments—they tell us to spend less. However, when they talk to us through their individual voices—as individual patients, family members, press reports, and lawsuits—they tell us to spend more. Depending on which voice you hear the most, that's what you'll tend to believe.

MHE: Which voice is right?

DME: I don't want to sound crass but, for the purposes of determining whether resources are limited, the voice that counts is the one that's paying the bills. We can discuss ideals, desires, rights, and demands all we want, but the bottom-line question is whether the people who have it in their power to allocate resources are willing to allocate more. If they say yes, then resources are not limited and cost-effectiveness analysis need not be used. If they say no, the unavoidable conclusion is that resources are limited.

MHE: What do they say?

DME: In some cases, such as Oregon's, the answer is pretty clear. When the taxpayers, the legislature, and the federal government were asked for more money, the answer was no. Business was willing to chip in, but only as part of a package deal that set priorities for services in the spirit of a cost-effectiveness analysis. Therefore, it's safe to say that resources for the care of the poor in Oregon are limited.

In other settings the answer is a bit less clear, but a definite pattern is emerging. If an HMO went to a corporation and asked whether it is acceptable to raise rates 15% next year, the response would probably be laughter. If a corporation went to its employees and asked them to accept a larger share of the premiums and higher copayments and deductibles, the response would probably be a strike. If the federal government went to taxpayers and asked for a special tax for health care, I suspect there would be a revolt. Indeed, if we just stopped laundering the costs of health care and got honest about the bookkeeping so that people could really see how much of their money was going to health care, I think they would be shocked.

But I'm getting off the topic. We don't have to settle the national debate about costs right now. All we're trying to do is understand why cost-effectiveness analysis causes a fuss. As I said before, cost-effectiveness analysis is caught in the middle of a national debate. We who do cost-effectiveness analyses aren't coldhearted accountants who take pleasure in depriving people of health care so we can flex our analytical muscles. We think that we are responding to a national call for help. We hear taxpayers, businesses, and governments crying out that health care costs are out of control. We hear the complaints about waste, inefficiency, and ineffective practices. We offer a tool to help solve these problems, and we run smack into a propeller.

MHE: Okay. Okay. You've got my sympathy. Now let's take stock of where we are. You've convinced me that, if resources are truly limited, cost-effectiveness analysis is a good tool for setting priorities. I'll also concede that there are some settings—Oregon might well be one of them—where resources are truly limited. But now I come back to a question I raised earlier, which you dodged at the time. However noble the attempts at cost-effectiveness analysis might be, the methodological and political problems you've described are real and, quite frankly, seem almost overwhelming. Is cost-effectiveness analysis up to it? Are the state of the art and the acceptability of cost-effectiveness analysis strong enough to justify applying it to real problems?

DME: I think I can answer that. But I need a break. Can we take that up next?

MHE: Sure.

My father, who was a general surgeon in solo practice in Bridgeport, Conn, died in 1987. While this conversation is hypothetical, it is based on memories of real ones.

❖ References

1. Eddy DM. What's going on in Oregon? *JAMA.* 1991;266:417-420 (Chapter 16).
2. Eddy DM. Oregon's methods: did cost-effectiveness analysis fail? *JAMA.* 1991;266: 2135-2141 (Chapter 17).
3. Eddy DM. Oregon's plan: should it be approved? *JAMA.* 1991;266:2439-2445 (Chapter 18).
4. Eddy DM. What do we do about costs? *JAMA.* 1990;264:1161, 1165, 1169-1170 (Chapter 10).
5. Hadorn D. Setting health care priorities in Oregon: cost-effectiveness meets the rule of rescue. *JAMA.* 1991;265:2218-2225.

❖ Source

Originally published in *JAMA.* 1992;267:1669-1672, 1674-1675.

Cost-effectiveness Analysis

Is It Up to the Task?

DAVID M. EDDY, MD, PHD: Let's see, where were we? I was going to try to answer the question of whether cost-effectiveness analysis, with all its problems, is ready for prime time.[1]

MAXON H. EDDY, MD: That's right. I agreed that *if* resources are limited, and *if* it's not possible to cover all treatments, then treatments should be given priority according to the amount of benefit they provide for their cost—what we were calling the cost-effectiveness ratio. I also agreed that there probably are some settings in which resources have reached their limit—Oregon being the most prominent example. But in the process of arriving at those conclusions, we generated a list of problems that, quite frankly, make cost-effectiveness analysis look pretty shaky. At this point, unless you can satisfy me that these problems can be overcome, I'm not yet convinced that cost-effectiveness analysis is solid enough to be used for real decisions, even in settings like Oregon.

DME: Keep an open mind until we've walked through all the problems. We described four main types—clinical, psychological, philosophical, and methodological. Before we discuss each of these, however, we should notice that they fall in two distinct categories, and call for different responses. Only the methodological problems affect how well cost-effectiveness analysis actually *works*—its actual effects on the health of patients. The other three problems affect how well cost-effectiveness analysis is *accepted*, and therefore, how well it will be implemented.

MHE: So let's do the methodological problems first. If they can't be solved, there's no point in discussing the implementation.

DME: All right. Where should we begin? The methods of cost-effectiveness analysis cover such a big area that we're only going to be able to skim the surface. There is a new introductory book on this topic that I really like,[2] but I suppose it would be inappropriate to plug it here. Perhaps the best way to proceed is to list a few of the most difficult methodological problems and describe how we might approach them.

MHE: I'll tell you the ones I want to hear about. The entire enterprise rests on being able to get complete and accurate estimates of benefits and costs. I want to know three things: How can you define a measure of benefit that captures all the important outcomes? Is the available evidence sufficient to estimate the effects of treatments accurately? And can you estimate costs accurately?

❖ Defining a Measure of Benefit

DME: Arrgh! Three arrows, right in the heart. Let's begin with the measure of benefit. To be suitable for a cost-effectiveness analysis, the measure must have several properties. Three are particularly problematic. The measure should capture all the necessary information about the nature, frequency, and desirability of all the important outcomes of the treatment; the measure should incorporate any additional features of the treatment or the patient that could affect the treatment's desirability; and the measure should be additive across patients.

MHE: To keep this from getting too abstract, can we use a real example?

DME: Sure. Let's set up a mini cost-effectiveness analysis. Imagine that you are a public health officer with a $5 million budget. To keep things simple, so we don't miss the forest for the trees, imagine that there are only two treatments for you to choose between: high-dose chemotherapy and autologous bone marrow transplantation (HDC/ABMT) for women who have stage IV breast cancer, and screening with 3-year Papanicolaou tests for women between age 20 and 75 years. (I'm going to use the words "treat" and "treatment" in very general senses that include screening.) Which would you choose?

MHE: Me? I thought you were going to set up the example. I don't know how to do a cost-effectiveness analysis.

DME: Actually, I think you do. It's all fairly intuitive. Give it a try.

MHE: Okay. Well, let's see. Both treatments are intended to reduce cancer mortality, so I suppose I should start there. But I don't really know the effectiveness of either treatment.

DME: I'll be your expert witness and research associate. Ask me any questions you want.

MHE: Well, let's begin with how each treatment affects the chance that a woman will die of cancer—breast cancer or cervical cancer.

DME: A fine start. There are no controlled trials showing that HDC/ ABMT for metastatic breast cancer improves survival compared with conventional doses, but let's be optimistic and assume that this treatment permanently cures 5% of women who would otherwise die from the disease. It's important to stress that this benefit has not actually been demonstrated,[3] but it's consistent with the assumptions made in a recent *JAMA* article on HDC/ABMT.[4] HDC/ABMT does have a relatively high treatment-related mortality—about 10%—but let's assume that the 5% cure rate takes that into account. As for cervical cancer screening, if an average-risk woman is never screened for cervical cancer, there is about a 1.2% chance she will die from cervical cancer. If such a woman is screened every 3 years from age 20 through 74 years, her chance of ever dying from cervical cancer would be decreased to about 0.2%, an absolute decrease of about 1% (1.2% – 0.2% = 1%).[5]

MHE: How about the cost?

DME: HDC/ABMT costs vary widely. Let's assume an average figure of about $125 000. (For convenience, I'll use "costs" for charges.) After taking into account all the Pap tests, office visits, possible workups, and possible treatment savings, 55 years of cervical cancer screening costs about $350 (present value, discounted at 5%).

MHE: So, compared with HDC/ABMT for metastatic breast cancer, cervical cancer screening has a lower benefit per person (1% vs 5%), but lower cost ($350 vs $125 000). Now what do I do?

DME: Keep going, you have $5 million to spend.

MHE: Five million dollars to spend. If I spend it on HDC/ABMT, I could treat about 40 women ($5 000 000 ÷ $125 000 = 40). If I spend it on cervical cancer screening, I could provide lifetime screening to 14 000 women ($5 000 000 ÷ $350 = 14 286).

DME: Which is better?

MHE: Well, if I used the money to treat 40 women who have breast cancer, I could expect to cure about 5% of them, which is two women (40 × 0.05 = 2). If I spend it to screen 14 000 women for cervical cancer, I'd decrease the chance of death from cervical cancer 1% for each of those women, which means I could expect to prevent about 140 deaths (14 000 × 0.01 = 140). Preventing 140 cervical cancer deaths clearly beats curing two women of breast cancer, by a factor of about 70, so I would have to spend the money on cervical cancer screening.

DME: You say this even knowing that the women with breast cancer will be pressing their physicians to do something, whereas the women to be screened will appear healthy, and the deaths you prevent there will be "statistical"?

MHE: Yes, even though I can't identify in advance which women will be saved by cervical cancer screening, they'd end up just as dead as if I could. I can't let 140 people die, to save two people, even if the 140 deaths are "statistical."

DME: You've just completed your first cost-effectiveness analysis.

MHE: It seemed too simple. I must have left something out. But I have to admit I think the conclusion is correct.

DME: Let's see how you handled each of the problems we listed. If you, who have virtually no experience with cost-effectiveness analysis, handled them correctly, then you'll have to agree that for at least some problems it is possible to define a suitable measure of benefit.

The first problem was that treatments usually have multiple outcomes, and the measure of benefit must "capture" the necessary information about all the outcomes. Multiplicity of outcomes is certainly a feature of this analysis. HDC/ABMT has at least four important outcomes: in addition to the chance of a cure, there is treatment-related mortality, treatment-related morbidity, and posttreatment quality of life. Likewise, cervical cancer screening has a major benefit that goes beyond preventing cervical cancer death: by finding a preinvasive lesion it can prevent a woman from ever getting invasive disease at all, which greatly reduces morbidity and increases quality of life. On the other hand, the screening examinations themselves are inconvenient and might detect a preinvasive lesion that might regress spontaneously. You didn't mention any of these. Why not?

MHE: Actually, I did think about them, but it happened so fast I didn't bother to mention them. Initially, I chose to focus on cancer death because it is an outcome shared by both treatments, and in my opinion, it is by far the most important outcome of either treatment. I considered the other outcomes briefly but decided there was no need to really worry about them for this decision.

DME: Why not?

MHE: The main reason was that, if anything, incorporating the other outcomes would have increased the gap between the two treatments. For cervical cancer screening, the benefits would have appeared much *greater* if I had included the decrease in morbidity associated with preventing the cancer altogether. The inconvenience and anxiety of the examinations and the chance that screening would have detected a lesion that would have regressed spontaneously would have diminished this somewhat, but I reasoned that at worst they would have done no more than balance out the decrease in morbidity. As for the other outcomes of HDC/ABMT, most of them work *against* that treatment. The 10% treatment-related mortality rate, while it was taken into account in the 5% cure rate, would have shortened a lot of lives. The rate of serious side effects is higher with HDC/ABMT than with conventional doses. And I don't believe anyone has really measured the quality of life after treatment.

My suspicions that the other outcomes wouldn't matter were confirmed when I saw that the effects of the two treatments on cancer death were going to differ by a factor of about 70. I decided that the other outcomes were very unlikely to be important enough to overturn this huge margin and cause me to change my mind.

DME: I like your reasoning. In fact, you succeeded in finding a measure of benefit—"chance of cancer death"—that was suitable for this problem.

MHE: But it didn't actually incorporate all the other outcomes. And the measure I chose didn't do anything fancy with life expectancy or adjustments for quality of life.

DME: It didn't need to. First, you found what we might call a "common, dominant outcome"—an outcome shared by both treatments, whose importance is so overriding that it's safe to base a guideline on it. A lot of cost-effectiveness analyses are based on dominant outcomes. Second, you left the outcome in its natural form—"chance of death." Because this took into account the effects of the treatment on mortality, there was no need to translate the outcome into life expectancy, and because you had finessed the issue of the nonmortal outcomes, there was no need to incorporate quality of life. There is an important lesson here. The measure of benefit doesn't have to be all-inclusive or fancy, in order to be useful. In general, you want to use the simplest and most understandable outcome measure required to solve the particular problem. In this case, the outcome you chose worked quite well.

MHE: Good for me. What about the second property that a measure of benefit should incorporate information about the nature of the treatment and the nature of the patients? What's the issue there, and how did I handle it?

DME: The issue there is that, whether right or wrong, some people feel that the value of a medical activity is a function of *who* is helped, and *how* they are helped, irrespective of the actual outcomes. For example, many people are excited by high-technology treatments for identifiable patients, such as a heart-lung transplantation for Mr Williams, and find them more desirable than mundane treatments for anonymous people, like antitobacco education for high school students. They feel this way even though for the same amount of money the latter would prevent far more deaths from chronic obstructive pulmonary disease than the former. It's amazing how irrational some of these choices can be, if we define "rational" as the choice that will actually provide the most health benefit.

MHE: I can tell you the psychological forces behind those choices. One is that new technology *is* exciting. It carries a sense of wonder about what scientists can achieve and provides hope for future achievements. There is also a strong association between "high technology," "state of the art," and "better." Although this is not always the case, new technologies usually improve on older technologies, and people assume that that pattern will apply to new medical technologies. With regard to the importance of *who* is treated, people find something much more desirable if they can identify with it. People can identify with a 38-year-old housewife who has terminal breast cancer, but they can't identify with an anonymous woman who never got cervical cancer because she was screened. People can identify with a suburban mother of three better than with a woman who is alone and poor. These psychological forces are real. I'm not certain you want to call them irrational.

DME: I agree with your assessment of the psychology. Whether choices based on these psychological forces are irrational or not depends on our objectives for health care: Are we trying to help people live longer with a higher quality of life, or are we trying to please spectators? And do we really want to place different values on different people based on their visibility and social circumstances? But we're getting off the topic—perhaps we'll talk about that some other time.

MHE: Well, whatever we conclude about the relative desirabilities of different types of treatments and patients, the fact is that I didn't take either of those into account. HDC/ABMT for metastatic breast cancer is surely an example of a high-technology treatment compared with cervical cancer screening, and HDC/ABMT affects "identifiable deaths," compared with the "statistical deaths" saved by cervical cancer screening. I ignored both those aspects of the treatments.

DME: I disagree. I think you took them into account; you just did it intuitively and subjectively. When you chose between the two treatments, you knew you were comparing two breast cancer deaths prevented by HDC/ABMT with 140 cervical cancer deaths prevented by screening. By framing the question in this way—that is, by including information about both the treatments and the diseases—you had the information you needed to consider the natures of the treatments (high-technology vs mundane) and the natures of the outcomes (breast cancer death vs cervical cancer death). You might also recall that I even asked you to reconsider your choice in light of the fact that HDC/ABMT affects identifiable deaths, whereas screening affects "statistical" deaths. Thus, the full descriptions of the outcome measures you used actually contained a lot of information about the patients and the treatments, and I wager they were in the back of your mind when you made your decision.

MHE: On reflection, you're right. For example, I was thinking that I might have tolerated a twofold or even a threefold difference in deaths because of the difference in "visible" vs "statistical" deaths—but not a 70-fold difference. Good for me again. Now, what did you mean by "additive across patients," and how did I handle that?

DME: Your use of the measure "cancer death" required that we believe that, for example, reducing the chance of death 1% for 100 people is equally desirable as reducing the chance of death 5% for 20 people. This is a reasonable assumption because in both cases we would expect to prevent one death ($100 \times 0.01 = 20 \times 0.05 = 1$). Achieving this additive property can be difficult for some other measures, however. For example, if we used life expectancy as the measure of benefit, that could require that we believe that adding 40 years of life expectancy to one person is equivalent to adding one year of life expectancy to 40 people. Or if we give "preventing death" a score of 1 and "tooth caps for pulp exposure" a score of 0.08, that could mean we consider it equally desirable to prevent one death as to provide 13 tooth caps.

MHE: So I managed to find a measure of benefit that worked for this problem. Frankly, it seemed so natural that I suspect you're downplaying the complexity of the problem.

DME: Yes and no. On one hand, the use of natural measures and dominant outcomes works well for a lot of cost-effectiveness problems. That approach is especially helpful when you are making head-on comparisons of similar treatments for the same disease or similar diseases. Examples from a different clinical area would be an analysis of different screening frequencies for hypertension, different drugs for hypercholesterolemia, and different thrombolytic agents for heart attacks. The head-on comparison—choosing which of two or more treatments is best—means that you do not have to determine exactly how much benefit each treatment offers; you only have to know which treatment offers the most benefit for the available resources. The similarity of treatments mutes the issue of the nature of the treatments, and focusing on one disease or similar diseases makes the outcomes directly comparable. When there is no single outcome that dominates all the others, the outcomes of a disease often move in synchrony, enabling an analyst to pick one to serve as a proxy for the others. For example, a comparison of treatments for hypercholesterolemia might focus on myocardial infarctions, with fair confidence that the results will also hold for sudden deaths, angina attacks, coronary insufficiency, and even angioplasties. Even when there are multiple outcomes that can't be finessed by choosing a dominant or proxy outcome, it is often possible to think of the outcomes as a group and let the package of outcomes serve as the measure, in the spirit of a balance sheet.[6] This works if you are comparing two treatments and can hold all the outcomes in your head.

MHE: If I'm following all this, it sounds as though this approach to measuring benefits is similar to the way I as a practitioner think through a complex decision involving several different outcomes. For example, if I'm weighing different initial treatments for breast cancer, I'll think of the benefits and harms of each treatment in the way I believe you are describing as a package of outcomes, and then weigh the packages.

DME: That's true. This approach to measuring the benefits of a treatment closely parallels, and indeed is modeled after, the way a practitioner thinks about the outcomes of a treatment. As we continue talking, I believe you'll see that much of cost-effectiveness analysis parallels clinical judgment.

MHE: Well, it can't all be that easy.

DME: You're right. Defining a measure of benefit gets much more difficult when the comparison involves a large number of very different treatments for very different diseases, each of which has a large number of different outcomes. For example, suppose you wanted to develop a cardinal ranking of in vitro fertilization, amniocentesis, a drug rehabilitation program, surgery for chronic low-back pain, and repair of a cleft palate.

MHE: How in the world would you do that?

DME: This type of cost-effectiveness problem does require that the analyst roll all the outcomes into a single measure. One measure that is commonly used for this purpose is the "quality-adjusted life-year," or QALY. The rationale for the QALY is the fact that all outcomes of any treatment have two basic dimensions—an effect on length of life and an effect on quality of life. In essence, the measure attempts to collapse these two dimensions into a single dimension—an equivalent length of life. The underlying supposition is that for any change in quality of life, it is possible to identify a change in the length of life that is equivalent in desirability. I don't believe that you want to hear everything there is to know about QALYs and other composite measures right now. Suffice it to say that it is possible to use measures like these, but doing so requires great care.

MHE: I do have one question. I sometimes see articles that are comparing similar treatments for the same disease, but they use life expectancy or QALYs as the measure of benefit instead of natural units. From what you said earlier, I would have thought that finding a dominant outcome or proxy outcome would have been simpler and more natural. Given that the authors were not trying to make comparisons across dozens of different disease, why did they use QALYs?

DME: In those cases, the authors really had two objectives. One was to compare the treatments that were the immediate target of the analysis, and it is true that natural measures would often have sufficed for that purpose. But another objective was to provide other analysts and decision makers with information about these treatments, for future use in comparisons with other treatments. If all analysts report their results using a common measure such as QALYs, we will slowly build an inventory of cost-effectiveness analyses that can be used for broader decisions.

MHE: So what's the bottom line? Is there a measure of benefit that can be used in any cost-effectiveness analysis?

DME: I don't think there is any single, practical measure that has all the desired qualities, for every problem, and about which every analyst agrees.

MHE: Aha! Was that the collapse of cost-effectiveness analysis I just heard?

DME: No. It just means that there is no general solution. The appropriate measure will depend on the particular problem.

MHE: Okay. I guess I'll have to take your word that it is *possible* to define suitable measures for specific problems, but that it requires considerable effort. What about the evidence? You're always talking about how poor the evidence is for most medical practices. Why doesn't that sink cost-effectiveness analysis?

DME: There is one final point I want to make about the measure of benefit. I don't want you to just take my word for it that appropriate measures can almost always be found. Let me try to convince you with the following insight. In general, if it's possible for a practitioner to draw conclusions about the benefits of a treatment, it should be possible for an analyst to use the same clues to develop a measure for those benefits. If it is not possible to develop any useful measure of the benefits of a treatment, you've got to wonder what practitioners are basing their decisions on.

MHE: Touché.

❖ Dealing With Incomplete Evidence

DME: Now, on to the evidence. First, there is no denying that the accuracy of the estimates of outcomes depends critically on the type of evidence that is available. Second, there are indeed lots of problems with the evidence available for most cost-effectiveness analyses. While there is sometimes good evidence that directly addresses the treatments you want to compare, more often than not the available evidence is not a direct hit on the problem you are trying to analyze. The evidence might involve a slightly different treatment (eg, a different screening frequency), or different patients (eg, high risk vs average risk), or different outcomes (eg, tumor response rates instead of survival). Or perhaps there is no direct evidence at all, and you have to use indirect evidence.

MHE: "Indirect evidence?" That sounds pretty flimsy.

DME: Actually, you use this type of reasoning all the time. For example, do you believe that treatment of hypercholesterolemia with lovastatin reduces the chance of sudden deaths and myocardial infarctions?

MHE: Yes.

DME: Why? Do you know of any direct evidence showing that?

MHE: Yes. There are several randomized controlled trials showing that lovastatin reduces low-density lipoprotein (LDL) cholesterol.

DME: But those studies didn't observe sudden deaths or myocardial infarctions. How do you know lovastatin will prevent those outcomes?

MHE: Because there's good epidemiological evidence that lowering LDL cholesterol will prevent sudden deaths and myocardial infarctions.

DME: So to make the connection between lovastatin and a decrease in sudden deaths and myocardial infarctions, you had to combine two bodies of evidence. One linked lovastatin to a decrease in LDL cholesterol; the other linked a decrease in LDL cholesterol to a decrease in sudden deaths and myocardial infarctions. That's indirect evidence.

MHE: All right, I'll accept the use of indirect evidence. But what do you do when there is virtually no evidence at all—either direct or indirect—or when the evidence is so messy and biased that you really can't trust it?

DME: There are several approaches. First, that's an important message in its own right. That is, the discovery that there is no good evidence of benefit for a treatment is an important result of a cost-effectiveness analysis. If there really is no evidence on which to base estimates of benefits, practitioners and patients should be told that. If the treatment is relatively new and not yet ingrained in practice, we could call it "investigational," and discourage practitioners from using it until its outcomes are better understood. If the treatment has been around for a long time—"time-honored," so to speak—practitioners might resist any efforts to stop them from using it, but we can at least tell them to be cautious about touting its benefits. Furthermore, a cost-effectiveness analysis showing there is no evidence of benefit for a treatment can be a powerful stimulus for better research.

But there is another way to approach a problem for which the evidence is incomplete. That is to make an a fortiori analysis, or to search for bounds. This technique is especially applicable to head-on comparisons and is the approach we took in the HDC/ABMT example. Recall that there are no controlled trials demonstrating that HDC/ABMT improves survival of women with metastatic breast cancer compared with conventional doses. We could have stopped the analysis at that point. I chose not to, however, because many oncologists believe that the treatment will eventually be shown to be effective—and indeed it might. Thus, I thought it would be interesting to determine how HDC/ABMT would compare with something like cervical cancer screening if the hopes came true. To determine that, we *assumed* that HDC/ABMT would cure 5% of patients who would otherwise die. If HDC/ABMT turned out not to be attractive based on an optimistic assumption about its benefits, it *certainly* would not be attractive if the lack of evidence of benefit was factored in. That is an a fortiori analysis.

MHE: What did you mean by "search for bounds?"

DME: That approach is an extreme example of an a fortiori analysis. The idea is that sometimes, even if you push an assumption about a treatment's effects to the extreme, the conclusion will still be obvious. Suppose an oncologist heard our assumption that HDC/ABMT has a 5% cure rate and argues that we're too pessimistic. Suppose the oncologist believes that the treatment will eventually be shown to cure 20% of women. Rather than engage in a fruitless argument about the cure rate—fruitless because there is no evidentiary basis for resolving it—we could push the benefits of HDC/ABMT to the extreme and see whether that would make any difference. For example, we could imagine that HDC/ABMT cured absolutely every woman with metastatic breast cancer. That's clearly an upper bound—you can't get any better than a 100% cure rate. A 100% cure rate would mean that for $5 million, you would save all 40 women who got HDC/ABMT ([$5 million ÷ $125 000] × 1.0 = 40). Saving 40 women from dying of breast cancer would still be less beneficial than preventing 140 women of dying from cervical cancer—by a factor of more than three.

While I'm on the topic, another tool analysts use to deal with incomplete evidence or uncertainty is sensitivity analysis. Sensitivity analysis involves varying the values of parameters about which there is uncertainty, to see if that will change any conclusions. For example, the cost of HDC/ABMT varies from institution to institution. What if it costs $75 000 at a particular institution? Would that change your conclusion? At a cost of $75 000, putting $5 million into HDC/ABMT might cure three to four women ([$5 million ÷ $75 000] × 0.05 = 3.3) instead of two women. That's a big improvement, but not nearly enough to wipe out the 70-fold difference with cervical cancer screening. Suppose we want to look ahead to anticipate the possible effects of colony-stimulating factors on the cost of HDC/ABMT. We don't yet know what its effect on cost will be, but we could ask how low the cost of HDC/ABMT would have to go to make it competitive with cervical cancer screening. In order to stretch $5 million to cure 140 people of breast cancer, HDC/ABMT would have to cost about $1750 ([$5 million ÷ x] × 0.05 = 140, solve for x). It's unlikely that colony-stimulating factor, or anything else, will accomplish that.

By the way, these comments illustrate an important point about cost-effectiveness analysis. Although you need excellent evidence to make precise estimates of outcomes, you often do not need excellent evidence to draw accurate conclusions. For many problems, the conclusion is clear even when the evidence is imperfect. We've already talked about the costs—our estimates of the benefits of either HDC/ABMT or cervical cancer screening could be off by a factor of more than 10 and the conclusion that cervical cancer screening is preferable would still be correct.

MHE: So how would you summarize the problem of poor evidence?

DME: I'm not going to claim that the evidence needed for cost-effectiveness analyses is great. But I can offer you another sobering insight. If a practitioner thinks there is enough evidence of benefit to justify using a treatment, then chances are an analyst has enough evidence to perform a cost-effectiveness analysis. On the other hand, if an analyst can't find enough evidence to estimate the benefits of a treatment, then once again you have to wonder what practitioners are basing their decisions on. Such a treatment might well be an example of the waste we are always looking for. But I also want to be perfectly clear about something: Even if sufficient evidence exists to make some judgments about a treatment, collecting and analyzing that evidence can be a very difficult task.

MHE: There's a pattern emerging here. These methodological problems might have solutions, but they're not easy. What about costs?

❖ Measuring Costs

DME: The problem of estimating costs is conceptually much easier than estimating benefits, although technically it can be more difficult. It is conceptually easier because we don't have to search around for a measure. There is an obvious measure—dollars. In rare cases the "scarce resource" will be some physical resource that cannot be manufactured, such as a kidney for transplantation, but for the great majority of analyses, dollars will do nicely.

There are other problems, however, that make the estimation of costs difficult. First, when estimating the cost of a treatment we need to know not only the immediate cost of the test or procedure, but also the long-term costs and savings. These are determined by the treatment's outcomes, which are usually probabilistic and delayed. Thus, to estimate the full costs of a treatment, an analyst usually has to estimate its outcomes and build some model that tracks the occurrence of outcomes over time. A second problem is that the reporting of costs is highly distorted. The most accessible numbers are not costs at all but rather charges, which can bear little relationship to actual

costs. A third problem is that both costs and charges can vary enormously
from site to site. Finally, depending on the perspective of the analysis, a cost
analysis might have to extend beyond medical costs to incorporate non-
medical costs.

MHE: At this point, I'm too tired to press you for details. I'll take your
word for it if you say that all those problems can be handled.

DME: In theory, they can. But once again, it's very difficult and must be
done on a one-by-one basis.

MHE: Does that cover all the important methodological problems?

❖ Defining Treatment/Indications

DME: Not quite. There is one more that greatly affects the
practicality of attempting a cost-effectiveness analysis like the one they
tried in Oregon. Cost-effectiveness analyses cannot be applied to a general
category of treatments like "breast cancer treatment." To be valid, a cost-
effectiveness analysis must be applied to treatments and patient indications
defined at a very high level of detail. This is necessary because if the description of the treatment or patient is too broad, there is no way to pinpoint the
expected outcomes.

MHE: I think I follow you, but I'm not sure.

DME: I can illustrate the problem with the example of metastatic breast
cancer. Suppose Mrs Smith asked you about her prognosis; what would you
tell her?

MHE: I couldn't tell her anything until I knew more about her. For
example: How long was she in remission before the disease metastasized?
How many metastases does she have, and where are they? Has she had any
prior chemotherapy?

DME: Exactly. Before you can estimate a patient's outcomes, you need
to specify a dozen or so characteristics that can affect those outcomes. We
sometimes talk loosely about the outcomes of a treatment or the cost-
effectiveness of a treatment as though they were *properties* of the treatment.
They are not. The outcomes, and therefore the cost-effectiveness of a treatment, depend critically on the characteristics of the patient to whom the
treatment will be applied. In similar fashion, I'm sure you can also appreciate that the outcomes of a treatment will also depend on the specific features
of the treatment, such as a particular drug regimen or screening frequency.
Thus, when we talk about the cost-effectiveness of a treatment, we are really
talking about the cost-effectiveness of a *very specific treatment* for a *very specific set of indications*—what we might call a "treatment/indication."

MHE: I can see that. But is that really a problem, provided that you do
define the indications carefully enough?

DME: It's not a conceptual problem, but it sure is a practical problem
because it tremendously increases the amount of work that has to be done. It
can also become a methodological problem if the indications aren't defined

in sufficient detail. For example, one of the services ranked by Oregon was "preventive services for adults with proven effectiveness/medical therapy." When I see that, I think of dozens of activities, such as antitobacco education, diet, exercise, screening, hypertension treatment, cholesterol treatment, flu vaccines—and the list goes on. And within each of these there can be a dozen items. For example, within screening there is screening for cervical cancer, for breast cancer, for colon cancer, for cholesterol, for hypertension, and so forth. Within each of these can be another dozen items. For example, screening for colon cancer can be done by digital examination, fecal occult blood test, rigid sigmoidoscopy, flexible sigmoidoscopy, colonoscopy, or barium enema. The tests can be given in any combination, at any frequency, starting and stopping at any age. The patients can have no risk factors, a history of adenomatous polyps, a family history of colon cancer, familial polyposis, and so forth. Just within colon cancer screening, there can be more than a hundred possible treatment/indications. Depending on which strategy is chosen, the cost-effectiveness can vary widely. Within "preventive services for adults," there could easily be more than a thousand treatment/indications, whose cost-effectiveness can range from virtually no effectiveness (eg, lung cancer screening) to great effectiveness (eg, antitobacco education).

MHE: What harm is done if you don't define the treatment indications in sufficient detail?

DME: If a category is too highly aggregated, it is virtually impossible to develop an accurate estimate of its effectiveness or its costs. For example, even if we restrict an analysis to "cervical cancer screening," the result will depend critically on whether we think of 3-year examinations (which are highly cost-effective) or 1-year examinations (which are highly cost-*ineffective* compared with 3-year examinations). Can you imagine what would happen if we tried to analyze "adult preventive services"? Furthermore, if you do manage to come up with an estimate of the benefit for a highly aggregated category of treatments and indications, the result would not apply accurately to every treatment/indication in the broad category, which would lead to many erroneous conclusions. For example, if the analysis of cost-effectiveness of "adult preventive services" was based on the benefits of 3-year Pap tests, that could erroneously scoop up baseline mammograms at age 35. And vice versa.

❖ Conclusions

MHE: Well, I've about had it with the methodological problems. Let's step back and see what we've done. I've gotten the message that the methodological problems have been thought about very hard, and that for at least some treatments—or should I say "treatment/indications"?—there are ways to overcome them. But I've also gotten the message that there is no general solution, that each problem must be hand-tailored, and that it can be very difficult.

DME: That's an accurate assessment. Actually, there is a helpful way to think about all these methodological issues. In many ways, the methods of cost-effectiveness analysis simply formalize many of the things that practitioners already do intuitively. Practitioners already sort patients into finely defined categories of indications when they choose an appropriate treatment. Practitioners already have ways of weighing the multiple outcomes of different treatments. And practitioners already have found ways to use incomplete evidence about the outcomes of a treatment to make their own decisions. These similarities mean that, in general, if a practitioner is able to draw a conclusion about a treatment, then a cost-effectiveness analyst will also be able to draw a conclusion. On the other hand, if the methodological problems are too difficult for a cost-effectiveness analysis, they are probably also too difficult for a practitioner.

There are five main differences between what an analyst needs or does for a cost-effectiveness analysis, and what a practitioner needs or does to make a decision about a patient, and it is instructive to review them. One big difference is that the analyst incorporates costs, whereas practitioners often ignore costs. It is probably this fact more than any other that leads to different conclusions. A second difference is that a practitioner's thinking is implicit and subjective, whereas an analyst's reasoning must be explicit and as objective as possible. A third is that a practitioner's reasoning is limited by the capabilities of the human mind. In contrast, an analyst can draw on tools such as computers that can handle much more complex problems. The fourth difference is that when a practitioner makes a decision, he or she is typically focusing on one individual patient, and lets the use of resources and the implications for other patients fall where they may. A cost-effectiveness analysis follows a set of principles and steps designed to use the available resources in the most efficient way to maximize the health of *all* patients. The final difference is that practitioners' decisions are virtually always limited to comparisons between a few treatments for the same disease—the disease their particular patient has. A cost-effectiveness analysis might try to rank scores of treatments for scores of diseases—as they did in Oregon.

❖ The Bottom Line

MHE: So, what do you say? Is cost-effectiveness analysis up to the task?

DME: It depends. If we're talking about comparing particular treatments, like HDC/ABMT for breast cancer and cervical cancer screening, the answer is yes.

MHE: Don't give me this "it depends" stuff. You know what we're talking about. Oregon was trying to use cost-effectiveness analysis to develop a list of all services, ranked by their cost-effectiveness ratios. Is the methodology up to that?

DME: No.

MHE: Wow! I never thought I'd hear it.

DME: You heard it right. I don't believe that the methodology or the evidence is sufficiently well developed to try to determine the effectiveness and cost of all the important medical treatments, for all their possible indications. Although in theory that might be possible, and although in principle it is the right thing to do, it is not a practical possibility yet.

❖ Implications for Oregon

MHE: So what does that mean? Did Oregon do the right thing?

DME: Oregon tried to do the right thing. As you and I have agreed,[1] when resources are limited and priorities must be set, the priorities *should* be based on cost-effectiveness. Oregon's leaders were correct in their thinking that ranking services by their cost-effectiveness ratios is vastly preferable to ranking people, which is the approach taken by the current Medicaid programs, or ranking services solely by the amount of benefit they provide without considering costs. So Oregon's leaders were definitely moving in the right direction and deserve our congratulations for that. The problem was that the task they were trying to do was just too big for the available data and methods. Oregon's leaders saw this after their first try and wisely retreated.

MHE: Does this mean their project should not be approved?

DME: No. As I said before,[7] the methods they eventually used, while by no means perfect, were good enough for their immediate purposes, and they were certainly superior to the methods (if you can call them that) that were used to design the current Medicaid program. Furthermore, their proposal goes far beyond the implementation of their priority list. They ended up cutting relatively few services. In my opinion, the major effect of their proposal is to extend coverage for the great majority of most beneficial services to about 450 000 people who currently have no coverage at all. That benefit is not affected by the details of the list.

MHE: If their plan is approved, what should Oregon's commission do about the list?

DME: Even though the current list was based more on effectiveness than cost-effectiveness, and even though it has some very broad categories, it is a reasonable starting point. I would encourage them to adhere to their original objective of giving priority to different treatment/indications according to their cost-effectiveness ratios. But instead of trying to rank all services all at once, which virtually forces them to use broad categories and crude measures, I would advise them to approach the problem in a more piecemeal fashion. Take the current list; look at services that are close to the cutoff point for coverage; also look at services that are highly aggregated and contain multiple treatments and patient indications; search for particular treatment/ indications that are currently covered but that are suspected to have low yields (ie, low benefit relative to costs); also search for particular treatment/

indications that are not currently covered but that are suspected to have high yields; and perform rigorous cost-effectiveness analyses of those problems, hand-tailoring the methods to fit each problem. The results can be used to improve the accuracy of the list—subtracting some currently covered treatment/ indications and adding some currently uncovered treatment/indications. That is, use cost-effectiveness analysis to tune the current list, starting with the most suspect or controversial items. I know this will be a much slower process, but I think it will be more accurate, acceptable, and defensible.

MHE: Fair enough. But I gather you still believe that cost-effectiveness analysis can be very helpful for solving particular problems.

DME: Absolutely. In fact, I think it is essential to good decision making in the circumstances that we described, where decision makers are constrained by costs and have to set priorities.

MHE: Well, then I guess we need to discuss the clinical, psychological, and philosophical problems that will impede the implementation of cost-effectiveness analysis.

Maxon H. Eddy is my father. Before he died in 1987, he practiced as a general surgeon in Bridgeport, Conn. Although this conversation is hypothetical, it is based on memories of real ones.

❖ References

1. Eddy DM. Cost-effectiveness analysis: a conversation with my father. *JAMA*. 1992; 267:1669-1672, 1674-1675 (Chapter 19).
2. Eddy DM. *A Manual for Assessing Health Practices and Designing Practice Policies: The Explicit Approach*. Philadelphia, Pa: American College of Physicians; 1992.
3. Eddy DM. High-dose chemotherapy with autologous bone marrow transplantation for the treatment of metastatic breast cancer. *J Clin Oncol*. 1992;10:657-670.
4. Hillner BE, Smith TJ, Desch CE. Efficacy and cost-effectiveness of autologous bone marrow transplantation in metastatic breast cancer: estimates using decision analysis while awaiting clinical trial results. *JAMA*. 1992;267:2055-2061.
5. Eddy DM. Screening for cervical cancer. *Ann Intern Med*. 1990;113:214-226.
6. Eddy DM. Comparing benefits and harms: the balance sheet. *JAMA*. 1990;263:2493, 2498, 2501, 2505 (Chapter 7).
7. Eddy DM. Oregon's plan: should it be approved? *JAMA*. 1991;266:2439-2445 (Chapter 18).

❖ Source

Originally published in *JAMA*. 1992;267:3342-3348.

❖ CHAPTER 21

Cost-effectiveness Analysis
Will It Be Accepted?

MAXON H. EDDY, MD: So. You don't believe the methods of cost-effectiveness analysis are strong enough to develop a priority list of all treatments, as they tried to do in Oregon.[1] However, you do believe that the methods are strong enough to estimate the benefits and costs of specific treatments. I will agree with those conclusions. But I cannot yet agree that cost-effectiveness analysis should be used routinely to set priorities for treatments. First, we need to resolve some of the nonmethodological problems that could block the successful implementation of a cost-effectiveness analysis.

DAVID M. EDDY, MD, PHD: Before we do that, I want to make certain there is no misunderstanding about my position on the use of cost-effectiveness analysis in Oregon. In circumstances like Oregon's, where budgets are limited and priorities must be set, in *principle* those priorities should be determined by the cost-effectiveness of different treatments, and in *theory* the methods can accomplish that. Thus, Oregon's attempt to apply cost-effectiveness analysis was correct, and the state should continue to pursue that goal. The problem is that the current methods and data for performing cost-effectiveness analyses are such that it is not *feasible* to apply cost-effectiveness analysis to rank *all* treatments. Attempting to do so forces analysts to aggregate treatments and indications to such a high degree, and to apply such crude measures of benefit and costs, that errors are inevitable, results become suspect, and the process is difficult to defend. I believe that, at this stage in its development, cost-effectiveness analysis must be applied to very carefully defined treatments for very specific patient indications, and that the methods must be hand-tailored to each particular problem.

MHE: We'll make sure the record states what you just said. So, from now on we'll be talking about the use of cost-effectiveness analysis for specific problems. Now let's examine some of the nonmethodological issues that will ultimately determine how cost-effectiveness analysis is received.

DME: Are you sure we need to do this? What ultimately counts is whether cost-effectiveness analysis will improve the health of patients, which is determined by its methods. If the methods are sound and the only issue is whether cost-effectiveness analysis is poorly understood or poorly received, our response should not be to discard cost-effectiveness analysis, but to help people understand it.

MHE: I agree. But I still think it's important to address the nonmethodological problems because successful implementation of the results will depend heavily on how people perceive the methods and objectives. All the methods in the world won't help, if people won't listen. Earlier,[2] we identified three groups of nonmethodological problems—you called them clinical, psychological, and philosophical. Let's start with the clinical problems.

DME: The main clinical problem was that the results of cost-effectiveness analyses are counterintuitive. A cost-effectiveness analysis will give priority to a less beneficial treatment over a more beneficial treatment, if the cost of the less beneficial treatment is low enough so that, for a fixed amount of resources, it can be provided to a large enough number of people to make its total benefit to the population exceed the benefit provided by the more beneficial but more expensive treatment.

MHE: Stop. That sentence was far too long.

DME: Point well taken. Let's describe the problem through the example we used earlier.[1] You'll recall that we were comparing high-dose chemotherapy and autologous bone marrow transplantation (HDC/ABMT) for metastatic breast cancer with cervical cancer screening. Although there is no good evidence to confirm this,[3] we assumed optimistically that HDC/ABMT would cure 5% of women who had metastatic breast cancer. We also estimated that 3-year Papanicolaou tests from age 20 to 75 years would decrease the chance a woman would die of cervical cancer about 1% (from about 1.2% without screening to about 0.2% with screening).[4] HDC/ABMT costs about $125 000 per patient, while the screening costs about $350 per woman (present value). When I asked you to picture yourself as a public health officer with a $5 million budget to spend and told you that you had to choose between the two activities, you chose cervical cancer screening.

MHE: That's correct. I reasoned that putting $5 million into screening would prevent about 140 cervical cancer deaths ([$5 million ÷ $350] × 0.01 = 143), whereas putting $5 million into HDC/ABMT would cure only two women of breast cancer ([$5 million ÷ $125 000] × 0.05 = 2). Cervical cancer screening won by a factor of about 70. No matter how much we varied the assumptions, we couldn't even come close to erasing that difference. Now what's the clinical problem?

DME: The clinical problem is that if I had let you think of yourself as a practitioner, I believe that you'd have given me an entirely different answer.

But let's confirm my suspicion. Here's the question. Suppose you have two patients. Mrs Smith is 38 years old, has metastatic breast cancer, and is a candidate for HDC/ABMT. Mrs Jones is 20 years old, she might get cervical cancer some time in the future, and she is asking about Pap tests. Imagine that you can treat only one woman. (I'm using the word "treat" in a general sense that includes screening.) Who will you treat? And when you answer the question for Mrs Smith and Mrs Jones, be aware that your answer will have implications for all women.

MHE: Well, I'd like to insist on treating both, but I know you won't accept that answer. If I could really treat only one woman it would have to be Mrs Smith, who has breast cancer. Although the potential outcomes are similar—breast cancer death and cervical cancer death—Mrs Smith's odds without the treatment are much worse than those of Mrs Jones, and treatment would provide greater benefit to Mrs Smith than to Mrs Jones.

DME: Does the cost of the HDC/ABMT bother you?

MHE: Of course, but in my opinion the greater benefit to Mrs Smith outweighs the higher cost. Besides, Mrs Smith already has her disease, she is standing in front of me asking for help, and I have to do something. Mrs Jones is healthy today; she might never get cervical cancer, and if she does, there is a good chance it can be treated successfully. The fact is that Mrs Smith has more to gain from the HDC/ABMT than Mrs Jones does from Pap tests.

DME: I have to admit that if I put myself in your shoes, I'd probably feel the same way. The question before us now is, how should we deal with this conflict between what the cost-effectiveness analysis says—give priority to cervical cancer screening over HDC/ABMT—and what our clinical judgment says—give priority to HDC/ABMT over cervical cancer screening? One option is to follow our clinical judgment and treat women with HDC/ABMT. If we do, we will make ourselves more comfortable as clinicians, but we will be delivering a lower overall amount of benefit to women. In this example, following our clinical judgment would allow a lot more women to die of cancer. Even though you probably won't see them in your practice, and even though no one will be able to track their deaths back to your decision, the suffering and deaths of these women will be real. On the other hand, if we reject our intuition and give cervical cancer screening higher priority, we will keep many more women alive, but we will make ourselves very uncomfortable. How would you handle this conflict?

MHE: Well, first I would have to confirm that I really believe the calculations. In fact, I do, especially after the a fortiori analysis and sensitivity analysis we walked through last time.[1] Therefore, I know I should accept the results of the cost-effectiveness analysis, and rearrange my clinical judgment. In the end, it's the patients' health that counts, not my comfort level. Okay, I'm prepared to say that the fact that cost-effectiveness analysis delivers counterintuitive results is not a reason to reject it. It's a reason to scrutinize the results very carefully, but not to reject them a priori. But doesn't this issue overlap with one of the philosophical problems—the choice between the practitioners' perspective and the population perspective?

DME: It does, and we'll talk more about that later. Now let's tackle the psychological issues. You'll recall that we had quite a list[2]: cost-effectiveness analysis is relatively new, which raises skepticism; it requires abstract thinking, which is difficult for some people to do, and therefore difficult for them to trust; it uses mathematics, which can create a barrier between practitioners and analysts; it creates winners and losers, which invites criticism; and it requires sharing control over decisions, which can be threatening.

MHE: Let me save you some time. Although I agree that factors like these will cause some people to resist cost-effectiveness analysis, I do not believe that they are reasons to reject the methodology. Everything is new when it is first introduced—that can't be a criterion for rejection or we would never make any progress. A lot of things in medicine require abstract thinking, such as the Krebs cycle, acid-base balance, and genetics. We've learned to deal with them, and the concepts behind cost-effectiveness analysis are no more complicated. With respect to mathematics I've been thinking about that since we last talked, and it's surprising how much we already rely on mathematics. Most modern medical technologies are based heavily on mathematics: electrocardiograms, radiation therapy, computed tomographic scans, ...

DME: But there's a difference between using mathematics to develop medical technologies, which you can use and interpret at your discretion, and using mathematics to determine the appropriateness of different treatments—the way cost-effectiveness analysis is intended to do. With cost-effectiveness analysis, we're talking about using mathematics to actually steer your decisions.

MHE: But that's not new either. We already use mathematics in ways that directly affect decision making. The most obvious example is that mathematics is the backbone of all the statistical methods used to design and interpret research. My colleagues and I don't begin to comprehend the theory behind most statistical methods, yet we accept them. I believe that over time, as we hear more about cost-effectiveness analysis, the barriers raised by newness, abstract thinking, and mathematics will slowly dissolve.

DME: So the solution to these problems is time?

MHE: Yes.

DME: How would you handle the criticism of the losers, those whose treatments receive low priorities?

MHE: That will happen. But if the analysis is methodologically sound and addresses the proper objective—and we still have to establish that—then I would hope the losers would understand the rationale for the results and accept them. If they criticize the method just because they don't like the results—that's like shooting the messenger because you don't like the message. The solutions to that problem are to make certain the analyses are airtight, and to write strong, understandable rationales.

DME: And what about the issue of sharing control? Use of cost-effectiveness analysis will add new members to the "old boy" network that traditionally has controlled medical priorities. And these new members might not have MD degrees.

MHE: We're not *that* stodgy. I'm not too troubled by the sharing of control, provided there is agreement on objectives, everyone understands and trusts the others' contributions, and all the participants are treated with respect. The way to avoid the territorial problem is to ensure that these ingredients are in place.

DME: I agree. Now, let's address the "philosophical" problem that we deferred earlier. Which perspective is correct—the practitioner's perspective, which focuses on an individual patient, or the population perspective, which tries to maximize the health of the entire population of patients? When we discussed this problem earlier,[2] you seemed to follow the logic for the population perspective. Are you still comfortable with that?

MHE: Comfortable? No. When the problem is presented in abstract terms, like "treatment 7," and "health benefit units,"[2] it's true that I can follow the logic. But I'm not sure how I'd feel about a real clinical problem.

DME: Well, we have a fairly real clinical problem in front of us—HDC/ABMT for metastatic breast cancer vs cervical cancer screening. How do you feel about that?

MHE: Torn. You've got me convinced that, depending on which perspective I use, I would assign different priorities to the treatments. But I'm still uncomfortable about which perspective is correct. This conflict is really the crux of the issue. It might well be the most important barrier to the acceptance of cost-effectiveness analysis. It is also the reason practitioners like me fight so vigorously against the idea that resources are limited. If we can hang on to the idea that resources are not limited, we won't have to choose between treatments, and the conflict will disappear. So you need to resolve this conflict for us. That would go a long way toward getting cost-effectiveness analysis accepted.

DME: Alas, I can't make the conflict disappear. It's inherent in any system with decentralized decision making. However, I can ask you some questions to help you decide once and for all which perspective is correct. Right now you're at an impasse. When you put yourself in the position of a public health officer, you decide one thing. When you put yourself in the position of a practitioner, you decide the opposite. We need a third opinion. Let's approach the problem in the following way. Imagine that there are two health programs. They are identical in every way with the sole exception that one program takes the practitioners' perspective and provides HDC/ABMT to women who get metastatic breast cancer, while the other program takes the population perspective and provides 3-year cervical cancer screening to women age 20 to 75 years. Our task is to determine which program is "best." The first question is, who should decide? The two obvious choices are practitioners or women.

MHE: That's easy. Women. It's their lives. As much as I like to think I control everything, I'm really here to serve my patients.

DME: I concur. Now we have to determine which women should decide. There are three main choices here: women who are destined to get breast cancer, women who are destined to get cervical cancer, and women who don't yet have either breast or cervical cancer but might get either disease some time in the future.

MHE: That's also easy: the third—women who don't yet have either disease. We can't use either of the first two for obvious reasons—they would have to be superhuman to ignore their selfish interests and choose anything but the treatment for their own diseases. A person with a particular disease will want to have all resources piled into that disease. If we want to determine which health plan is best for women in general, we must pick a "general" woman.

DME: I concur again. Your 20-year-old granddaughter fits that description. She doesn't have either cancer, but she might develop one or both in the future. Should we let her provide the third opinion that will break the tie between the public health officer and the practitioner?

MHE: Fair enough. I'll abide by what's best for her.

DME: The choice of your granddaughter is also good because she is in an "original position" with respect to these two diseases.[5]

MHE: What?

DME: Sorry. Let's just say that our choice of your granddaughter to resolve this conflict fits with current theories of distributive justice.[5]

Now here's the ultimate question. Imagine that your granddaughter has to choose between the two programs and comes to you for advice. Which program do you think is best for her—the one that allocates its limited resources to HDC/ABMT for breast cancer, or the one that allocates its resources to cervical cancer screening?

MHE: The program that offers cervical cancer screening. She is much more likely to be one of the 140 women who will be saved from cervical cancer than she is to be one of the two women cured of breast cancer.

DME: So you agree that if you can offer only HDC/ABMT for breast cancer or cervical cancer screening, but not both, women in general are better off if they are screened for cervical cancer?

MHE: It sure looks that way. But wait a minute. The calculation of two breast cancer deaths and 140 cervical cancer deaths was based on the fact that I had $5 million to spend. To answer your question of what I'd recommend for my granddaughter, don't I need to take into account the probabilities she will get either breast cancer or cervical cancer? Breast cancer is almost 10 times as frequent as is cervical cancer. That might mean she'd get more benefit from the program that offered HDC/ABMT.

DME: Well, as we discussed briefly before,[2] if you are going to set priorities across a lot of treatments, the cost-effectiveness ratio is all you need. The prevalence of a disease won't affect its ranking. However, when you are comparing only two treatments, you might indeed want to know the frequencies of the diseases, so here they are. Your granddaughter has about a 10% chance of getting breast cancer some time in the rest of her life, and about a 5% chance of developing terminal metastatic disease.[6] Let's assume optimistically that every woman who gets terminal breast cancer is a candidate for HDC/ABMT. So the effect of having access to HDC/ABMT, which we are assuming will give her a 5% chance of a cure if she should be unfortunate enough to develop breast cancer, is to decrease her chance of dying from breast cancer by 0.25% ($0.05 \times 0.05 = 0.0025$). As we've already said, having access to cervical cancer screening will decrease her chance of death from that disease by 1%. Calculation of the costs gets a bit complicated because of the fact that both treatments will occur in the future. I won't go through the calculations here, but a rough estimate is that in terms of the costs of the two health programs, your granddaughter would have to pay at least about four times as much to have access to HDC/ABMT than to have access to cervical cancer screening.

MHE: So my granddaughter would pay more money, but would get less benefit if she chose the plan that took the practitioner's perspective and offered HDC/ABMT instead of cervical cancer screening. Any way I slice it, I have to conclude that if only one treatment can be offered, it should be cervical cancer screening.

By the way, will an example like this always come out indicating that the population perspective is preferable? What if we had chosen different treatments to compare; would my granddaughter always agree with the public health officer?

DME: No matter what clinical problems you choose to compare, your granddaughter (assuming that we stick to diseases that affect only women over age 20) will make the same choices as the public health officer. It is instructive to examine why this is true. Our objective is to determine how limited resources should be distributed between two treatments. In this example, the fact is that putting the resources into screening will prevent more deaths than putting the resources into HDC/ABMT. The question is why the public health officer and your granddaughter both see that, while the practitioner does not. The answer lies in the breadth of perspectives. The public health officer and your granddaughter both have broad perspectives, whereas the practitioner usually has a narrower perspective. There are three possible directions from which to look at a resource allocation problem: from the top down, from the bottom up, and from the middle. The public health officer looks at the problem from the top down—he or she is searching for what is best for the population as a whole. Your granddaughter views the problem from the bottom up—she is searching for what would be best for the individual. Although at first thought those two perspectives appear to be quite different, they are really very similar because they both have to consider all the possible diseases a woman might get—in this case, both breast cancer and cervical cancer. The public health officer has to determine which will prevent more deaths, cervical cancer screening or HDC/ABMT for breast cancer. Your granddaughter has to determine which will improve her odds more, cervical cancer screening or HDC/ABMT for breast cancer. They both come to the same conclusion because, in essence, they are asking the same question. The only way you could arrive at a different conclusion is if you looked at the resource allocation problem from the middle, so to speak. If, instead of looking at the problem from the top down or from the bottom up, you look at the problem from the point of view of a woman who *already* has breast cancer, you will immediately want all resources to be allocated to the treatment of that disease. You will barely even consider cervical cancer screening. However, this is obviously an inappropriate position from which to make a decision about how resources should be allocated across treatments, because the choice has already been narrowed down to one treatment—that is, there is no choice left. Now, where do practitioners fit in? Unfortunately, practitioners see decisions like this from the middle, because their contact with the decision is through their individual patients who already have particular diseases. In essence, it is because practitioners see allocation decisions through the eyes of patients who *already have* particular diseases that they do not have the breadth of perspective necessary to determine how resources should be allocated *across* diseases.

MHE: I'll try not to take offense at that.

DME: Believe me, no offense was intended. It's not the practitioners' *fault* that they see patients who already have diseases; indeed it's their *job*. Nonetheless, one consequence of that job is that practitioners have a narrow perspective, which limits their ability to determine what is best for the population as a whole, or for your granddaughter. The plain fact is that the practitioner's particular role in delivering health care virtually precludes him or her from being able to make resource allocation decisions accurately.

MHE: Well, I'm still tempted to act offended. However, I have to admit that what I chose as a practitioner was not what I thought was best for my own granddaughter. That's a pretty sobering thought.

I have one more question on this topic. Did the example you picked work out the way it did because we were comparing a preventive service against a treatment? What if we were comparing two treatments, or two preventive services, or different treatments and preventive services?

DME: The appropriateness of using the population perspective does not depend on the types of treatments we choose to compare. Just to put to rest the issue of prevention vs treatment, I can assure you that if we had compared, say, setting a fractured femur vs lung cancer screening, setting the fracture would have won. Another important point is that the population perspective and the practitioner's perspective are not always in conflict. The conflict occurs only when a practitioner's perspective is narrowed down so far that he or she can't see the other treatments that might deserve priority. The more specialized a practitioner is, the more likely it is that his or her perspective will be in conflict with the population perspective. An oncologist has a narrower perspective than an internist, who has a narrower perspective than a family practitioner, and so forth.

MHE: Despite that last bit of encouragement, I don't particularly like the way this is going, but I don't see any way out. Once I accept the premise that resources are limited and choices have to be made, it seems I'm going to be forced to accept the fact that I won't be able to do everything I want to do.

DME: That's true. It's really very simple, to the point of being a tautology: If we don't have enough resources to do everything we want to do, we won't be able to do everything we want to do. Let's call that the "fundamental law of limited resources."

MHE: Don't be cute. This discussion is depressing enough as it is. Now that we understand which perspective is best, how do we solve the problem that practitioners, and even most patients, won't like it?

DME: I think this problem has to be solved the way you proposed to solve the other problems—with airtight analyses, good explanations, compassion, and time.

MHE: It's also going to take a great deal of leadership. The idea that practitioners' instincts might not be the best way to allocate limited resources to medical treatments challenges one of the most basic assumptions of American medicine—that "doctor knows best." Reshaping that assumption will require not only solid methods and time; it will require the strong support of the thousand or so people who shape the ideas in our profession.

Let's move on to the other philosophical problem that affects cost-effectiveness analysis—the disagreement about whether resources are truly limited. Actually, I think that we can pass that one pretty quickly because everything you've said about cost-effectiveness analysis has been based on the premise that resources are limited. You agreed that in settings where there are no limits on resources, there is no need for cost-effectiveness analysis and I can give every treatment I want. Frankly, this is the fine print that keeps me happy, because I think there are in fact very few settings in which resources are truly limited.

DME: Actually, there is a very important point we need to discuss about limits on resources. And you're not going to like it. Up to this point we've talked as though the issue of limits was neat and clean—budgets were either limited or not. In fact, the distinction is not that clear-cut. There are intermediate positions: budgets can be "tight," resources can be "scarce," the federal government can push increased costs into the deficit. It's helpful to distinguish between two types of limits. One is a "hard" limit. It acts like a steel wall. The budget is absolutely fixed and cannot be raised, no matter what. An example might be a state cancer control program. When a program faces a hard budget limit, the need for cost-effectiveness analysis is absolutely clear. A more common situation, however, is a "soft" limit. This acts more like a rubber band than a steel wall. There is a budget, and everyone growls when it is exceeded, but it is possible to exceed the budget. Money can be spent against a soft limit, but doing so requires stretching the rubber band, and each expenditure stiffens resistance against further increases.

Here is the point you are not going to like. Virtually every health care budget in the country is up against at least a soft limit. I can't think of a single health care program that doesn't care about its costs. State Medicaid programs *can* expand, but at the expense of welfare, education, highways, and the like. States can raise their taxes, but it is political suicide. Insurance companies and health maintenance organizations can raise premiums and rates, but their customers will threaten to go elsewhere. Businesses can pay more for health care, but they will have to raise their prices, which will make them less competitive. People can pay higher out-of-pocket expenses, higher insurance premiums, and higher taxes, but they sure don't want to. The fact is that while we *can* raise health care costs, doing so requires pulling money from other activities, and no one wants to do that. What we really have to appreciate is that all activities—health and nonhealth—are under a single budget, and that that budget has a hard limit. I hate to tell you this, but this means that cost-effectiveness analysis really should be applied to everything.

MHE: What?! That's not fair. If I accept that little sleight-of-hand—forgive me, *big* sleight-of-hand—you'll get to apply cost-effectiveness analysis to everything in health care. I appreciate that budgets can have what you call soft limits, but I won't agree that all of them are so tight that they can't be expanded at all. You can't claim that just because most people don't want to pay more, they can't or won't pay more. There must be an intermediate position between restricting cost-effectiveness analysis to state cancer control programs, and applying it to everything.

DME: I have to agree with you. There is. While the economic theory can get quite complicated, I believe the following practical test will indicate when it is appropriate to consider a budget sufficiently limited to justify the use of cost-effectiveness analysis. Whenever a decision maker—whether it is a state legislator, a hospital administrator, a medical director of a health maintenance organization, or a chief of service—finds himself or herself contemplating an activity and saying something like, "We can't handle these costs; we're going to have to set some priorities," that is an indication that cost-effectiveness analysis is needed. Cost-effectiveness analysis is a tool for setting priorities. Whenever a decision maker does not have enough resources to do everything he or she wants to do and has to set priorities, then cost-effectiveness analysis is needed.

MHE: That helps somewhat. But I'm still uncomfortable. It seems that I've lost every point in this discussion.

DME: Not really. Along the way, you've extracted several important conditions from me. I agree that cost-effectiveness analysis need not be used unless the budget is so tight that decision makers determine that they must set priorities. I agree that practitioners should not be asked to give up an effective practice unless there is a solid rationale demonstrating that there are other activities that deserve higher priority, and there is a plan to actually implement those higher priority practices.

MHE: Won't you also agree that we shouldn't use cost-effectiveness analysis at all until we've eliminated all our sources of waste?

DME: I will agree that we want to give first priority to eliminating waste. But to me that doesn't mean we should postpone applying cost-effectiveness analysis, for two reasons. First, I consider the elimination of waste to be one of the main services cost-effectiveness analysis will perform. Remember that an integral part of a cost-effectiveness analysis is an examination of a treatment's benefits. To say that a treatment is truly wasteful means that it has no benefit. A cost-effectiveness analysis will determine that fact and put the treatment at the top of the list of things to be eliminated. The second reason is that eliminating waste is a never-ending task. Even while we take steps to identify and eliminate waste, our resources will still be limited and we still have to set priorities. Choices will always have to be made and cost-effectiveness analysis is the best way to make them.

MHE: I need to ask one more question that's been bothering me. If things are as bad as you say, how in the world did medicine get this far without thinking anything was wrong? Everyone was comfortable until cost-effectiveness analysis came along and told us we should be uncomfortable. That makes me suspicious that you're finding problems where they don't exist.

DME: I do not agree with you that *everyone* has been comfortable. I agree that most practitioners have been comfortable, but that is because they have a rather selective and privileged view of our health care system. First, their attention has been focused on people who seek their care (their patients), and what happens to them after they seek care. Second, because practitioners have historically had enormous control over how health care resources are used, they have generally been able to obtain whatever resources they felt they needed to provide care to those people. In contrast, people who have different positions in the health care system have not been nearly as comfortable. For example, people who view our health care system from the population perspective have been uncomfortable for a long time about the fact that there haven't been enough resources to do a lot of things that should be done for people *before* they see physicians. They have also been uncomfortable that a lot of people do not get to see physicians at all, or not until it's too late. Another group that has been uncomfortable is the people who have been paying the costs. In fact, if you are looking for a trigger that has initiated all these challenges to the way you practice medicine, it would not be cost-effectiveness analysis; it would be the costs themselves. Until fairly recently, the people who pay the bills have tolerated the increases in costs. The rubber band was being stretched, but it hadn't reached the snapping point. Now it has. Patients, employers, unions, and taxpayers are no longer willing to accept the inexorable increases in costs, and they are demanding that costs be controlled. It is this fact more than any other that is forcing the changes in how medicine is practiced. Remember, cost-effectiveness analysis is just a tool. It didn't create the cost problems; it's just a method offered to help solve them.

MHE: As I said before, it's all pretty depressing. But I still have to wonder whether this is not all pretty theoretical. Most of the cost-effectiveness analyses I read seem to come out of academic settings and end up saying something like "decision makers can take these results into account when determining the appropriate use of (some treatment)," or even "these results must be confirmed with controlled trials." It's difficult to tell if the cost-effectiveness analyses that are published are actually attached to real decisions. Can you show me a real example where a real health care delivery organization made a real decision that actually recommended *against* the use of a treatment that everyone agreed was effective, strictly because a cost-effectiveness analysis indicated it was too expensive?

DME: You sure know how to go for the jugular.

Maxon H. Eddy is my father. Before he died in 1987, he practiced as a general surgeon in Bridgeport, Conn. Although this conversation is hypothetical, it is based on memories of real ones.

❖ References

1. Eddy DM. Cost-effectiveness analysis: is it up to the task? *JAMA*. 1992;267:3342-3348 (Chapter 20).
2. Eddy DM. Cost-effectiveness analysis: a conversation with my father. *JAMA*. 1992; 267:1669-1672, 1674-1675 (Chapter 19).
3. Eddy DM. High-dose chemotherapy with autologous bone marrow transplantation for the treatment of metastatic breast cancer. *J Clin Oncol*. 1992;10:657-670.
4. Eddy DM. Screening for cervical cancer. *Ann Intern Med*. 1990;113:214-226.
5. Rawls J. *A Theory of Justice*. Cambridge, Mass: Harvard University Press; 1971.
6. Eddy DM. Screening for breast cancer. *Ann Intern Med*. 1989;111:389-399.

❖ Source

Originally published in *JAMA*. 1992;268:132-136.

❖ CHAPTER 22

Applying Cost-effectiveness Analysis
The Inside Story

MAXON H. EDDY, MD: I understand the principles of cost-effectiveness analysis,[1] and I feel fairly comfortable that the methods will work for at least some clinical problems.[2] I can also appreciate your argument that in settings where resources are limited and priorities have to be set, cost-effectiveness analysis is an appropriate way to do that.[3] But I still have this nagging feeling that no one would actually use it. That is, I have a difficult time imagining that anyone who actually takes care of patients would withhold a treatment that is known to be effective, just because of its cost. I'm not talking about armchair doctors like you who live in a nice clean world of numbers; I'm talking about practitioners or organizations that really face the heat. Can you give me an example of cost-effectiveness analysis being applied in a real health care organization?

DAVID M. EDDY, MD, PHD: Does what they did in Oregon fit your criteria?

MHE: Technically speaking, the Oregon Medicaid program is a third-party payer, not a health care delivery organization. But beyond that, what happened in Oregon might be the exception that proves my point. Oregon's leaders took so much criticism for their decisions, and so few people stood up for them, that you have to wonder if this approach has any real advocates outside of academics and economists.

DME: I agree with you that cost-effectiveness analysis is a lot easier to accept in principle than it is to apply in practice. But there are some examples of real applications. Here's one.

❖ A Guideline for Contrast Agents
for Radiologic Procedures

Approximately 10 million radiographic procedures using iodinated contrast agents are performed in the United States every year. Until
recently, agents having a relatively high osmolality, called "high osmolar contrast agents" (HOCAs), have been used for these procedures. They have excellent diagnostic properties but can cause discomfort and adverse reactions
due either to the high osmolality or to allergic reactions. The side effects and
reactions range from a sensation of heat and mild flushing, to nausea and
vomiting, to severe circulatory or respiratory collapse.

Although HOCAs have been considered safe and effective by the medical
community and the Food and Drug Administration for decades, the possibility
of reactions led investigators to search for alternative agents that have lower
risks. In late 1985 and early 1986, a new set of agents that have lower osmolality, called "low osmolar contrast agents" (LOCAs), were approved by the Food
and Drug Administration. Because most of the LOCAs are nonionic com-
pounds, they are also called "nonionic agents," and the older contrast agents
(HOCAs) are called "ionic agents." As expected, LOCAs did cause fewer reactions related to osmolality. Unexpectedly, they also appeared to cause fewer
allergic reactions. Unfortunately, depending on the institution, they cost 10 to
20 times as much as do HOCAs. This raises the crucial questions: Are the lower
risks of nonionic agents worth their costs? And what are the appropriate indications for the different types of agents?

Organizations and individual authors addressing these questions have
acknowledged that use of the more expensive LOCAs might be restricted to
high-risk patients, and that HOCAs might be appropriate for low-risk patients. However, professional societies have been ambivalent about actively
recommending such a policy. A resolution issued by the American College of
Radiology (ACR) is illustrative:

> Some radiological facilities have decided to use Lower Osmolality Con-
> trast Agents on all patients. Other radiological facilities have decided on
> the selective use of LOCA. In these institutions radiologists should give
> consideration to the use of LOCA and utilize . . . guidelines (to identify
> high-risk patients).[4]

This guideline clearly implies that it can be appropriate to use HOCAs in
patients who do not have high-risk characteristics, but also clearly stops short
of recommending such a practice. In essence, the ACR invites each health care
organization to develop its own policy.

Earlier this year, Kaiser Permanente Southern California Region (KPSC),
a large group practice health maintenance organization, developed a practice
guideline for the intravenous use of contrast agents. It recommended that unless a patient has risk factors indicating a higher than average chance of a
reaction, HOCAs should be used. Although LOCAs are known to cause fewer

adverse reactions, even in low-risk patients, KPSC determined that this benefit did not justify the higher cost.

The following is a brief description of the guideline and rationale. Because I have served as an adviser to KPSC since 1991, I will use the pronoun "we" when describing the project.

Methods

To develop the guideline we used an explicit approach[5,6] that involved four basic steps: (1) analyze the evidence about the occurrence of reactions with HOCAs vs LOCAs; (2) estimate the actual rates of different types of reactions in low-risk patients who receive the agents intravenously; (3) estimate the costs of the agents; and (4) determine if the differences in reaction rates are worth the difference in cost.

Definitions

To be consistent with most of the studies of reaction rates with different agents, we defined a reaction to be "mild" if it required no treatment (eg, flushing, nausea, mild urticaria, slight difficulty breathing, or slight facial edema). A reaction that required some treatment but that otherwise was not serious (eg, vomiting, difficulty breathing, moderate facial edema, or transient drop in blood pressure) was called "moderate." A reaction was considered "severe" if it was potentially life-threatening and required immediate treatment (eg, cardiovascular collapse).

Our definition of a low-risk patient was derived from Palmer,[7] the author of the largest study that published results separately for low-risk patients. By this definition, a person is considered low-risk if he or she does not have any of the following: a previous reaction to contrast agents, asthma, a significant history of allergies to agents other than drugs, renal or cardiac impairment, poor hydration, diabetes mellitus, myelomatosis, sickle cell anemia, or young age (infant or small child). In Palmer's study, approximately 85% of patients were low-risk by this definition.

Review of Evidence

A literature search identified approximately 60 articles that contained primary data about the rates of various types of reactions with HOCAs or LOCAs. We limited our analysis to those studies that involved intravenous use of contrast agents, that included internal comparisons of HOCAs vs LOCAs, and that reported results separately for the different categories of reactions. Four studies[7-10] were particularly important because of their size or because they were conducted at a KPSC facility and therefore provided "local" data.[9] They are summarized in the form of an evidence table (Table 22.1).

TABLE 22.1   Studies Comparing Rates of Mild, Moderate, and Severe Reactions in Patients Receiving Ionic and Nonionic Contrast Agents

Source, y	Design*	Sample Size†	Results-Reaction Rates, %			
			Mild	Moderate	Severe	Very Severe
All Patients						
Palmer,[7] 1988	NSP	(I) 79278	3.32	0.35	...	0.09
		(N) 30268	1.04	0.099	...	0.02
Low-Risk Patients						
		(I) 77910	3.25	0.31	0.085	...
		(N) 15188	0.97	0.092	0	...
High-Risk Patients						
		(I) 1368	7.24	2.71	0.37	...
		(N) 15080	1.12	0.11	0.033	...
Katayama et al,[8] 1990	NCP	(I) 169284	14.84‡	...	0.22	0.037
		(N) 168363	3.24‡	...	0.042	0.0036
Kent,[9] 1988	NSP	(I) 2650	3.25	0.19	...	0.080
		(N) 3182	0.53	0.03	...	0
Wolf et al,[10] 1989	NSP	(I) 6006	2.50	1.20	0.40	...
		(N) 7170	0.58	0.11	0	...

*NCP indicates nonrandomized sequential prospective, and NSP, nonrandomized concurrent prospective.
†I indicates ionic contrast agents, and N, nonionic contrast agents.
‡Calculated from number of reactions (not number of patients).

Estimation of Probabilities of Reactions

Based on this evidence, we estimated the probabilities that a low-risk patient receiving agents intravenously would have various types of reactions with HOCAs or LOCAs. The results are shown both as decimals and as fractions in the form of a balance sheet (Table 22.2). While there is uncertainty about each of these numbers due to such factors as sampling, imperfections in study designs, and differences across studies, these are the best estimates that we could make based on the available evidence.

The fourth column of Table 22.2 gives the differences in probabilities of reactions if a patient receives a HOCA instead of a LOCA. For example, the entry in the last row and last column of Table 22.2 can be read as, "If a low-risk patient is given a HOCA instead of a LOCA intravenously, the chance that the patient will have a severe reaction is increased 0.094%." Or, "Of 1064 patients who receive contrast agents, one additional patient can be expected to have a severe reaction" ($1 \div 1064 = 0.094\%$).

A controlled trial by Lasser et al[11] has shown that the rates of reactions can be reduced by about a third if patients are pretreated with corticosteroids. Perhaps more important, class III reactions (comparable to our "severe" category) were reduced 62%. Thus, the probabilities of reactions shown in Table 22.2 would overestimate the actual probabilities for patients who are pretreated. To be conservative (favoring LOCAs), we continued to use the estimates shown in Table 22.2 for our subsequent comparisons of benefits and costs.

Deaths have occurred with both agents. However, they are very infrequent with either agent (on the order of 1 in 100 000), they are not always directly attributable to the agents,[8] and there is no evidence yet that the probability of death is higher with one type of agent or the other.[12,13]

Estimation of Costs

In KPSC, LOCAs cost approximately $90 more than HOCAs, per patient. The savings from a lower rate of reactions with LOCAs could

TABLE 22.2   Rates of Mild, Moderate, and Severe Reactions in Low-Risk Patients Receiving High Osmolar Contrast Agents (HOCAs) and Low Osmolar Contrast Agents (LOCAs)

Reaction Type	Reaction Rates, %		
	HOCAs	LOCAs	Difference*
Mild	3.19 (1/31)	0.75 (1/133)	+2.25 (1/44)
Moderate	0.32 (1/313)	0.085 (1/1176)	+0.23 (1/435)
Severe	0.097 (1/1031)	0.0037 (1/27 027)	+0.094 (1/1064)

*Rate with HOCAs minus rate with LOCAs.

reduce this difference by less than $8 per patient, leaving a net increase in cost with LOCAs of about $82 per patient.

Comparison of Benefits and Costs

In our judgment, the lower risks of LOCAs (Table 22.2) did not justify the increased costs ($82 per patient). We determined that reallocating the resources to other activities would produce considerably more benefit to our Health Plan members. More specifically, we determined that for the same amount of money that would be required to provide LOCAs to low-risk patients, we could provide 10 to 100 times greater benefit if we allocated the resources to such activities as cervical cancer screening or breast cancer screening.

Guideline

We recommended that for procedures involving intravenous administration, patients who can be determined to be at low risk of having a reaction should receive HOCAs. Patients who have risk factors for a reaction should receive LOCAs. The full guideline contains more details about specific risk factors and pretreatment with corticosteroids.

❖ The Inside Story

As most readers can appreciate, the actual history of this guideline is not nearly as clean as this description implies. In essence, the organization has been struggling with the appropriate use of contrast agents ever since the first LOCAs were approved in 1985.

Kaiser Foundation Health Plan of Southern California is a nonprofit health maintenance organization that provides care to more than 2.2 million members, primarily through 12 large medical centers located from San Diego to Bakersfield. The total annual budget is more than $3 billion. Physician services are provided by the Southern California Permanente Medical Group, which is a professional partnership legally independent of but under contract to the Health Plan. The Medical Group has an elected medical director, as well as a variety of officers, such as an associate medical director for clinical services, an associate medical director for operations, and associate medical directors for each of the 12 medical centers. Each of the medical centers has a staff of radiologists, led by an appointed chief. The chiefs of the 12 centers meet periodically as the "radiology chiefs group." The main forum for the development of this guideline was the radiology chiefs group, in consultation with the associate medical director for clinical services.

Like other radiologists around the country, before LOCAs were introduced in 1985 our radiologists were accustomed to using HOCAs for all their patients. However, the opportunity to reduce our patients' discomfort and risks was clearly desirable, and use of LOCAs began to increase soon after they became available. The main brake on expanded use was the cost. In our organization, even after negotiation of a substantial discount, LOCAs cost about 20 times more than HOCAs. This difference could not help but raise questions about whether the benefits justified the costs.

Although some early reports and marketing by vendors indicated that reaction rates were lower with LOCAs, in the early years of use there were no definitive studies describing the magnitudes of the reaction rates with the two agents. Lacking such evidence, our radiologists did not believe a definitive guideline could be developed, and the guidelines that existed in the first several years of use were more descriptive than prescriptive. For example, in January 1987 the radiology chiefs group advised that LOCAs should be used when "medically appropriate." This flexible stance was repeated at a subsequent meeting in October 1987, when the radiology chiefs group recommended that LOCAs "should be used selectively" and "the decision should rest with the patient's physician."

During the next 2 years, several important articles were published, but they still left some uncertainty about the appropriate roles of different agents. In 1988, Palmer[7] published a study from Australia showing lower reaction rates with LOCAs. However, the potential impact of this study in favor of LOCAs was dulled by publication a few months earlier of a controlled trial showing that pretreatment with corticosteroids could cut reaction rates with HOCAs about in half and bring them into alignment with the rates observed with LOCAs.[11] An editorial that accompanied the latter study concluded that "in most patients whose conditions are stable and uncomplicated, conventional agents (HOCAs) should be used." An additional factor was that the ACR was contemplating a large-scale, multi-institutional trial to provide definitive information. The fact that such a study was being designed implied that all the answers were not yet in. Thus, despite continuous heavy marketing by manufacturers of LOCAs, our radiologists believed that more evidence was needed before a stronger guideline could be justified.

This "wait and see" position ended in 1989 when the ACR published in its bulletin a preliminary review of a huge study from Japan by Katayama et al.[8] After noting the enormous size of the study and the clear reductions in reaction rates with LOCAs, the ACR announced that it considered the results to be sufficiently definitive to permit conclusions, and that as a consequence it was dropping its plans to conduct its own study. While some might question the ACR's motives, the message from the ACR was clear: All the information needed to make decisions was available, and the time for a definitive guideline had come.

Endorsement by the ACR of the study by Katayama et al put everyone on notice that risks were definitely lower and therefore quality of care was higher with LOCAs than with HOCAs. The only remaining issue was the cost. Although many authors had raised the issue of costs, no definitive position had yet emerged. To resolve this issue, the chairman of the radiology chiefs group met with the associate medical director/physician manager of operations, who in essence said, "If you think LOCAs are medically indicated, then we should use them." He asked only that the radiologists estimate the expected use of LOCAs so he could budget for it. With that green light, the radiology chiefs issued the following "directive" at their September 1989 meeting: "As of 1990, all IVP [intravenous pyelogram] and CT [computed tomography] examinations will be switched to nonionic contrast agents (LOCAs) exclusively."

During 1990 the use of LOCAs increased markedly in most of the KPSC medical centers. Interestingly, however, despite its strong wording, the directive did not take hold uniformly. Use of LOCAs varied from center to center, from radiologist to radiologist within centers, and from procedure to procedure (eg, IVP vs CT scan). The overall use of different agents would probably have stabilized in a mixed pattern like this except for two events in late 1990 and early 1991.

The first event was a dramatic change in the financial climate. The nation was entering a recession, and Los Angeles was (and still is) one of the hardest-hit areas. Our largest and most important corporate customers, although they had always been concerned about costs, began to tighten the pressure on us to control costs. They also became very explicit about the fact that they wanted more "value" for their money. The idea of "value" contained two concepts. One was that there should be an appropriate balance between quality of service (eg, member satisfaction), quality of medical care (eg, health outcomes), and financial costs. The other was that there should be an appropriate balance between providing slight improvements in care for a few individuals vs providing greater improvements in care for the entire membership. Thus, the idea of value recognized the need to allocate finite resources to maximize health and quality of care for the group as a whole.

The second event was that following the 1990 directive to use LOCAs, the actual amount we were spending on contrast agents greatly exceeded the amount we had expected. A utilization study revealed that our radiologists were using LOCAs far more than was originally anticipated. Because the decision about contrast agents was still fairly fresh, the associate medical director for clinical services decided to take this opportunity to reexamine the basic question of the indications for LOCAs in light of the new financial realities. Suspecting that a concerted attempt to use LOCAs only in high-risk patients might free up resources that could be put to better use elsewhere (that is, achieve greater "value"), he asked the radiology chiefs to revisit the issue of contrast agents in early 1991.

The radiology chiefs group appointed a smaller work group to update the literature review and to summarize the current recommendations of other organizations. The work group confirmed the evidence that LOCAs cause fewer reactions, agreed with the findings that there was no evidence of higher mortality with HOCAs, and noted the position statements of the ACR and others that it was reasonable to use HOCAs in low-risk patients. They decided to recommend that position as a formal guideline.

However, the radiology chiefs as a whole were very reluctant to reverse the directive they had just issued a year earlier. They saw four main problems. One was their instinctive concern for the quality of care of their patients, and their knowledge that reverting to HOCAs, even for low-risk patients, would increase discomfort and cause more reactions. Another was the fact that, if a reaction occurred, they would bear first responsibility for treating it. A third was a sense of exhaustion about having to revisit a decision that took several years to make, and that they liked. The fourth problem was a vague fear that even if some money could be saved by using HOCAs for low-risk patients, there was no guarantee that the savings would be reallocated to increase value. Thus, from their point of view, nothing was broken, so why fix it? At a political level, the decision process was deadlocked.

The process was also deadlocked at a scientific level. Everyone knew that the risks were higher with ionic agents, but there was uncertainty about how much higher. Everyone also agreed that nonionic agents cost about $90 more than ionic agents per patient, but there was a debate about whether these costs would be offset by savings from not having to treat as many reactions. Without knowing just how much safety was being bought with how much money, there was no rational way to determine if the trade was worthwhile.

To try to break both deadlocks, we decided to try an approach based on the principles of conflict resolution.[14] The process involved separating the problem into its components, identifying specific points of disagreement, resolving the disagreements one by one, and then reconstructing a solution. The first step would be to use the evidence to estimate the actual magnitudes of the increases in reaction rates in HOCAs. The second would be to estimate the difference in costs. The third would be to compare the difference in reaction rates with the difference in costs. The last step would address any remaining issues, such as lawsuits.

Evidence Analysis

The analysis of evidence was fairly straightforward, with four exceptions. First, while there were several large comparative studies, none of them was randomized. This raised the possibility that in some of the studies, practitioners might have recommended particular agents for patients based on their perceptions of each patient's risk of a reaction. Unfortunately, there were reasons to believe that if this bias existed, it would be most likely to affect the largest study, that by Katayama et al.[8] Other aspects of this study's methods had also been questioned.[15] This created a methodological dilemma. The study by Katayama et al was by far the largest and most widely cited, and for that reason alone it was impossible to ignore. On the other hand, there was little we could do to determine whether this potential bias existed, and if it did exist, what its magnitude was. If we chose to include the study we knew we could use the ACR's "endorsement" of it to defend our decision, but the comfort this provided was more political than methodological.

We decided that we would continue with the analysis taking the results of Katayama et al at face value, and then see whether the results were out of line with the results of the other studies. If so, we would decide at that time how to deal with the study.

The second set of problems is a generalization of the first, and affects every attempt to interpret the medical literature: Virtually every study has something wrong with it. There might be some small flaw in the design or execution. There might be differences between studies, such as slightly different definitions of reaction categories. Or the study designs might not match local conditions perfectly. One option was for us to be purists, declare all the evidence invalid, and discard it. But that would leave us with no evidence at all. We believed that, despite the imperfections, the evidence had some value, and the best option was to use it, albeit cautiously. We would let the sensitivity of the conclusions to any uncertainties about individual studies determine how much work we had to do to delve into the minute details of each study.

The third problem with the evidence was that only one study, that by Palmer,[7] described reaction rates separately for low-risk and high-risk patients. This forced a methodological decision about what to do with the evidence from all the other studies that reported results for a combined group of "average-risk" patients (a mixture of low-risk and high-risk patients). We decided to try two approaches and hope that they gave the same answers. One was to calculate reaction rates using only Palmer's results for low-risk patients, and ignore all the other evidence. The other was to use Palmer's results to estimate the ratio of reaction rates in low-risk vs average-risk patients, and then use this ratio to adjust the overall reaction rates observed in the other studies. Although this approach required some assumptions that, although reasonable, had no objective evidence, it was the only way we could think of to incorporate the results of all the other studies. Fortunately, both approaches gave very similar results. This spared us from having to decide which approach was more likely to be correct. To be conservative, for the subsequent steps of the process we used results that slightly favored LOCAs.

The fourth problem concerned the rate of mild reactions with HOCAs. The rate observed in the study by Katayama et al[8] (approximately 15%) was considerably higher than the rate observed in the other studies (about 3%).[7,9,10] Because the Japanese study was so large, its results, if taken at face value, would dominate the rates observed in the other three studies. However, we concluded that there were several reasons to discount the rate of mild reactions observed in Japan. The reasons related to the definitions of reaction types, the patient population, the subjective nature of mild reactions, and reporting methods. To determine the transferability of the Japanese results to our population, we decided to use as an anchor the study by Kent,[9] because it was done locally at one of our medical centers. Some statistical tests indicated that the differences between Kent's and Katayama's results for mild reactions were very unlikely (with a probability of less than 1 in 10 million) to be explained by sampling error, and were very likely to represent real differences in definitions, patients, or reporting methods. We therefore excluded the results of Katayama et al for mild reactions. Katayama's results for severe and very severe reactions were similar to the results of other studies and were not affected by this decision. Although this approach was not perfect methodologically, it was the best we could do.

Estimation of Costs

The direct costs of HOCAs and LOCAs were easy to estimate from our pharmacy records. A more difficult question was how much money would be saved by the fact that fewer reactions would occur with LOCAs, which would lower the cost of treating reactions. A full analysis of this issue would be time-consuming and expensive. For example, to estimate the cost of a moderate reaction such as nausea and vomiting, we would have to conduct time-motion studies to determine how long an episode of vomiting ties up a radiological suite, and the cost of janitorial service. Rather than conduct a detailed study of the costs of various types of reactions, we decided to make some conservative estimates of treatment costs (favorable to LOCAs) and see if the savings made much of a difference. If they did, we could always return to this step and refine the numbers. Thus, for the first draft of the analysis we allowed $100 for the cost of a mild reaction (eg, itching), $500 to treat a moderate reaction (eg, nausea and vomiting), and $5000 to treat a severe reaction. When these numbers were combined with the estimated differences in probabilities of reactions (Table 22.2), the expected savings from decreasing the probabilities of reactions was about $8 per patient. This left a net increase in cost of at least $82.

Comparison of Benefits and Costs

The choice of a contrast agent for low-risk patients depends on whether the benefits of LOCAs listed in Table 22.2 are worth their higher costs, and on whether the costs could deliver greater benefits if they were allocated to other activities. We explored three main ways to make this determination: global subjective judgment, direct assessment of patient preferences, and indirect comparisons.

By far, the most common method used historically to compare health outcomes and costs is global subjective judgment: The people who are designing the guideline—in this case, the chiefs of radiology and the associate medical director for clinical services—simply think hard and make the judgment. Despite the fact that this is the traditional and time-honored approach used by the profession for centuries, it is very difficult to defend from a methodological point of view, for obvious reasons. Furthermore, when we tried to apply this method, we simply could not come up with a convincing answer. The issues were just too complex to solve in our heads. If possible, we very much preferred to find some beacon to guide our decision.

One obvious beacon was the preferences of the people who would actually receive the agents, suffer the risks, and pay the costs—the members of our Health Plan. To learn how they felt about the risks and costs of the two agents, we decided to try to assess their preferences directly through a questionnaire or poll, in the spirit of rationing by patient choice.[16,17] Before launching a large survey, however, we wanted to test the feasibility and accuracy of this approach by conducting focus groups with our members.

Here is the type of question we wanted our members' opinions about. (The actual wording of the question for our members contained more explanations and included several variations.) You, the reader, can play along. Imagine that you need an IVP. You can choose to have either a HOCA or a LOCA. The risks of the two agents are described in Table 22.2. For example, if you choose a LOCA, the chance of having a severe but nonfatal reaction is reduced about 1 in 1000. However, if you choose to receive a LOCA, you will have to pay for it. The amount of money you would have to pay depends on your income. Our members can think about $82. However, because you, the reader, probably have a considerably higher income than our typical Health Plan member, I will have to adjust the cost that you should think about. Take your annual family income (eg, $80 000), divide it by $10 000 (eg, $80 000 ÷ $10 000 = 8), and multiply the result by $25 (eg, 8 × $25 = $200). This calculation will cause you to think about an amount of money (eg, $200) that will cause you as much financial pain as $82 would cause our typical health plan member. The question to you is: Are you willing to pay that amount of money to receive the lower risks of a LOCA?

Unfortunately, this strategy did not work. Although the focus groups provided good information about how our members thought about the risks and costs of contrast agents, they did not yield a clear answer to the question of whether the lower reaction rates of LOCAs were worth the amount specified. For example, when members were asked the question I just asked you, they overwhelmingly indicated that they would *not* be willing to pay the higher costs of LOCAs in order to receive the lower risks. (I get the same response when I pose the question to large professional audiences at conferences.) However, when members were asked to imagine themselves as healthy people who might some day need an IVP or CT scan and were asked whether they were willing to pay a slight increase in their monthly premium to receive LOCAs and their lower reaction rates (a mathematically equivalent but psychologically different question), they overwhelmingly said they *would* be willing to pay for LOCAs. There are theoretical reasons to discount the answers to the second question because it involves numbers that are so small as to be nearly incomprehensible. ("Are you willing to pay 13¢ a month to decrease your chance of a severe reaction by 1 out of 56 000?") Nonetheless, the inconsistency was disconcerting. More troublesome was the fact that when we examined some questions that were built into the process to determine whether the participants truly understood the issues, we discovered that many of them did not. For example, after they had read an information sheet saying that LOCAs cost about $82 more than HOCAs, they were asked which agent cost more money. Several participants answered "HOCAs." While this exercise suggested that the benefits of LOCAs were not worth their costs, we decided that the methods were too shaky to justify a definitive conclusion. This outcome was a considerable disappointment to me personally because I have recommended this approach as a general method for making rationing decisions.[17] While I believe the problem we encountered can be resolved with refinements of the technique, I cannot escape the fact that it did not work for this case.

The third method for comparing benefits and costs involves making comparisons across different medical activities. The reasonableness of this approach depends on how limited resources are. If resources cannot be expanded, then resources spent on one activity will not be available for other activities, and it is not only reasonable but desirable to compare the amounts of benefit that could be gained by allocating the existing resources to different activities. To apply this approach, we could examine the benefits that would be gained if resources were spent on LOCAs instead of HOCAs, and compare those benefits with the benefits that would be gained if the same resources were used to provide other health care activities or treatments. But before we could use this approach, we had to satisfy ourselves that it was really not possible to increase the budget to accommodate the higher costs of LOCAs—that is, we had to answer the question my father and I struggled with at the end of the last chapter.[3]

This is a very difficult determination to make in realistic settings. On the one hand, in an organization with an annual budget that exceeds $3 billion, it is always possible to add a few more million dollars. On the other hand, if that reasoning were applied to every activity, the budget would blow up by a much larger amount, which would be unacceptable. We needed some sign from above that our budget had truly hit the point at which additional increases could not be tolerated and priorities had to be set.

By coincidence, just at the time we were trying to decide how tight our budget was, we received such a sign. On January 14, 1992, one of our largest contracts, the California Personnel Employment and Retirement System (CalPERS), called our top officers to Sacramento to ask us to lower our 1992 rates to a level below the 1991 rates. Because of its budget deficit, the state had had to limit salary increases and benefits for its employees, and wanted to pass the reductions on to its contractors, such as us. Although we were very much in sympathy with the state's budget problems and the plight of its employees, we could not agree to their request because it would have required us to increase the rates for our other employer groups, which we thought would be unfair. We offered to develop for PERS a package with reduced benefits at a lower cost—our benefit package was already more comprehensive than the packages provided by our competitors—but PERS rejected this option. The discussions ended in a stalemate. In response to our not freezing our rates for PERS, PERS decided to freeze us by not permitting any new members to join our Health Plan in the coming year. Although this event affected only one of our customers, that customer was not only one of our largest, but one with which we historically have had a very close relationship. Furthermore, the pressures faced by PERS, and passed on to us, were symbolic of pressures that we knew were affecting all our customers and members. The sign was unmistakable; our customers were telling us that the time had come for health care providers like us to make some tough choices.

We therefore stopped thinking about whether our rates could accommodate the cost of LOCAs, and proceeded to analyze the cost-effectiveness of LOCAs in low-risk patients. We estimated that we perform approximately 42 000 procedures using intravenous contrast agents in low-risk patients every year. Given the rates of reactions per patient shown in Table 22.2, using HOCAs instead of LOCAs in these 42 000 patients could be expected to increase the number of mild reactions each year by approximately 1000 patients, increase the number of moderate reactions by approximately 100 patients, and increase the number of severe reactions by approximately 40 patients. We had no reason to believe that there would be any increase in deaths with HOCAs. In return, using HOCAs instead of LOCAs in low-risk patients would free up approximately $3.5 million each year. The crucial question was whether there were other activities to which we could allocate the $3.5 million to deliver greater benefit to our members. There were. For example:

- Nationally, at least one fourth of women between the ages of 50 and 65 years are not being screened for breast cancer. We estimated that despite a strong commitment to prevention, there are still many women in our organization in that age group who have not yet been screened. Spending $3.5 million to aggressively identify and screen those women annually would prevent about 35 deaths from breast cancer.[18] A 2-year frequency would yield even greater benefit. These calculations include the increased cost of identifying and bringing in these hard-to-screen women.
- Nationally, approximately 10% of women have never received a Papanicolaou test. We estimated that allocating $3.5 million to aggressively identify and screen previously unscreened women with Papanicolaou tests every 3 years would prevent about 100 deaths from cervical cancer.[19]
- If $3.5 million were spent on a cholesterol treatment program for people at highest risk, approximately 13 sudden deaths, 105 heart attacks, and 250 cases of coronary insufficiency, angina, and other coronary artery disease events could be prevented. Furthermore, after the program was up and running for a few years, the reduced costs of treating sudden deaths, heart attacks, and other coronary artery disease events would just about completely offset the $3.5 million in drug costs (D. M. Eddy, MD, PhD, and S. Sarma, PhD, unpublished data, 1992).

When we compared 40 severe but nonfatal reactions with 35 breast cancer deaths, 100 cervical cancer deaths, or 13 sudden deaths and 100 heart attacks, the conclusion was obvious; spending money on LOCAs for low-risk patients instead of on other activities like these harms the quality of care for our members. The more comparisons we looked at, the more confident we became that our members would be better off if we diverted resources from LOCAs to other activities.

As a final check, I did some back-of-the-envelope estimates of willingness to pay and quality-adjusted life-years (QALYs). In order for the lower reaction rates with LOCAs to justify the higher cost, our typical member would have to be willing to pay about 2 years' household income (about $87 000) to avoid a severe but nonfatal reaction ($82 ÷ 0.00094 = $87 234). It is highly doubtful anyone would be willing to pay that much. In terms of QALYs, in order to get the cost per QALY to $50 000, which is still a high level, a person would have to be willing to give up about 1.75 years of life expectancy in order to avoid one severe but nonfatal reaction ($82 ÷ ($x \times 0.00094$) = $50 000, solve for x). To put this in perspective, 1.75 years of life expectancy is about 10 times the life expectancy gained by screening for cancer of the cervix or breast. Thus, by either of these measures, using LOCAs for low-risk patients is not a good buy.

Law, Politics, and Public Relations

The last step was to examine the nonscientific and nonfinancial issues. They boiled down to three questions: Would we be sued? If we were, would we lose and, if we did, would the costs and bad publicity wipe out the gains we thought we could make by reallocating resources? On the first question, a search revealed that to date there has not been a major problem with litigation regarding reactions to contrast agents. On the other hand, based on published numbers,[12,13] we could expect a death to occur in patients receiving contrast agents about once every 2 years, no matter which contrast agent we used. Even though our actual experience was a far lower frequency of deaths, it was inevitable that some deaths would eventually occur. In addition, any one of the 40 severe but nonfatal reactions that could be expected to occur each year could become a lawsuit. Putting all this together, we had to acknowledge that it was possible we would be sued.

Would we win? We concluded that we should win. Our guideline was developed by a process that was careful, accountable, and truly motivated by the health of our members. Everything we had read about guidelines and malpractice indicated that this should be an effective defense.[20,21] Furthermore, there was already a school of thought supporting our decision, and we could cite prestigious groups such as the ACR.

What if we lost? Given the relatively low probability of being sued and the defensibility of our guideline, the number of cases we would lose should be very small, if any, and the direct costs of lawsuits should not seriously drain the savings we planned to reallocate to other activities. The nonfinancial

costs of bad publicity, however, would persist no matter what the legal outcome was. While this troubled us, we felt it was outweighed by a principle
that was at stake. If we thought the guideline truly served the interests of our
members, we believed we should stand up for it. To fail to make what we
think are medically correct choices because of a fear of lawsuits would be to
abrogate our overriding responsibility to our members.

Design of the Guideline

Although the radiology chiefs group still felt uneasy about the
fact that the quality of care of their patients receiving HOCAs would suffer,
they agreed that the quality of care of our members as a whole would increase. The guideline was clear; we had to recommend HOCAs for low-risk
patients.

❖ From Theory to Practice

In theory, this application of cost-effectiveness analysis should
have been about as simple as any application of cost-effectiveness analysis
ever could be. First, the clinical problem itself had several features that made
this application comparatively easy. There were only a few health outcomes
to consider, and they all pointed in the same direction—toward LOCAs. This
spared us having to weigh benefits against harms and allowed us to focus on
the comparison of benefits and financial costs.

This example was also relatively simple methodologically. The outcomes
occur rapidly and are fairly easy to measure. The evidence about outcomes
was direct and fairly complete, and the analysis was fairly straightforward.
Perhaps the biggest methodological boon was that the gap between the cost-
effectiveness of contrast agents and other activities such as cancer screening
was very wide. This freed us from having to nail every number down tight.
There was a lot of room for uncertainty without threatening the conclusion
that other activities could provide much greater benefit. Finally, the value
judgments, although they appeared so difficult when they were presented in
qualitative terms, were really quite obvious once they were described with
numbers. Who could fail to choose to prevent 35 to 100 cancer deaths over
40 severe but nonfatal reactions?

This example even had some desirable political characteristics. A recommendation to use HOCAs for low-risk patients is not a radical move. The
ACR and others[22] have clearly acknowledged the appropriateness of such a
position. Furthermore, this is by no means the first guideline that has recommended against a beneficial treatment because of its cost. Medicine is filled
with lines and thresholds that cut off beneficial treatments. Examples are the
ages to begin or stop screening, the frequencies of screening and surveillance
tests, indications for diagnostic tests, laboratory values that trigger workups,
and indications for treatments. Behind all these commonly accepted practices

there is an implicit decision that just on the other side of the threshold, the benefits of the treatment are not worth their costs. Treatment of cholesterol is recommended for patients with LDL (low-density lipoprotein) cholesterol levels over 4.14 mmol/L and two or more risk factors[23]; does anyone really believe treatment has no benefit in patients who have only one risk factor, or who have two risk factors but LDL cholesterol levels of 4.01 mmol/L? A decision to use risk factors to draw a line between HOCAs and LOCAs should be in good company.

So, by all these measures, this decision should have been easy. Why then did we agonize over this guideline for more than a year?

Several issues concerned us. Most important was that this guideline was the first instance in which this organization explicitly estimated the consequences of reallocating resources from an activity acknowledged to be beneficial, to other activities. Although health maintenance organizations have led the profession in the efficient practice of medicine, they have traditionally done it by improving the *processes* of care—reducing hospitalizations, improving the efficiency of operations, and negotiating with vendors—not by altering the *content* of care. This decision about HOCAs was different. Here we deliberately based a recommendation on an explicit analysis of costs and effectiveness. Here we actually estimated the number of patients who would have "avoidable" reactions if HOCAs were used, and made a conscious choice that there were better ways to use the resources. It might be true that there are decisions like this buried in every threshold, but that is just the point—they have always been buried, invisible. With very rare exceptions, the thresholds that pervade medicine are not the result of any explicit estimation of either costs or effectiveness. Rather, most of them have evolved through an implicit, anonymous process. Few people even realize that they contain implied judgments about cost-effectiveness. In short, the precedent these "standard and accepted" thresholds create is not obvious.

A second concern was the one felt directly by the radiologists, and vicariously by all of us. The radiologists are the ones who will see the patients face-to-face, pick up the syringe, and inject the agent into their veins. They are the ones who will know that a reaction might occur, and who will be the first on hand to treat it. From this perspective, it is small consolation to know that this guideline will redistribute resources to improve the quality of care for our members as a whole. Appreciating that requires a broad perspective that spans beyond the immediate concerns of a particular group of practitioners.

Third, as a methodologist, I was concerned about some inconsistencies. For example, this guideline is directed to low-risk patients, and recommends HOCAs for that group on the logic that the chance of reactions is too low to justify the cost. For high-risk patients, we recommend LOCAs. But Palmer's data (Table 22.1) indicate that the risk of a reaction in patients with risk factors such as asthma or a history of a previous reaction is only about four times higher than for low-risk patients—instead of a 1 in 1000 chance of a severe reaction, they have a 4 in 1000 chance. With corticosteroid pretreatment, the chance would drop to about 2 in 1000. I will not go through the mathematics here, but if we recommended *HOCAs* for *high*-risk people and put the savings into screening for cervical cancer, we would increase the number of severe reactions by about 36, but would prevent 40 more deaths from cancer. Thus, a good case can be made that we should have recommended HOCAs for most high-risk people as well. I did not recommend that because I thought we had pushed rationalism about as far as we could on this problem. Words like "high risk" have a psychological impact far beyond their actual numbers, the ACR did not bless HOCAs for high-risk people, and we were approaching burnout. In short, we did not pursue this because of timidity and fatigue. These are not particularly defensible reasons.

Finally, while reactions to contrast agents have not attracted lawsuits in the past, and while we are confident we can defend our guideline, there is always the possibility of a suit and even the experience of winning it would be unpleasant.

In light of these concerns, this guideline seems crazy.

❖ The Bottom Line

Why then did we do it? We did it because of three convictions. First, we are convinced that our customers really do want us to control costs, and really do want us to maximize the quality of care we provide within the constraint of costs. Second, we are convinced that this guideline will accomplish these objectives. We have already initiated plans to reallocate resources to beef up our preventive activities such as cancer screening; for the few people who will face a very small increase in risk, hundreds will be helped. This guideline is clearly in the best medical and financial interests of our members as a whole. Third, although the decision is an uncomfortable one, if health care organizations back off whenever there is a tough decision that requires reallocating resources to increase overall quality of care, our country will never make headway against the problems of high cost and inefficient allocation of resources. Achieving a balanced approach to health care will require some people to step forward. If we are not willing to do that, how can we expect others to?

MHE: So does this story have a moral?
DME: It has four morals. Although the principles of cost-effectiveness analysis are sound and the methods can work for specific problems, cost-effectiveness analysis is not easy to implement. Bear in mind that this is probably the simplest analysis I have been involved in, yet still it is messy. This example provides a feeling for the art of applying cost-effectiveness analysis—the types of methodological issues that can arise, some techniques for handling them, the judgments and compromises that must be made, and the imperfections that persist in any application. Second, cost-effectiveness analysis is not just done by cold-hearted economists and mathematicians who bear no primary responsibility for patients. It is being done by real practitioners and real health care organizations that pride themselves on providing the

highest quality care, but who are trying to respond to changing social demands. Third, as a society we are very poor at applying cost-effectiveness analysis to medical problems. Society is still sending out mixed signals, and we in the profession still have mixed emotions. Even very disciplined organizations struggle when they face problems like this. But the fourth moral is much more hopeful. As this example illustrates, by suggesting how resources can be reallocated, cost-effectiveness analysis offers tremendous opportunities for improving the quality of care while controlling costs. In this example, a few more people will face higher risks of a reaction, but scores of deaths will be prevented. This is an improvement by anyone's measure.

MHE: I have two questions. How did you sell this to the practicing radiologists? And were your corporate clients pleased?

DME: The short answers are "with difficulty," and "I hope so, but I don't know for sure." However, those two questions push us face-to-face against two of the most perplexing problems in medicine today—redefining the role practitioners should play in providing health care, and developing a partnership with our customers. They deserve more discussion.

❖ Update

On September 2, 1993, the Health Benefits Advisory Council (HBAC) of CalPERS studied this article and concluded that KPSC's decision was "a reasonable and appropriate response to the CalPERS Board's call for more cost reduction, while maintaining a high level of quality, and that CalPERS should accept responsibility for the consequences of its actions." On November 17, 1993, the CalPERS Board adopted this resolution:

It is the responsibility of the health plans to manage high cost care that yields small marginal benefits. It is also the responsibility of the health plans to determine which procedures are not proven to be safe and effective and which guidelines might be appropriate because they raise quality. . . . It will be necessary and appropriate for health plans and care providers to make value-for-money decisions in cases in which the costs of health care practices are high in relation to the benefits produced. Such decisions are a useful tool, along with continued efforts to encourage efficiency and appropriate medical treatments, in an effort to provide the best quality and value to PERS members. Clinical policies based on the principle that health resources are unlimited are not realistic, and are not consistent with the best interests of PERS members or Californians in general.

❖ References

1. Eddy D. Cost-effectiveness analysis: a conversation with my father. *JAMA.* 1992; 267:1669-1672, 1674-1675 (Chapter 19).
2. Eddy D. Cost-effectiveness analysis: is it up to the task? *JAMA.* 1992;267:3342-3348 (Chapter 20).

3. Eddy D. Cost-effectiveness analysis: will it be accepted? *JAMA*. 1992;268:132-136 (Chapter 21).
4. American College of Radiology. Resolution regarding the use of contrast agents. Memorandum, September 1990.
5. Eddy D. *A Manual for Assessing Health Practices and Designing Practice Policies: The Explicit Approach*. Philadelphia, Pa: American College of Physicians; 1992.
6. Eddy D. Practice policies—guidelines for methods. *JAMA*. 1990;263:1839-1841 (Chapter 5).
7. Palmer F. The RACR survey of intravenous contrast media reactions: final report. *Australas Radiol*. 1988;32:426-428.
8. Katayama H, Yamaguchi K, Kozuka T, Takashima T, Seez P, Matsuura K: Adverse reactions to ionic and nonionic contrast media: a report from the Japanese Committee on the Safety of Contrast Media. *Radiology*. 1990;175:621-628.
9. Kent B. *Ionic and Non-ionic Iodinated Contrast Agents: A Comparison of Reactions and Cost*. Fontana, Calif: Kaiser Health Plan at Fontana Medical Center. Unpublished report.
10. Wolf G, Arenson R, Cross A. A prospective trial of ionic vs nonionic contrast agents in routine clinical practice: comparison of adverse effects. *AJR Am J Roentgenol*. 1989;152:939-944.
11. Lasser E, Berry C, Talner L, et al. Pretreatment with corticosteroids to alleviate reactions to intravenous contrast material. *N Engl J Med*. 1987;317:845-849.
12. Curry N, Schable S, Reiheld C, Henry W, Savoca W. Fatal reactions to intravenous nonionic contrast material. *Radiology*. 1991;178:361-362.
13. Caro J, Trindade E, McGregor M. The risks of death and severe nonfatal reactions with high- vs low-osmolality contrast media: a meta-analysis. *Am J Radiol*. 1991;156:825-831.
14. Eddy D. Resolving conflicts in practice policies. *JAMA*. 1990;264:389-391 (Chapter 9).
15. Gerstman B. Epidemiologic critique of the report on adverse reactions to ionic and nonionic media by the Japanese Committee on the Safety of Contrast Media. *Radiology*. 1991;178:787-790.
16. Eddy D. Connecting value and costs: whom do we ask, and what do we ask them? *JAMA*. 1990;264:1737-1739 (Chapter 11).
17. Eddy D. Rationing by patient choice. *JAMA*. 1991;265:105-108 (Chapter 12).
18. Eddy D. Screening for breast cancer. *Ann Intern Med*. 1989;111:389-399.
19. Eddy D. Screening for cervical cancer. *Ann Intern Med*. 1990;113:214-226.
20. Hall M. The defensive effect of medical practice policies in malpractice litigation. *Law Contemp Probl*. 1991;54:119-145.
21. Hirshfeld E. Practice parameters and the malpractice liability of physicians. *JAMA*. 1990;263:1556-1562.
22. Evens R. Economic impact of low-osmolality contrast agents on radiology procedures and departments. *Radiology*. 1987;162:267-268.
23. Expert Panel T. Report of the National Cholesterol Education Program Expert Panel on detection, evaluation and treatment of high blood cholesterol in adults. *Arch Intern Med*. 1988;148:36-69.

❖ Source

Originally published in *JAMA*. 1992;268:2575-2582.

Chapter 23

Broadening
the Responsibilities
of Practitioners
The Team Approach

The previous chapter described how a large health maintenance organization (HMO), Kaiser Permanente of Southern California (KPSC), developed a guideline for the use of intravenous radiographic contrast agents for low-risk patients.[1] The principal issue was whether the lower rates of reactions with low osmolar contrast agents (LOCAs) were worth their higher costs compared with high osmolar contrast agents (HOCAs). After estimating the magnitudes of the risks and costs, KPSC determined that they were not; the same resources could provide greater overall benefit to its members if put into other activities, such as screening for cancers of the cervix or breast. The final guideline stated: "For procedures involving intravenous administration, patients who can be determined to be at low risk of having a reaction should receive HOCAs. Patients who have risk factors for a reaction should receive LOCAs." The full guideline contains more details about specific risk factors and pretreatment with corticosteroids.

DAVID M. EDDY, MD, PHD: Well, you've had an opportunity to study the guideline and its rationale.[1] What do you think?

RADIOLOGIST: I don't like it. I know that some of my colleagues accept this approach. But I also know a lot of other radiologists who feel the way I do—very uncomfortable.

DME: Then you're the one I want to talk to. Why don't you like it?

R: It's very difficult for me and, I would suspect, for any physician to consciously withhold a treatment that has known benefit because of its cost. It runs counter to my personal principles, to everything I was taught, and to what my patients expect of me. Despite the arguments you make on paper,[1] I

219

don't like the idea of cutting quality to save money. It's your right to try to do it, but it's my right to fight back.

DME: I can understand all those concerns. However, I was hoping that they would be balanced by the fact that this guideline will cause resources to be allocated in a way that will provide much more overall benefit to the members of the HMO. Doesn't this overcome your objections?

R: Not much.

❖ Defining the Problem

DME: Why? Let's try to find the point of disagreement.[2] Do you agree that resources are limited?

R: Yes. Or at least I agree that in the environment in which KPSC had to make its decision, with their customers demanding that rates be held down, resources were limited.

DME: And do you agree that when resources are limited, it's not possible to do everything that might have benefit, that tradeoffs have to be made, and that priorities have to be set?

R: Yes.

DME: Do you also agree that when priorities are set, guidelines should be designed to maximize the health of *all* the members of the HMO,[3] not just a particular group of patients who happen to be candidates for a particular treatment?

R: In general, yes. I do agree with that.

DME: And do you agree that shifting resources from LOCAs to screening hard-to-reach women for cervical cancer will offer more benefit to the HMO members as a whole? More specifically, do you agree with our estimates that using HOCAs in low-risk patients might increase the number of severe but nonfatal reactions by about 40 a year, but would also free up about $3.5 million a year, which could be used to prevent about 100 cervical cancer deaths a year?

R: I can't vouch for those exact numbers, but I'm willing to take your word that those are the approximate outcomes. Put it this way: I can't find any errors in your analysis of the literature or calculations.[1]

DME: That's good to hear. And finally, do you agree that it is preferable to prevent 100 women from dying of cervical cancer than to prevent 40 severe but nonfatal reactions?

R: Yes, I do.

DME: Then what's the problem?

R: Well, I suppose I just don't think that the hypothetical benefit to other patients overrides my responsibility to my patients.

DME: I see two parts of your statement that we need to discuss: the notion that the benefit is "hypothetical," and the idea that your responsibility to your patients overrides what happens to other patients.

❖ Are the Benefits Hypothetical?

Let's begin with "hypothetical"—what do you mean by that? The dictionary defines a hypothetical thought as a tentative assumption or conjecture. The connotation is that it might well not be true. I often get the impression that some people try to attach the label "hypothetical" to an idea they don't like, on the belief that that will invalidate it. So let's address this issue straight on: When you say the benefits are hypothetical, are you actually retreating from your previous answer that the guideline should prevent about 100 cervical cancer deaths in return for about 40 severe but nonfatal reactions?

R: No, I don't really mean that. I guess I'm using "hypothetical" to capture three thoughts. One is that the estimates are based on mathematical calculations rather than tangible observations, which makes them suspicious. A second is that the cancer deaths to be prevented are in the future, whereas my patients are now. Who knows what will happen in the future? The third is that I'll never see the women whose cancer deaths will be prevented, whereas my patients are right in front of me. In fact, no one will ever be able to identify any particular women who didn't die of cervical cancer because of that guideline. For all intents and purposes, they're invisible. All these diminish the psychological impact of your estimates.

DME: I'm tempted to tackle each one of those one at a time. But we might be able to save some time with the following question. You're a radiologist. Do you believe women should be screened for breast cancer?

R: Yes.

DME: Do you realize that the benefits of mammography screening are "hypothetical" in the three ways you just described: the projected benefits are based on mathematics, they will occur in the future, and they will be unobservable to you?

R: I see that now. . . . So why am I confident about the benefits of screening when I'm advocating a mammography program but nervous about the benefits of screening when I think about the guideline for contrast agents?

I'm a bit embarrassed to admit this but I guess that the feature of the two cases that bothers me is that in the first case—when I'm advocating mammography screening—I'm on the receiving end. I'm gaining resources for my patients. Whereas in the second case—when I'm troubled by switching resources from LOCAs to cervical cancer screening—I'm on the losing end. That might sound like a double standard, but there is a consistency to my reasoning. In both cases I'm trying to do what is best for my patients.

DME: That's certainly a valid concern. And it coincides with the other problem you described, your sense of responsibility for your patients. But if that's the problem, let's deal with it directly, and avoid the connotation that comes with the word "hypothetical."

R: Fair enough.

DME: Now let's home in on the real source of your discomfort—the feeling that if you support this guideline you will be abrogating your responsibility to your patients, even though the guideline offers greater total benefit to the group.

R: Before we do that, I've thought of a few other things about this guideline that make me uncomfortable that you haven't asked about.

DME: Let's address them now.

❖ Emergencies, Lawsuits, and Conflicts of Interest

R: One has to do with the act of giving the agents to patients, and the possibility of a reaction. You have to understand that it's very difficult to stand there and inject into your patient's vein an agent that you know has an appreciably higher chance of causing a severe reaction than that of another available agent. I hate life-threatening emergencies. I haven't had to manage an emergency code since my internship, and I don't ever want to see one again. Indeed, one of the reasons I went into radiology was to get away from medical emergencies.

DME: I can understand that. I left clinical practice for similar reasons. But let me ask you this. Do you believe that your distaste for emergencies, as understandable as it is, is a sufficient reason to let 100 women die from cervical cancer? We also need to consider the fact that in order to avoid causing 40 radiologists the stress of severe reactions, we will be causing 100 other physicians to suffer the stress of 100 women dying from cervical cancer. Then we could compare the stress in the families of the patients. . . .

R: Stop. I'll yield on this point. But it's back there in my mind somewhere. All these sources of discomfort add up.

DME: That's true. It's helpful to sort out the different sources of discomfort so that you can deal with them separately. Are there any other issues that are important, before we talk about responsibilities?

R: Yes, malpractice. I don't want to be sued.

DME: Neither would I. But you understand, don't you, that the risk of a suit is extremely small, and the probability that you'd lose it is even smaller.

R: How small?

DME: Under pessimistic assumptions, the chance of getting sued is in the range of one in a half million. As for the outcome of the suit, you'd have the protection not only of a carefully developed guideline, but of the fact that there are other health care delivery organizations as well as professional societies with similar policies. Perhaps most helpful is that the American College of Radiology guideline clearly permits the use of HOCAs in low-risk patients. In other words, although many people do use LOCAs for low-risk patients, there is unquestionably an established school of thought —which is what I believe the courts look for—that HOCAs are appropriate for those patients. Another point to consider is the potential for lawsuits if we *fail* to screen women for cancer of the breast or cervix. The probabilities are much higher there, and there is no school of thought that recommends against such screening. If your concern is lawsuits, you should be in *favor* of transferring resources to cancer screening. A final point to consider is that in an HMO like KPSC, it is the group that is sued, not the individual practitioner. This doesn't eliminate the stress, but it does eliminate the financial risk.

R: Okay, I'll admit that this issue is another one that is more emotional than real, but it's real emotion. If we are adding up "discomfort points," lawsuits are a big item.

DME: I know what you mean. Anything else?

R: Yes . . . forgive me for asking this, but I understand that you helped KPSC develop this guideline. Do you personally benefit from this guideline? That is, is your salary or any bonus tied to how much money a guideline saves the HMO?

DME: No. But suppose my income, or even my professional job satisfaction, did depend on the outcome of a guideline I helped design. Would you think that was inappropriate?

R: It would severely discredit the guideline.

DME: Then does it bother you that many guidelines are produced by professional societies whose members' incomes and satisfaction *are* directly affected by the guidelines they produce?

R: Well, now that I think about it, it does bother me when another specialty writes a guideline that affects my practice.

DME: You've identified a very important issue that deserves more discussion, but it would require more time than we have now. And it really doesn't affect this guideline, which was designed with the radiology chiefs. Should we move on?

R: Yes.

❖ Who Is Responsible for What?

DME: All right, let's talk about your sense of responsibility. It's worth spending some time on this. Ironically, the practitioner's sense of responsibility to his or her individual patients is probably the most important barrier to the responsible use of health care resources. My first question is whether the focus on your patients indicates that you are not concerned about other patients.

R: Of course not.

DME: But do you consider yours to be more important in some way?

R: Well, they're more important to *me* in the sense that I know them personally. I have an emotional attachment to them. But please understand, my desire to help my patients is not based on any conviction that they are "worth" more than other patients in any absolute sense. When I say I feel a responsibility for my patients, the emphasis is not on "my patients," but on "my responsibility."

It boils down to this. I believe that the reason American medicine works so well is that every individual practitioner assumes responsibility for each patient under his or her care. I think of the responsibility a practitioner feels for his or her patients as a tent that stands over the patients and protects them, in the sense of making certain that they get what they need. I picture the patients as a huge crowd of people in a rainstorm. Each practitioner has a tent, and the patients under their care at any time are under their tent. So the way our system works is that I look after the patients under my tent, other practitioners look after the patients under their tents, and all the patients end up being covered. If each of us provides the best possible care to each of our patients, then all patients get the best possible care.

DME: I can see the appeal of that idea. It allows for both autonomy and synchrony—autonomy because each practitioner can follow his or her personal sense of responsibility; synchrony because all the individual responsibilities work together to maximize everyone's health. I also like your analogy of the tents. Patients can move around in the crowd, seeing a variety of practitioners throughout their lifetimes, but, according to the theory, they will always be covered by someone's tent.

R: You've got it. That's the way medicine has worked for as long as I can remember, probably forever. If it isn't broken, why fix it?

DME: Well, if that theory is true, you should indeed carry on as you have been. More specifically, you should continue to fight this guideline. So let's think about it very carefully.

I'm worried about two things. First, I fear there are rather large gaps in this system of tents. That is, I don't believe that everyone actually has a practitioner who feels responsible for them at all times. One obvious example is the people who are outside the medical system because they lack insurance. But without denying the importance of that problem, I'm inclined to set it aside for now because it isn't an issue in an HMO such as KPSC. An example that is more pertinent to this guideline is that even in an HMO, people are under a tent only when they are actually seeking the care of a practitioner who feels directly responsible for them. Indeed, that type of gap is the main rationale for this guideline. You yourself said that the women who might be saved from dying from cervical cancer are invisible. Women who appear for screening are under someone's care, but this guideline is designed to help women who aren't currently seeking care because they feel perfectly well. They will become visible only *after* they get cervical cancer, and then it's too late. So my first question is, who is responsible for them?

R: In an HMO such as KPSC, I assume it's the medical director or some high-level task force like a guidelines committee.

DME: If we restrict our discussion to managed care organizations, the existence of someone like a medical director would indeed solve the first problem that concerned me about your theory. Let's use "medical director" as a general term to describe some person or committee that has an overview and that feels responsible for the entire group of people covered by a health care organization. So part of your theory is that, in addition to the individual practitioners who feel responsible for the patients currently under their care, there is also a "medical director" whose responsibilities span *all* the members of the HMO, both those who are currently under someone's care and those who are not.

R: That's right. The medical director is part of the system of overlapping tents.

DME: And the medical director's tent is broader than the tents of the individual practitioners because it covers more people. It's like a "super tent." Should we call it the "superdome"?

R: This analogy is beginning to get out of hand, but that's right. So everyone is covered by at least one tent, and some patients might be covered by several tents.

DME: And what happens when the medical director, whose responsibilities span all patients, wants to do one thing and practitioners like you want to do something else? It sounds as though you are willing to allow the medical director to intrude in the decisions of practitioners.

R: No, we don't want that, because that would undo the autonomy that is such a desirable feature of this system. I'm assuming that the medical director can discharge his or her responsibilities without affecting what I do for my patients. As you said, all the responsibilities work in synchrony.

DME: That's the *theory*. What we're doing now is testing the theory. And my fear is that while that theory might have worked in the past, it doesn't work now.

R: Why not?

❖ Conflicting Responsibilities

DME: Because the choices you make as an individual practitioner are often in conflict with the decisions that a medical director makes on behalf of the group as a whole. This conflict is the second aspect of your theory that worries me. And this guideline is a good example. The medical director, in order to fulfill his responsibility (I'll use the masculine pronoun because in this case the medical director was a male), determined that more health benefit will be delivered to the HMO's members if resources are shifted from LOCAs to cancer screening. But this conflicts with your sense of responsibility to maximize the care you provide to your patients. I believe that the words you used earlier were, "It's your right to do it, but it's my right to fight back." In fact, this type of conflict is very common. The reason is not that either party is dumb or hardheaded. It is simply a consequence of the fact that as they are currently perceived, the responsibilities of the two parties are frequently in conflict.

R: I have to agree that that happened in this case. But I'm not certain why conflicts like this should be common.

DME: They will occur commonly because of the differences in the breadth or scopes of the responsibilities of the two parties. Compared with a practitioner who is focusing on an individual patient, the medical director sees the effect of a guideline on a broader range of patients. In this example, the medical director can see both the effect of HOCAs on your patients who need a contrast agent *and* the effect of cervical cancer screening on women who are currently underscreened. On the other hand, *you* see the effect of the guideline only on your patients who need a contrast agent. It's not your fault that you aren't aware of what's happening with cervical cancer screening; it's just a consequence of the different job descriptions—your span of responsibility and therefore your "vision" are just narrower than the medical director's.

The medical director's perspective is also broader in another way. Because he is higher up in the management chain, he is more likely to deal with the people who are paying the bills—corporations and representatives of member groups. This means he is more likely to appreciate the financial constraints. Many practitioners still don't quite believe that resources are limited or that trade-offs have to be made. Medical directors *know* that resources are limited and that tradeoffs are unavoidable.

R: So what should we do to resolve these conflicts in responsibilities?

❖ Whose Responsibility Deserves Priority?

DME: Actually, you already answered that question when you agreed earlier that the overall objective is to provide the most health care possible to the entire patient population. It is the medical director's responsibility that coincides with that objective. That means that when the responsibilities and decisions of the medical director conflict with the responsibilities and decisions of individual practitioners, the medical director's responsibilities and decisions have to take priority. Just like the hierarchy of tents, there is a hierarchy of responsibilities. The position in the hierarchy is determined by the scope of the responsibilities—the span of the tent.

R: So the responsibilities of all the parties do not work in synchrony after all.

DME: I'm afraid that's true, as this guideline illustrates. *Either* there is no one who takes responsibility for the group as a whole, in which case there are gaps. *Or* there *is* someone who has that responsibility, in which case there will be conflicts between that broad responsibility and the narrower responsibilities.

R: You said that the approach I described used to work. What did you mean by that? When did it work, and what changed?

DME: In general, the theory you described would work if two conditions held: first, everyone would have to be under the care of at least one fully accountable practitioner at all times. By "fully accountable," I mean someone who is looking out for every aspect of his or her patients' health care at all times—not just when they are seeking care. Second, there would have to be no limits on resources.

R: It's easy to see how practitioners like me would believe the theory. From our point of view, those two conditions have pretty much existed for the last half century. Insurance took care of the second condition. And while the first condition might not have held, we weren't aware of the gaps because we were thinking only of the patients under our care, and, by definition, they are all under someone's care. Our attention is focused on what happens inside our tents, so we don't see the gaps between the tents.

DME: That's an excellent explanation of why so many practitioners *think* the theory works. Your next question asked about what's changed. Two things have changed: First, we have recently become much more concerned about the uncovered people, both those inside the health care system (ie, insured but not currently under anyone's care), and those outside the system (ie, the uninsured).

Second, the people who pay the bills—business, government, taxpayers, and premium payers—just aren't willing any more to provide unlimited money in the way they used to. This places practical limits on resources that make it impossible for both you and the medical director to get what you want to fulfill your responsibilities as you perceive them.

❖ What Is the Practitioner's Responsibility?

R: Well, then, if maximizing the care for my individual patients is an inappropriate act on my part, what is my responsibility?

DME: Your responsibility is to provide the best care possible to your patients, consistent with the overall objective of using resources in the most effective way to maximize the care for the entire group.

R: "Consistent with . . . "—that sounds pretty fuzzy. What does that mean in practical terms?

DME: It means that the actions you can take to maximize care for your individual patients will be constrained—limited—by guidelines that are designed to maximize care for the group as a whole. A trivial analogy is that your ability to perform a computed tomographic scan is constrained by the waiting list for use of the equipment. You are used to physical constraints like that. Guidelines are more cerebral constraints. They steer you *toward* doing certain things, and *away* from doing other things. In practical terms, the guideline we've been discussing will mean that when you are performing a procedure on a patient who requires contrast agents, you will want to do everything possible to minimize the chance of a reaction, *except* offer LOCAs to patients who have no risk factors. Things you *would* do include taking a good history to ensure that the patient has no risk factors, pretreating with steroids if indicated by the guideline, explaining the procedure carefully to alleviate anxiety, having a crash cart handy, keeping up to date on resuscitation techniques, and so forth.

R: But you're saying it's *not* my responsibility to give LOCAs to low-risk patients?

DME: I'll go further than that. I'll say that it *is* your responsibility to *not* give LOCAs to low-risk patients, because to do so would pull resources from other activities that would provide greater benefit.

R: Wow! That's a switch. Now it's my responsibility to do something that *harms* my patients.

❖ A Broader Responsibility: The Team Approach

DME: If you look at your responsibility narrowly, that's true. But there is a better way to look at your responsibility. In fact, guidelines like this represent an *increase* or *broadening* of your responsibilities rather than a narrowing. To appreciate what this means, step back for a moment from the fact that you are a radiologist, and drop your current perception that you are responsible only for your individual patients. Imagine that you are part of a multispecialty team that is responsible for the health of *all* the members of the group.

R: I already think of myself like that—I'm a member of a multispecialty group.

DME: Not a *group*, a *team*. A "group" implies a collection of people, each one going about his or her responsibilities as he or she sees fit. A "team" implies something quite different. It implies working in coordination with other people to achieve a common goal. It implies that there is a coach, in this case the entity we're calling the medical director, who is coordinating the actions of the individual team members. And it implies that the team members suppress their personal objectives in favor of the team's objectives. Being a member of a team will mean that you won't always be able to do everything you want to do—just as a star running back, no matter how talented, won't be given the ball on every play. And when he is given the ball, he will try to follow the playbook, ad libbing only when necessary. Being a member of a team will also mean that you will be asked to help others do what they need to do—just as running backs sometimes block for other runners.

R: "Broadening" is a pretty sneaky way to describe this idea you're trying to sell. It makes us feel good. And I appreciate your attempt to cast this in terms a Super Bowl fan can understand. But it's pretty easy to see through your verbal legerdemain and macho analogies. Whatever you call this, it is really a narrowing of responsibilities—I'm doing *less* for my patients, and I'm not actually *doing* anything more for anyone else's patients.

DME: I'll withdraw the football analogy. But I'm going to keep the word "broadening." First, I didn't claim that your *actions* would necessarily broaden—in the sense that you'll be doing more x-ray procedures. I claimed that your *responsibilities* have broadened. The idea is that when you make a decision about what to do, or not do, to one of your patients, you will also consider the effect of that decision on *other* patients. Furthermore, you will feel some obligation—responsibility—to balance the implications of the decision for your patients against the implications of the decision for other patients. I think of that as a broadening of responsibility. The rationale for this broadening of responsibility is that the limits on resources create a link between every practitioner. Everything one practitioner does affects what every other practitioner can do. The effect might be small or large, depending on how tight the resource limit is and on how many resources the practitioner's actions consume, but the link is there. This linkage is a relatively new feature of medicine. Before resources were limited, it was reasonable for each practitioner to act as an independent agent. Now, because all practitioners are linked together by the need to share resources, it is no longer responsible to think that way.

A second point I would make about whether the idea I am selling will narrow what you do is that under the team approach you *will* be doing some additional things—both for some of your patients, and for the patients of other practitioners. The reason is that shifting resources doesn't necessarily mean you'll always be on the giving end—unless everything you are currently doing is wasteful. To the extent that you currently lack resources for some high-priority activities, you will also be on the receiving end. An example is mammography screening; this very guideline we've been talking about highlights the need to increase mammography screening in women older than 50.[1] So that's an example of an action you will pick up.

You will also be doing some additional things that, although they might not be actions in the physical sense of the word, are extremely important to the health of the group. A good example is helping identify opportunities to save resources. Obviously, when searching for ways to control costs, everyone's first choice is to weed out any practices that are truly ineffective or unnecessary, and to find ways to streamline processes. Specialists like you are in a particularly good position to do this. I'm sure you can think of some x-ray-ordering practices of primary care practitioners that, although well intended, provide little or no benefit.

R: I can think of one immediately—magnetic resonance imaging (MRI) for knee pain. You wouldn't believe how many patients are in our waiting rooms for that procedure. I'm convinced that a 6-week trial of conservative management would solve the problem in a high proportion of cases, either because the knee pain resolves or by making arthroscopy the next obvious step.

DME: I don't know much about MRIs or knees, but from the way you're talking, that sounds like a great example. You are confirming my point that simply by suggesting potential topics for guidelines you can do a lot to improve both the quality and efficiency of care. And those guidelines are the best kind because, although they might put the referring practitioners on the defensive, they tend to be noncontroversial from a scientific point of view, and they do not harm quality at all.

R: Well, I'm happy to offer up suggestions like that. But I still see the restrictions on what I can do for my patients as a narrowing of something that I don't want to have narrowed—whether you call it a broadening of responsibility or not. And I can tell you that primary care physicians will not like it if I or you or the medical director tell them they are ordering too many MRIs. These changes violate our right to manage our patients as we see fit.

❖ A Physician's Right to Autonomy

DME: "Our right to manage our patients as we see fit. . . ." Now you've pushed one of *my* buttons. For starters, I could ask, who gave physicians that right? Did we get it when we were accepted into medical school, or when we took the Hippocratic oath, or passed the board exams?

R: Let's see. It's certainly not written in any constitution, and the public never voted on it. But what about the doctrine of the captain of the ship? We *were* taught that. Doesn't the responsibility that comes with being the captain of the ship carry with it the right to make all the decisions?

DME: Not *all* the decisions. Indeed, the captain of a ship is a great analogy for what we've been talking about. The captain is certainly in charge of the day-to-day management of the ship. But captains follow guidelines, and ships are part of a fleet. In short, the captain of a ship is responsible for doing the best possible job of managing the ship, but *within* the constraints defined by the ship's orders, port regulations, instructions from the owner or fleet commander, international maritime law, and so forth. In similar fashion, you are the captain of the ship in the sense that you are responsible for the moment-to-moment management of your patients. But you already exercise this responsibility within a wide variety of constraints that range from implicit constraints like "standard and accepted practice," to rigid rules like using sterile technique in the operating room. Many practitioners try to fight these constraints because they'd rather have complete freedom. Who wouldn't? But the "captain of the ship" doctrine provides little support for that position.

R: You seem to feel strongly about that.

DME: I get sensitive whenever I hear about *any* group claiming a right to do whatever it pleases. That position can be very destructive. For example, if physicians can declare that right for themselves, can everyone else also claim a similar right? Imagine the chaos if every administrator, nurse, and respiratory therapist did whatever he or she pleased?

R: I guess we avoid that chaos now because physicians staked their claim first and now we won't let anyone else in.

DME: I tend to agree. But let's drop this discussion of rights because it gets tied up in turf battles and ego trips. Instead, let's address the real issue, which is whether it is in the best interests of patients to have physicians free to do whatever they please, without concern for the implications for other patients, or to accept some constraints on their actions, as called for by the team approach. To address this issue, I'd like to flip the problem around. Suppose the medical director concludes that the indications for a particular drug for treating acute myocardial infarctions should be tightened because the money could provide greater benefit if used to buy—let's pick something that you want—a new MRI unit. And let's imagine that the cardiologists are balking. They are doing everything they can to subvert the guideline, and they continue to use the drug. Because of their resistance you can't get your MRI unit. What would you say about that?

R: I would say the cardiologists are being hogs.

DME: But the cardiologists will give you all the arguments about the number of patients who die from heart attacks, their responsibilities to their patients, the fact that the benefits of the MRI unit are "hypothetical," the fact that they might be sued if they don't use the drug, and so forth.

R: I get your point. But if it can truly be determined that I could put the resources to better use, I'd expect them to act in good faith and carry out the guideline.

DME: Would you say they're being irresponsible if they don't?

R: Yes.

DME: Would you go so far as to say it is their responsibility to *not* use the drug, even though it might have offered their patients some benefit?

R: Why do I feel like a calf being corralled into a corner?

DME: And how about this? Would you say that if a patient is harmed because he or she couldn't get an MRI because the resources were—I'll use your word—"hogged" by the cardiologists, that the cardiologists bear some responsibility for the harm?

R: Given that all the rest of us agreed it was best to buy the MRI unit, I'd say they bear major responsibility for the harm.

DME: Then their span of responsibility is broader than their individual patients?

R: Yes.

DME: Bingo. Now all we have to do is apply the golden rule. In the same way that they have a responsibility to assist you when the guideline goes in your direction, you have a responsibility to support someone else when a guideline goes in their direction. That's teamwork. And that's what I mean by a broadening of responsibilities. In the case of LOCAs vs HOCAs, your responsibility as a team member is to follow the guideline in good faith, knowing that it is designed to maximize the health of the HMO's members.

❖ Building Trust

R: That phrase you just used—"knowing that the guideline is designed to maximize the health of all the members"—that knowledge is going to be a key in actually pulling off this team concept. Before they'll even consider changing their practices, practitioners are really going to have to *believe* that the guideline really will provide more benefit than harm.

DME: I agree. That's why I spent so much time asking you what you meant by the benefits of the guideline being "hypothetical." I wanted to make certain you truly understand and believe that the guideline for contrast agents will provide greater benefit to other patients. If you hadn't believed that, I would have spent a lot more time on that issue.

By the way, this introduces another role you will have to play as a member of a team. The medical director, or whatever entity in the organization has the broad responsibility for the group, will need your help to design the best guideline. In fact, a medical director per se won't even try to make a decision like this by himself or herself. The design of a guideline itself must be a team effort. This guideline for contrast agents is a real example—the lead group was the radiology chiefs.

Now, having said that practitioners have an important role to play in the design of a guideline, it is important to describe that role. Their role is *not* to act as advocates fighting for a particular position. Rather, their role is to provide the expertise needed to ensure that the guideline team has accurate information about the consequences of different options. In particular, practitioners will act as experts about the aspects of the guideline that affect their patients. The guideline team must then put that information together with the effects of the guideline on other patients, to determine what is best for the group as a whole.

R: That helps a little bit. Are there any other positive aspects of this approach that might help boost our sagging morale?

❖ Identifying With the Success of the Team

DME: I'll tell you one that would give me great satisfaction if I were still practicing. There is absolutely no question in my mind that organizations that develop a team approach will be able to provide the best care at the lowest cost. This is due to two facts. First, they are by far in the best position to allocate their resources to achieve those objectives. Second, they can avoid the enormous waste and low morale that come with all the territorial squabbles that occur with the current system. Given this, I can imagine practitioners deriving great pride from knowing that they're an integral part of the success of such an organization.

R: You know, everything you say about responsibilities and teamwork makes sense intellectually. My mind—at least the left side of my brain—is beginning to agree with you. But I just can't get over this gut feeling of discomfort when I think about not using LOCAs.

DME: I can certainly understand that. In fact, if I were in your shoes I would feel exactly the same way . . . for a while.

R: "For a while"?

DME: Here's how I try to deal with the discomfort that occurs with situations like this. It might be helpful to you, or it might not.

❖ Dealing With the Discomfort

There is no doubt that discomfort is a very powerful feeling that can have a profound effect on our actions. All of us have strong built-in instincts to avoid actions that cause us discomfort. Furthermore, I believe that discomfort can serve a useful purpose. It can act as a homeostatic mechanism that keeps us from doing things that might cause us harm—like the discomfort we feel if we get too close to the edge of a cliff. However, it also seems that discomfort is not always an accurate indicator of what is truly best. I believe that the level of discomfort we feel in medical practice has far more to do with *change* than with what is actually right. That is, each of us develops particular patterns of behavior. We become comfortable with those behaviors, and we get uncomfortable when we're asked to change them. But, in my case at least, discomfort can't discriminate very well between various types of change. In particular, it tends to resist *proper* change—behavior changes that are required to respond to a changing environment—almost as forcefully as it resists *im*proper change. For example, practitioners can cling to a "time-honored" practice, like diethylstilbestrol for pregnant women, long after trials have shown it doesn't work. So when I feel discomfort about an impending change, I view it as a signal that I should be cautious and think carefully. It's as though my stomach is alerting my mind to switch into high gear. But I don't let the discomfort control my actions. I give my mind priority over my stomach. It takes me some time to bring my stomach around, but it does come around eventually and the discomfort goes away. Does that make sense?

R: In general, yes. But how does that translate to this guideline?

DME: This guideline is responding to a profound and rather sudden change in the environment in which medicine is practiced. The idea that resources are limited calls for rather sharp changes in our behavior. Hence the discomfort. How should practitioners deal with it? They should examine changes in the environment, examine the guideline, and then assure themselves that the guideline is in fact an appropriate response to the changing environment. If so, they should thank their discomfort for signaling the need for caution, but not let it get in the way of change. Eventually the discomfort will go away, and the new way of practicing will become the comfortable one.

R: Okay. Then help me intellectualize the need to accept this change. To do this, I'd like to try an approach that might seem backward. I want *you* to identify what you consider to be the *weakest* points of your argument. So I'll pose the question this way. Suppose I wanted to undo this whole thing and get my autonomy back; what are the key parts of your argument that I should try to destroy?

DME: That's a great question. I would identify the two main premises on which the team approach is based. One is that resources are limited. If there are limits, we can't do everything we want to do and we have to make choices.

R: I won't argue with that premise. All I have to do is read a newspaper or turn on a TV.

DME: The second premise is that the objective is to maximize the quality of care for the entire group. That premise did several things. First, it highlighted the importance of making someone responsible for people who are not currently under anyone's care, like women who need cervical cancer screening. Second, it created the medical director's authority to be responsible for the entire spectrum of patients. Third, it answered the question about whose responsibilities deserve priority—the medical director's or the practitioner's. This premise says that the broader the responsibility, the higher the priority.

R: I remember how in one of your previous chapters, your father decided that for his granddaughter he would recommend a health care organization that maximized care for the group as a whole.[3] I asked myself the same question about my family, and I came to the same conclusion.

DME: Then let's try this right now. You are about to join an HMO. You are considering two, and they both charge the same rates. One of them has a guideline that prevents 40 severe but nonfatal reactions to contrast agents, but lets 100 women die from cervical cancer. The other prevents the cancer deaths, but has 40 more reactions. Which HMO would you join?

R: Clunk. There's no question—the latter. Okay, I'll agree with the second premise. I guess that means that I agree with the team approach. Then here's the bottom line. Whatever the merits of the team approach, do you actually believe that any organizations will achieve it?

DME: Because the idea of physician autonomy is so deeply entrenched, I fear that the transition to teamwork will be a fairly painful process. But I am confident of three things. First, it *will* happen, because the changing environment demands it. Second, the organizations that first succeed in developing a team approach will be the ones that will thrive in the new environment. Third, the organizations that fail to achieve the team approach will dwindle.

R: Well, the next few years should be very interesting.

DME: Indeed.

This conversation is hypothetical, based on conversations with several radiologists and other practitioners.

❖ References

1. Eddy DM. Applying cost-effectiveness analysis: the inside story. *JAMA.* 1992;268: 2575-2582 (Chapter 22).
2. Eddy DM. Resolving conflicts in practice policies. *JAMA.* 1990;264:389-391 (Chapter 9).
3. Eddy DM. Cost-effectiveness analysis: will it be accepted? *JAMA.* 1992;268:132-136 (Chapter 21).

❖ Source

Originally published in *JAMA.* 1993;269:1849-1855.

❖ CHAPTER 24

Three Battles
to Watch
in the 1990s

However the debate on national health system reform comes out, and whatever strategies are eventually used to achieve the seemingly incompatible goals of providing universal access, improving quality, and controlling costs, one thing is certain: The day-to-day decisions of those who actually provide health care will be put under ever-increasing stress. Reform will not solve the problems that have been causing the pressure on physician decision making over the last decade; to the contrary, it will rely on *increasing* the pressure to force practitioners and health plans to solve the problems.

We know this will occur for several reasons. Begin with the fact that of the three main goals of health care reform—access, quality, and cost—the driving force is cost. To be more precise, the driving force is the *rate of increase* in costs—the fact that health care costs have been rising at about twice the rate of inflation. It is this feature of health care that has transformed it from a stable and predictable, albeit large item in business and government budgets into an uncontrollable item that is consuming larger and larger amounts of resources. As it keeps busting out of its budget, health care pushes other programs to the side, and forces managers and legislators to raise additional funds to cover the deficits it leaves in its trail. It is this "excess" rate of increase in health care costs that has brought on the current health care crisis, and the pressures for health care reform either at the national or local level will not rest until that feature has been controlled.

The next fact is that no matter how ingenious policymakers and politicians are in designing systems for financing care, reform of financing alone will not solve the cost problem. Whether we end up with managed competition, single payer, all payer, "pay or play," vouchers, national health insurance, state autonomy, or anything else, all that financing systems can do is

235

reroute the payments; they cannot make them go away. For example, expanding employer-based financing through "pay or play" might appear to bury the cost problem in the deep pockets of business. But as far as health care is concerned, business is not a money tree; it is a money conduit. In the end, the costs "paid" by business will have to resurface to be paid by the public through the equivalents of sales taxes (if business covers the costs through price increases), payroll taxes (if business has to cut back employees' salaries or other benefits), capital gains taxes (if the costs come out of profits), and/or unemployment (if the costs affect market share and foreign competition). A similar story can be told for all the other financing systems that have been proposed.

This is not to say that it makes no difference which financing system is ultimately chosen. The chosen system will determine who gets hit first with the costs and therefore who feels the greatest need to solve the problem (eg, consumers, business, state governments, the federal government). It will also affect how the costs will be distributed when they eventually filter down to be paid by the public—how progressive or regressive the payments will be (eg, direct payments, sales taxes, income taxes, social security taxes). Perhaps most important for achieving cost control, whatever financing system is selected will determine the range of incentives, the instruments, and the amount of pressure that can be applied on various parties to solve the real problem. The pressure points and techniques for controlling costs available to businesses are very different from those available to governments. But the fact remains that no matter how hard we try to launder health care costs, there is no magic financing formula that will make them go away. Solving the cost problem will require going to its source—to the factors that are generating the excess rate of growth.

This leads to the third fact. No attempt to control the excess increase in health care costs will be successful over the long term unless it addresses the decisions physicians make about treatments. (I will use the word "treatment" very broadly to include any type of health care intervention, ranging from primary prevention through support care.) According to the Congressional Research Service, about 42% of the growth in health care expenditures is general price inflation, and another 9% is due to the growth and aging of the population.[1] These factors are beyond the control of health care reform. Of the remaining 49%, about 17% is due to medical price inflation in excess of general price inflation. Although that is potentially controllable and will be an obvious target for reform, even if it were totally eliminated it would correct only a portion (about a third) of the excess increase. The remainder, 32% of the total increase in costs but a full two thirds of the controllable portion, is due to other factors, primarily increases in the volume and intensity of services that exceed anything explained by demographics. If the fight to control health care costs is to be successful, it will have to address this aspect of health care. Efforts to reduce administrative costs, schedule operating rooms more efficiently, streamline cafeterias, and root out obvious waste and inefficiency are important ways to set costs back, release some pressure, and buy some time. These steps should definitely be taken, but they will not permanently reduce the excess rate of increase that is at the heart of the cost problem.[2] Until something is done to control the volume and intensity of services, the expansive growth in costs will eventually reappear to demand attention.

The facts are clear. Sooner or later, one way or another, the solution to the cost problem will have to address practitioners' decisions about treatments. Unless physicians can somehow solve the problem on their own, or unless the country makes an about-face and decides to give health care whatever portion of any budget it wants, the forces being reflected in health care reform will inevitably collide with one of the most cherished features of clinical practice—control over day-to-day decisions about how patients should be treated. This collision will not be an unintentional by-product of reform; it will be one of the main *instruments* of reform. The changes in structures and incentives that are being proposed are not designed to solve the cost problem directly; they are designed to create incentives to force health plan administrators, medical directors, and practitioners to solve the cost problem.

Unfortunately, the result will be battles—battles over what practitioners do, and how they do it. Three in particular will be especially important to watch as the decade unfolds, because they will address the intellectual core of physician decision making. Those battles will be over evidence, costs, and physician autonomy.

❖ Evidence

The question here is: How much evidence is needed to say that a treatment is "appropriate," that it should be used, and that it should be paid for? Traditionally, a decision to use a particular treatment could be justified by little more than a claim that it was "standard and accepted," or that the individual physician believed that it was in the patient's best interest, or simply that no other treatment was available. However, the credibility of clinical judgment, whether exercised individually or collectively, has been severely challenged by observations of wide variations in practices, inappropriate care, and practitioner uncertainty.[3] The presumption that if a treatment is widely used it must have *some* benefit has been shaken not only by reports that many common treatments have no supporting evidence of effectiveness,[4] but by actual trials that have overturned some common beliefs, such as the value of encainide and flecainide for heart attacks[5] and steroids for acute optic neuritis.[6] The response has been a gradual but persistent movement to require documentation beyond the testimony of experts and the existence of a consensus, and to require empirical evidence of benefit before recommending that a treatment be used.[7-9] Despite the fact that this trend is quite consistent with the Hippocratic maxim of "First do no harm," it will be fought. Some will fight it as an insult to physician judgment, or a threat to physician control. But even those who concur with the principle that decisions should be backed by evidence might balk when that principle uproots one of their favorite treatments.

What Evidence Is Needed to Be 'Sufficient'?

The battles over evidence will cover three main issues. The first concerns just how much and what type of evidence is "sufficient" to justify a treatment's coverage and use. Examples of specific questions include: What end points must be demonstrated in a clinical trial? Are actual health outcomes needed, such as survival or quality of life, or will intermediate outcomes do, such as normalization of serum enzyme levels or the disappearance of a tumor on x-rays? Whatever end points are used, do studies have to be controlled, or will stacks of uncontrolled clinical series be persuasive? Must the designs be prospective or can they be retrospective or historical? Indeed, if enough experts agree that a treatment is effective, is it necessary to have any empirical evidence at all? (And just how many experts are "enough"?) These issues are well illustrated by several current problems.

How Many Studies Are Required?   The Minnesota randomized controlled trial of the fecal occult blood test, which began almost two decades ago, has finally been reported.[10] It showed a statistically significant 33% reduction in mortality (from about 9 per 1000 to about 6 per 1000). It is the only study of fecal occult blood tests to show a significant reduction in mortality from colorectal cancer. Although others have shown a shift in stage or nonsignificant trends, they have not yet shown a mortality reduction.[11] Is the result of this single trial sufficient to justify a recommendation that all adults between the ages of 50 and 70 years (about 43 million people) be screened annually with fecal occult blood tests, at a risk of a 9% false-positive rate and an annual cost of about $4 billion?

Will Retrospective Designs Suffice?   Although there are good theoretical reasons to believe that sigmoidoscopy should reduce mortality from colorectal cancer, that belief has never been confirmed in any prospective controlled trial. The best evidence to date consists of a single retrospective case-control study, involving 261 cases and 868 controls.[12] It showed that screening at intervals up to 10 years can achieve a 60% reduction in mortality for cancers within reach of the scope. Is that sufficient to advocate screening millions of people?

Are Intermediate Outcomes Acceptable?   Several randomized controlled trials have shown that a 6-month course of interferon alfa reduces transaminase levels in a statistically significant proportion of patients with hepatitis C (about 20% of patients in the treated group had normal transaminase levels 6 months after termination of treatment).[13] Clinical common sense would indicate that this is a desirable result. However, as encouraging as it is, it tells us little about the effect of interferon on the actual outcomes that patients care about, such as whether they will die of cirrhosis or liver failure 5 or 10 years from now. Expectations for the effect of interferon alfa on these outcomes are muted by several factors. A recent study of patients with non-A, non-B hepatitis who were not treated with interferon alfa had no higher overall mortality after 18 years of follow-up.[14] The difference in deaths due to liver deaths was small (1.8%), which puts an upper bound on the potential effectiveness of interferon alfa. The long-term effects of the treatment on the immunological system are unknown. Finally, normalization of enzymes at 6 months does not guarantee that the disease would not reactivate any time in the future. So the question is, does improvement in the short-term intermediate outcome with interferon alfa justify use of this treatment?

If Enough Experts Testify, Do We Need Evidence at All?   Interest in screening men for prostate cancer with prostate-specific antigen (PSA) is sweeping the country. However, a hard look reveals that the evidence of effectiveness for this screening test is weaker than for virtually any other screening test that has been widely recommended. Not only are there no prospective controlled studies showing a reduction in prostate cancer mortality, there are barely any studies showing an improvement in intermediate outcomes. The evidence consists solely of observations that the test can detect occult prostate cancers.[15] But even that is clouded by uncertainty about the natural history and clinical significance of those lesions. In fact, the "evidence" that is actually driving this national campaign is the testimony of some experts and the visibility of prominent individuals who have had lesions detected by PSA. Is this sufficient to justify a false-positive rate of about 13%, a lot of unnecessary surgery or radiation, and billions of dollars in costs?

These issues might seem dry and methodological, but they have profound practical and therefore political implications. Because the quality of evidence for different treatments varies so widely, the resolution of these seemingly methodological issues could swing the doors of coverage open, or could clang them shut for hundreds of treatments.

Who Has the Burden of Proof?

The second main issue that will arise in battles over the quality of evidence is this: Who bears the burden of proof? Is a treatment considered "investigational" until someone produces sufficient evidence that it is effective and appropriate (however we end up defining "sufficient")? Or is a treatment assumed to be effective and appropriate until someone shows it is not? As a country, we have a long history of wanting it both ways on this issue. The Food and Drug Act is based on the premise that a new drug is assumed to be investigational for an indication until it is shown in "multiple, well controlled studies" to be effective. On the other hand, once a drug is approved to be marketed for any one indication, physicians are legally free to use it for any other indication without any additional evidence. Hundreds of diagnostic tests, devices, procedures, and services are currently used and paid for without any evidence of effectiveness for any indication.

This issue is well illustrated by the long-standing debate over recommendations to screen women younger than the age of 50 years with mammography. The battle lines were drawn about 15 years ago when the National Cancer Institute (NCI) held the first consensus conference and concluded that there was not sufficient evidence to recommend screening in this age group. With this finding, the NCI implicitly put the burden of proof on those who want to recommend mammography. However, in 1983, the American Cancer Society (ACS) reversed its position. This move was not justified by any dramatic change in evidence. The only new evidence was indirect and uncontrolled.[16] What this new position really represented was a shift in the burden of proof. The ACS reasoned that, given the frequency and seriousness of the disease, unless there was proof mammography was *not* effective, policymakers should assume that it was. In subsequent years questions grew about the effectiveness of screening the younger age group as more and more trials began to publish their results.

There were just as many equivocal or negative studies as positive ones. In 1988, the public position of the ACS was reinforced by nine other organizations. They apparently agreed with the ACS that the burden of proof should be on those who want to not recommend mammography. But other groups, such as the US Preventive Services Task Force and the American College of Physicians, held to the position that, given the very high stakes (there are about 15 million women between the ages of 40 and 50 years), the burden was to have good evidence of effectiveness before a recommendation to screen should be made. The issue came to a head again this winter with the publication of the Canadian trial[17]—the only trial specifically designed to determine the value of mammography in this age group. Although not statistically significant, it found an *increased* mortality in the group that was offered screening. As might be expected, the study's design and results were challenged by mammography's proponents, but a blue-ribbon panel of the NCI recently confirmed that there is no evidence of benefit in this age group. So the battle lines are drawn again. The ACS continues to recommend screening women age 40 to 50 years, saying that there is still no proof it is not effective, while the US Preventive Services Task Force and the American College of Physicians are no doubt even more confident that there is no proof that it is.

It is difficult to overstate the importance of this issue. The less one knows about the effectiveness of a treatment, the more important the burden of proof becomes. In a field filled with uncertainty and doubt, the difference between "when in doubt, do it" and "when in doubt, stop" could easily swing $100 billion a year.

Old vs New Treatments

A related issue pertains to the evaluation of "old" vs "new" treatments. Currently, the overwhelming proportion of research funding and administrative attention goes to new treatments. The Food and Drug Administration requires evidence of effectiveness for new indications for drugs before they can be marketed. Insurers concentrate on new treatments when they make coverage decisions. In the meantime, hundreds of "old" treatments that have been grandfathered in during a period when the threshold for "sufficient evidence" was much lower, continue to be marketed, used, and paid for. This is the famous 80% to 90% of treatments that have not been adequately evaluated with controlled studies.[18]

In essence, different burdens of proof have evolved for new vs old treatments. But there are no theoretical reasons—medical, economic, or ethical— that old treatments should not be held to the same standards as new ones. The reasons they are not have more to do with logistics and a fear of professional and public outcry than with any logic or theory. Nobody has the resources to systematically examine all existing treatments. Even if they did, if modern standards of evidence were applied to all medical practices, a huge proportion would be thrown into limbo, hundreds of "standard and accepted" practices would be disrupted, and medical practice would be in chaos.

On the other hand, if we are really serious about rooting out ineffective treatments, eliminating waste, and controlling costs, why should old treatments be exempt? Even if there are not enough resources to study all old treatments, it is certainly possible to scrutinize some of the most important ones.

Lack of Evidence for Old Treatments. A recent example of a very common and important old treatment for which there is no definitive evidence of benefit (over doing nothing) is surgical or radiation treatment for early prostate cancer.[19] A sense of how representative this problem is can be gained from the following anecdote. At a workshop on methods for evaluating medical practices for specialty societies, groups of participants reviewed the evidence that supported various treatments that were important to their specialties.[20] The treatments included such things as tympanostomy for otitis media, prenatal screening for the human immunodeficiency virus infection, prophylactic lidocaine for patients with chest pain, in-hospital rehabilitation for women with hip fractures, arteriography for patients with pulmonary embolism, and pulse oximetry for patients undergoing conscious sedation. For each of these problems, the participants classified the existing evidence as "excellent," "good," "fair," "poor," or "none." For only one problem was there excellent evidence that compared the effectiveness of the treatment on an important outcome. For 18 of the problems, the evidence was "poor" or "none." For two problems, there was "good" evidence. Unfortunately, for those problems the evidence *contradicted* current practices.

Like the previous issues relating to evidence, this issue has very important implications for what treatments physicians can offer their patients and what they will be paid for. Like the other issues there is no way to estimate precisely what the potential impact really is—we do not even know how much we do not know. But one thing is certain; the stakes again are high.

❖ Costs

Virtually everyone now recognizes that the cost of health care is a major national problem that must be solved. Over the long run, the excess rate of increase can be controlled only by addressing its main source—increases in the volume and intensity of services. The cost problem cannot be separated from the content of clinical care—from the decisions practitioners make about their patients.

Drawing Lines Between Quality and Cost

Like the battles over evidence, the battles over costs will take place on several fronts. The most familiar will be issues relating to where to draw the lines for the intensity of a treatment or for the patients to whom it should be applied.

Drawing the Lines on Treatments.   A wide variety of clinical decisions involve a treatment that can be applied with different degrees of intensity. This raises an obvious question: Which level of intensity is appropriate? For one example, screening tests can be offered at virtually any frequency. As the frequency is increased, the benefits increase, but so do the costs, and with each notch up in the frequency, the amount of benefit gained gets smaller and smaller as the "flat of the curve" is approached. Some of the most visible debates include 1-year vs 3-year Papanicolaou tests and 1-year vs 2-year mammograms, but this type of problem is surprisingly common. For example, how frequent should follow-up visits be scheduled for a patient on antihypertensive medications? How long should interferon alfa be given to patients with hepatitis C—6 months, 1 year, forever? What is the appropriate dose of lovastatin—20 mg, 40 mg? How long should a patient with chronic knee pain be managed conservatively before arthroscopy is indicated?

Drawing the Lines on Patients.   There are also many examples of treatments that can potentially be given to a broad range of patients defined by some continuous variable. Virtually everyone agrees that moderate and severe hypertension should be treated; what about mild hypertension? If you believe that glaucoma treatment is effective, what level of intraocular pressure justifies the treatment to prevent glaucoma? If screening colonoscopy should be reserved for high-risk patients, what is the line that defines high risk? The National Cholesterol Education Program (NCEP) recommends drug treatment for people with two or more risk factors who, after a trial of diet, have low-density lipoprotein cholesterol levels higher than 4.14 mmol/L (160 mg/dL). Why not 3.88 mmol/L (150 mg/dL), or 4.40 mmol/L (170 mg/dL)?

Questions like these present some of the best opportunities for controlling the cost of health care. They are also extremely common—so common that we tend to forget that they involve trade-offs between quality and cost. But they do, and as the screws tighten on costs, these types of questions will arise more and more frequently, and will become more and more contentious.

Sibling Treatments

The second type of battle over costs will occur when there are two treatments for the same problem that differ slightly in benefit, but differ a lot in cost—what I will call "sibling treatments."

Similar Benefit but Different Costs.   The recent debate over ionic and nonionic contrast agents in low-risk patients is one example.[21] But a newer battle has just reached the horizon. The Global Utilization of Streptokinase and Tissue-type Plasminogen Activator (t-PA) for Occluded Arteries (GUSTO) trial showed that t-PA can shave an additional 1% off the short-term mortality compared with streptokinase (30-day mortality is about 7% with streptokinase vs about 6% with t-PA), but at a cost of more than $2000 per patient (Eric J. Topol, unpublished data, April 30, 1993). Is $2000 too much to pay for a 1% greater chance of surviving past the 30-day mark?

In short, wherever there is a choice of drugs (eg, for antihypertensives, antibiotics, diuretics, antiarthritics), or diagnostic tests (eg, plain films, computed tomographic scans, magnetic resonance imaging), or treatment sites (eg, hospital, outpatient, home), or any other aspect of a treatment, trade-offs will have to be made between quality and cost, and battles will arise.

It's Not Much, but It's All We've Got

As difficult as the problems raised by sibling treatments might be, they have several features that soften the emotional impact. In particular, the disagreements will be about differences in benefit that are relatively small and probabilistic. Instead of switching a patient from "cure" to "no cure," the effect of choosing the less expensive treatment will be only to change the *probability* of some event by a small amount. Furthermore, because this type of battle always involves another option, even if a decision is made to use the less expensive, less effective treatment, the practitioner will still have something to offer.

A more difficult case arises when there is only one treatment to offer the patient. This greatly increases the perceived value of the available treatment, even if its benefits are still small and probabilistic compared with no treatment at all. The patient will usually be acutely aware that there is no alternative, and there is no way for patients or practitioners to retreat to the comfort of knowing that at least something was done. Even if the actual improvement in outcomes is just a few percent, as far as the patient is concerned, the treatment itself is all or nothing.

Small Benefit but No Alternative

This type of problem is well illustrated by "last hope" cancer treatments. Suppose high-dose chemotherapy with autologous bone marrow transplantation is eventually shown to increase 5-year, disease-free survival by 8% in women with metastatic breast cancer. Does that justify $50 000 to $150 000? If so, how about 4%, or 2%?

It's All We've Got and It's a Lot

The fourth type of battle raises the stakes one more level. Like the case of "last hope" treatments, this controversy arises when there is no alternative treatment, but it adds the element that the treatment's effect is large and certain, not small and probabilistic.

No Alternative and Big Benefit

This case is well illustrated by enzyme replacement treatment for Gaucher's disease, a rare genetic lysosomal storage disease caused by a deficiency of glucosylceramidase. An infantile form is characterized by severe neurologic involvement and early death. An adult form is much milder, with the diagnosis often being made as an incidental finding of splenomegaly or thrombocytopenia. There is no neurologic involvement, but pathologic fractures, bone pain, pulmonary infiltrates, and moderate liver dysfunction can occur. The clinical course is variable and many patients live a full life. Until recently, treatment was symptomatic and relatively unsatisfactory—such as bone marrow transplants for thrombocytopenia. But now a replacement for the enzyme has been developed that for all intents and purposes corrects the disorder. The problem is that the enzyme costs between $200 000 and $400 000 a year, depending on the dose. Depending on the severity of a patient's symptoms and where one draws the line, it could be required for the rest of the patient's life. Is that too much to pay?

If you want to contemplate a more intense debate, imagine that investigators succeed in developing lung or heart-lung transplants to the point that they can prolong the lives of patients with terminal lung disease. Now think of the thousands of smokers who die of emphysema every year.

Futile Care

The final type of battle over cost is the most public: How much do we want to spend on futile treatments—treatments that do not have any reasonable probability of providing a quality of life that would be satisfactory to the patient?[22] By definition, these treatments offer little or nothing to the patient. Their main purpose seems to be to satisfy the family's desire that everything possible be done, and to satisfy a social value that it is unacceptable to give up, even when the effort is clearly futile. Although precise estimates are impossible, a conservative one is that tens of billions of dollars could be saved and reallocated to provide much greater benefit to other patients. But making the switch will be controversial to say the least.

❖ Viewpoints for Watching the Battles

Those who want to watch the battles over evidence and costs should keep their eyes on two main sites: coverage exclusions and practice guidelines.

Coverage Exclusions

Coverage exclusions are an integral part of any benefits package. Benefit packages, like the one being developed as part of President Clinton's proposal for health care reform, begin by describing general categories of treatments that will be covered, such as in-hospital care, preventive services, and emergency services. But within these categories are broad ranges of treatments that vary from highly beneficial to unknown to downright harmful, and health plans will have to determine which are which. To handle this problem, benefit packages also contain criteria for excluding specific treatments. This creates the circumstances for at least two types of battles. The first involves the language that specifies the exclusion criteria. The second arises when plans apply that language to individual treatments.

On the first point, the exclusion criteria that will emerge from health care reform will include such terms as "investigational," "medically necessary," "reasonable," "appropriate," and "judicious." Depending on how these terms are defined, billions of dollars worth of treatments will be swept to one side or the other. As the nation moves toward health care reform, there will be several opportunities to define these terms. First in line to assume that task will be those who draft the legislation. They can try their hand at developing precise, operational definitions. However, with precision comes controversy, so it is easy to imagine that legislators will decide to leave the language vague. If they choose not to be precise, the next opportunity to write the language will fall to those who write the regulations that implement the legislative language. However, they too can leave the language imprecise. This pattern can be repeated, with the responsibility for developing specific criteria being passed to states, to health insurance purchasing cooperatives, or to health plans themselves. Even the plans can leave the language vague, in which case the task of interpreting whatever words exist will fall to the individual committees in each plan, where the need for interpretation will reoccur every time another treatment comes up for a decision.

Sooner or later, the criteria will have to be defined, and whenever and wherever that happens, there will be controversies. Things to watch for will be the definition of "investigational"—the quality of evidence it requires, how it will be applied to old vs new treatments, and who will have the burden of proof. Also important will be any language that indicates how costs should be incorporated in the decisions. Options range from not mentioning costs at all, to addressing only the least controversial cases (eg, similar benefit, dissimilar costs), to tackling a comprehensive set of criteria. Finally, it will be important to watch not just *what* the details of the criteria say, but *where* each detail is added—at the national, state, purchasing cooperative, plan, or committee level. The level at which the details are written will determine how consistent the criteria will be across plans, and the amount of fairness vs turmoil that will result. There are compelling theoretical reasons to be as specific as possible at the national level, but there are also compelling political reasons to pass the responsibility to the next layer down.

After the language is written a whole new set of controversies will arise when it comes time to actually apply whatever language is developed. Those controversies will also occur at several different levels. National policies could be set by a national board, regional policies could be developed by states or purchasing cooperatives, and plans will address the remaining issues. For a variety of reasons, such as allowing for local autonomy as well as avoiding national controversies, the great majority of the coverage decisions will probably be made by individual health plans. This means that every committee in every plan will face a potential battle every time it tries to apply the criteria to another treatment.

Guidelines

The second main place where battles will occur is guidelines. Exclusion criteria are fairly blunt instruments for controlling the use of treatments. Generally they are applied to entire treatments, such as basal metabolic rates or surgical treatment for obesity. They can also be applied to particular indications for a treatment, but that usually occurs only when there are clear lines between indications. For example, coverage of high-dose chemotherapy and autologous bone marrow transplantation might be granted for Hodgkin's disease and acute lymphocytic leukemia, but not for breast cancer. Coverage exclusions are usually too blunt to distinguish between, say, 3-year vs 1-year Papanicolaou tests, giving t-PA only within 4 hours of the patient's heart attack, or a particular dose of glucosylceramidase for Gaucher's disease depending on the severity of the patient's symptoms. That type of fine-tuning requires guidelines and related instruments for steering clinical decisions (eg, formulary decisions, clinical protocols, preutilization criteria, and quality review criteria).

As with the battles over coverage policies, battles over guidelines can be fought over both the language and its application. In this case the language will address the principles and methods that should be used to design a guideline. The language should define the key terms and provide instructions for evaluating evidence; estimating outcomes; incorporating expert judgment; balancing benefits, harms, and costs; and incorporating logistical restrictions. As abstract as this might seem, the definitions and instructions can have tremendous leverage over the guidelines that come out the other end.

The battles over guidelines will only begin with the methods. Every time a new guideline problem is encountered, the language will have to be applied to actual evidence in actual settings. The interpretations are almost never clearcut, and every new problem is likely to have some special feature that cannot be anticipated or captured in a terse set of instructions. Developing guidelines for these problems will require judgment, interpolation, and negotiation. If all the parties agree on the goals and principles, the process can go smoothly. But if just one or two do not, a battle will arise.

Both these types of battles—the language and the applications—can be fought at each of the political levels. A national board could specify preferred methods and could recommend or even impose some national guidelines. States and purchasing cooperatives could add details to the language and write some regional guidelines. But as with coverage exclusions, most of the responsibilities will fall on health plans. Indeed, guidelines will probably be one of the main factors on which health plans will compete as they try to maximize the value they can provide for their budget. Because guidelines are so pervasive and because they do the fine-tuning that touches the physician and patient most closely, they will probably be the most visible and personal manifestations of the battles over evidence and cost.

❖ Physician Autonomy

Many physicians will not like these trends. Indeed, many of them will be volunteering for duty to fight the battles. The reasons are obvious. These trends threaten what has historically been one of the most desirable features of medical practice—the autonomy of physicians to make their own decisions. Until very recently, the mandate to physicians has been to apply their best judgment to provide the best possible care to their individual patients as they see it. Both components of that mandate are under scrutiny—the quality of their judgments, and the idea of maximizing services for an individual patient without concern about the effects on the health of others.

Many practitioners will see the efforts to address evidence and costs as a badly needed step to help solve the problems of uncertainty, variations, and inappropriateness, and to help correct the inconsistencies and questionable outcomes they bring. These practitioners will understand that it is no more insulting to use a guideline than it is to get help from any other source, such as reading a journal or calling a colleague. But others will have a different view. At the extreme, some practitioners will see the efforts to shape medical decisions as insulting, as an usurpation of control, and as a retraction of their perceived right to do as they please. They will be sorely tempted not only to fight the changes, but to ignore the coverage policies and guidelines that result.

And they could well succeed. The very nature of a guideline is that it is intended to be advice, not an order. Although guidelines are less blunt than coverage policies, they are still too blunt to be applied categorically to all patients in a computer-like fashion, with no interpretation, judgment, or tailoring by practitioners.[23] To be at their best, guidelines must be applied flexibly by informed, sensitive practitioners. But wherever there is flexibility, there is the potential for manipulation. If a practitioner wants to subvert a guideline, he or she can do it. Practitioners can be provided incentives, sent reminders, and given feedback, but in the end no one can force them to apply a particular treatment.

Herein we find the last battle. Practitioners who are determined to block the implementation of a guideline will be able to do so, as innumerable studies of unsuccessful implementations have shown. Guidelines are easy to sabotage by any number of techniques, ranging from filibustering committees, to behind-the-scenes politicking, to finding loopholes in the wording, to simply ignoring the guideline.

Practitioners who choose this course will be involved in two battles. One will be the visible battle with administrators, medical directors, and colleagues on committees, as they tie up efforts to reach agreement. The other will be more subtle. When resources are limited, the activities of all practitioners are connected.[24] Practitioners who consume resources for uses that please them will be depriving resources from other practitioners for other uses. Ideally, practitioners as a team will agree on the best ways to use the resources. Those who deviate from the team's decisions will be undermining their colleagues' efforts to make the best out of an uncomfortable situation. This battle will not only undermine the intended effect of their colleagues' decisions on patient care, it will also sap the spirit of cooperation that will be essential to developing a successful response to the demands of health care reform.

❖ The Future

In many respects, the future of medical practice—both in technical terms of what treatments can be offered and in more abstract terms of practitioners' quality of life—will be determined by how these battles over evidence, cost, and autonomy are fought and resolved. Questions about how much evidence is needed to justify an action, how those actions should be constrained by costs, or the practitioner's right to follow his or her own instincts go to the heart of clinical practice. Given the forces that are affecting medicine today, some change is inevitable. Also inevitable is some disagreement about how to accomplish that change. The challenge is to channel disagreements away from destructive personal fights into a constructive force that helps locate the best solution to an admittedly difficult problem. A key to accomplishing this is to agree in advance on the principles that should guide the debates. Without agreement on the principles, discussions can easily spin off into contention, bitterness, and bad decisions. *With* agreement on the principles, the discussions can become positive exercises that focus on the true merits of the different positions and that find solutions to very difficult problems.

❖ References

1. Congressional Research Service. Analysis of national health expenditure data. In: Committee on Ways & Means, US House of Representatives. *Health Care Resource Book, April 16, 1991*. Washington, DC: Congressional Research Service; 1991.
2. Eddy DM. Health system reform: will controlling costs require rationing services? *JAMA*. 1994;272:324-328.
3. Eddy DM. The challenge. *JAMA*. 1990;263:287-290.
4. Institute of Medicine. *Assessing Medical Technologies*. Washington, DC: National Academy of Sciences; 1985.
5. Akiyama T, Pawitan Y, Greenberg H, Kuo C, Reynolds-Haertle R. Increased risk of death and cardiac arrest from encainide and flecainide in patients after non-Q-wave acute myocardial infarction in the Cardiac Arrhythmia Suppression Trial. *Am J Cardiol*. 1991;68:1551-1555.
6. Beck R, Cleary P, Andreson M Jr, et al. A randomized controlled trial of corticosteroids in the treatment of acute optic neuritis. *N Engl J Med*. 1992;326:581-588.
7. Eddy DM. Practice policies—guidelines for methods. *JAMA*. 1990;263:1839-1841.
8. Evidence-Based Medicine Working Group. Evidence-based medicine: a new approach to teaching the practice of medicine. *JAMA*. 1992;268:2420-2425.
9. Sox HC, Woolf SH. Evidence-based practice guidelines from the US Preventive Services Task Force. *JAMA*. 1993;269:2678.
10. Mandel J, Bond J, Church T, et al. Reducing mortality from colorectal cancer by screening for fecal occult blood. *N Engl J Med*. 1993;328:1365-1371.
11. Winawer S. Colorectal cancer screening comes of age. *N Engl J Med*. 1993;328:1416-1417.
12. Selby J, Friedman G, Quesenberry C Jr, Weiss N. A case-control study of screening sigmoidoscopy and mortality from colorectal cancer. *N Engl J Med*. 1992;326:653-657.
13. Davis G, Balart L, Schiff E, et al. Treatment of chronic hepatitis C with recombinant interferon alfa: a multicenter randomized, controlled trial. *N Engl J Med*. 1989;321:1501-1506.
14. Seeff LB, Buskell-Bales Z, Wright EC, et al. Long-term mortality after transfusion-associated non-A, non-B hepatitis. *N Engl J Med*. 1992;327:1906-1911.
15. Mettlin C, Lee F, Drago J, Murphy GP. The American Cancer Society National Prostate Cancer Detection Program: findings on the detection of early prostate cancer in 2425 men. *Cancer*. 1991;67:2949-2958.
16. Baker L. Breast Cancer Detection Demonstration Project: five-year summary report. *CA*. 1982;32:194-225.
17. Miller A, Baines C, To T, Wall C. Canadian National Breast Screening Study, I: breast cancer detection and death rates among women ages 40 to 49 years. *Can Med Assoc J*. 1992;147:1459-1476.

18. Office of Technology Assessment, US Congress. *Report on Assessing Efficacy and Safety of Medical Technologies*. Washington DC: Office of Technology Assessment; 1978.
19. Fleming C, Wasson J, Albertsen P, Barry M, Wennberg J. A decision analysis of alternative treatment strategies for clinically localized prostate cancer. *JAMA*. 1993; 269:2650-2658.
20. Eddy DM. Uncertainty, outcomes, and the quality of medical care. In: *Proceedings: Cornerstones of Health Care in the Nineties: Forging a Framework of Excellence*. September 16-18, 1990; Hot Springs, Va. Sponsored by the Joint Commission on Accreditation of Healthcare Organizations and The Prudential Insurance Company of America.
21. Eddy DM. Applying cost-effectiveness analysis: the inside story. *JAMA*. 1992;268: 2575-2582 (Chapter 22).
22. Lundberg G. American health care system management objectives: the aura of inevitability becomes incarnate. *JAMA*. 1993;269:2554-2555.
23. Eddy DM. Designing a practice policy: standards, guidelines, and options. *JAMA*. 1990;263:3077, 3081, 3084 (Chapter 8).
24. Eddy DM. Broadening the responsibilities of practitioners: the team approach. *JAMA*. 1993;269:1849-1855 (Chapter 23).

❖ Source

Originally published in *JAMA*. 1993;270:520-526.

Principles for Making Difficult Decisions in Difficult Times

In the last chapter I described several issues or "battles" that will be particularly contentious in the coming decade.[1] They relate to the evidence needed to justify use of a treatment, to the need to balance a treatment's benefits against its costs, and to the autonomy of physicians to answer these questions for themselves. (I will use the word "treatment" very broadly to encompass any type of health intervention.) One way or another, these issues will be resolved in the next few years. Setting aside for a moment the actual solutions that are developed, the process by which these issues are addressed will provide one of the most visible displays of how the medical profession manages itself and responds to an urgent social need.

The main battlefield on which these issues will be resolved will be debates over coverage and guidelines for individual treatments. These debates will occur in every organization that is responsible for providing health care to a population—ranging from individual health plans, to state Medicaid and public health programs, to Medicare. The debates will occur over each new treatment as it is introduced, as well as over scores of old treatments that have been taken for granted for decades. The debates themselves will be unavoidable. The question is not whether they will occur, but how they will be conducted and the quality of the conclusions.

The key to ensuring that these debates will be resolved in an orderly fashion is to begin by agreeing on the principles that should guide them. If the principles are addressed in advance and in the abstract, the discussions can focus on the important medical, ethical, and economic issues. On the other hand, if there is no agreement on the principles at the beginning, each debate will quickly get mired in the details of the specific treatments and the narrow objectives of particular constituencies.

Ideally, there should be national agreement on a single set of principles. Whether health system reform will provide this type of leadership remains to be seen. However, the fact that no current proposal for national health system reform contains any such principles makes it unlikely that this will occur. In the absence of national leadership, every health care organization will need to create its own set of principles.

To assist this process, this chapter proposes 11 principles that should guide debates over evidence and costs in organizations that must allocate shared or public resources to serve a defined population. "Shared" or "public" resources are accounts built from the contributions of many individuals—through such mechanisms as insurance premiums, health maintenance organization (HMO) dues, and state and federal taxes—to be spent on particular individuals who need treatments. If an individual is paying for a treatment by himself or herself, many of the principles, especially those dealing with costs, become moot.

When they are presented in the abstract, many of the principles will seem obvious, even trivial. However, applying them consistently will require some major shifts in our traditional ways of thinking and will have far-reaching consequences that will make many people uncomfortable. My hope is that health care organizations will debate each of the principles and either will agree with the ones I have proposed or will develop better ones. I also propose that, after it has reached agreement within itself, each organization should make its principles public. This should help achieve "informed consent" among providers, payers, consumers, and patients, and should help all parties develop realistic expectations.

Despite their apparent simplicity, each of the principles begs questions about the best methods for implementing them. A full discussion of the methods is beyond the scope of this chapter. It is important to understand, however, that the validity of a principle does not depend on its ease of implementation. For two obvious examples, the principles "all men are created equal" or "turn the other cheek" are not invalidated by the difficulty of their implementation.

Finally, because the pressure of applying the principles will be most intense for the practitioners who actually provide the treatments, I will sometimes discuss the principles from their point of view. However, the applicability of the principles to all decision makers should be apparent.

❖ The Principles

The first principle deals with costs, because that is the main driving force behind the current changes in medical practice. It is really a premise.

1. The Financial Resources Available to Provide Health Care to a Population Are Limited.

It is crucial that every health care organization reach some conclusion on this premise, because all else follows from it. If this premise is false—if an organization truly faces no limits on the financial resources it has available for treatments—then the remaining principles become simple. In that case, it is acceptable for practitioners and patients to use any treatment they believe offers any hope of benefit. There is no need to determine that the treatment really does provide benefit (unless it also has harms), no need to consider its costs, and no need to make difficult tradeoffs. The only remaining issues are to ensure that any harms of a treatment are outweighed by its benefits and, if more than one treatment is available for a particular health problem, to determine which treatment offers the greatest net benefit. Debates will be relatively peaceful because hardly anyone will be denied what they want.

The position that there are no limits on the amount of money that can be spent on health care treatments will be very popular. Not only do most of us have strong psychological, medical, and financial incentives to behave this way, but it is also a fact that until fairly recently there really were no practical limits on the amount of money available for health care. This is the traditional view, and it is the view that prevailed when most current treatments evolved into common use.

Unfortunately, there is strong empirical support for the premise that, whatever might have been true in the past, financial resources today are limited. Anyone working under capitation or prospective payment is obviously working under limits. Another impressive piece of evidence is the president's proposal for health system reform. It includes not only the limits imposed through the marketplace by competition, but an explicit, enforceable requirement that by 1999, the increase in a health plan's per capita premiums must be kept to the general rate of inflation. Even if this feature of the president's bill is eliminated in the congressional debates, its existence recognizes that the amount of money available for health care is limited. But the acid test for whether financial resources are limited is to simply ask those who are responsible for the budgets of health plans whether they have enough money to do everything everyone wants to do. If not, then the budget is limited.

If it is agreed that there are limits on the financial resources available to a health plan, there still might be disagreement over whether there are limits on the resources available for treatments. Some might feel that it should be possible for a health plan to respond to the financial limits by finding savings in administrative costs and hotel-type services, without having to impose any limits on the use of treatments. In the next chapter, I will argue that it will not be possible to meet the limits imposed by the medical marketplace and health system reform through administrative efficiencies alone and that the limits must affect the use of treatments. In the meantime, it is important to understand that the issue is not whether it should or should not be possible to meet the limits on resources without affecting the use of treatments. The critical question is whether the limits do affect the use of treatments. The presence of such things as precertification, utilization review, case management, fee schedules, restrictive formularies, and guidelines are all indications that the limits are affecting treatments. However, the acid test again is to ask those who are actually responsible for the budgets. Can they find all the savings they need from administrative efficiencies alone, or are they also looking at things such as drug utilization, use of expensive diagnostic tests, referrals to specialists, and expensive procedures? If they are, then the resources available for treatments are limited.

If it is agreed that the financial resources available to an organization for treatments are limited, or if an organization wants to prepare for the day when that will be the case, then it is important to examine the consequences of the first premise. Although there should be little debate about the next three items, because they follow directly from the limits on resources, it is important to state them explicitly.

2. Because Financial Resources Are Limited, When Deciding About the Appropriate Use of Treatments It Is Both Valid and Important to Consider the Financial Costs of the Treatments.

3. Because Financial Resources Are Limited, It Is Necessary to Set Priorities.

4. A Consequence of Priority Setting Is That It Will Not Be Possible to Cover From Shared Resources Every Treatment That Might Have Some Benefit.

One does not have to think very hard to realize that these three principles raise the specter of rationing, which dictionaries define as the "distribution of scarce resources." This is obviously a very unpleasant idea to accept. But the only way to avoid it is to go back and reject the opening premise. Assuming that there is agreement on that premise, the next issue that arises is how the resources should be distributed and how priorities should be set. Most people will agree that the distribution should be equitable in some sense (although some advocacy groups for particular diseases or populations might prefer an unequal distribution in their direction). If we agree that the available resources should be distributed equally, the operational question is, how do we achieve that? This forces us to define the primary objective of health care.

5. The Objective of Health Care Is to Maximize the Health of the Population Served, Subject to the Available Resources.

This principle has enormous importance. In many ways, it is the fundamental principle that underlies the entire health care enterprise. On its face, it seems straightforward. However, as will become clear in a moment, it can be in conflict with another possible objective that we all cherish, which is to maximize the care we provide to every individual. Indeed, principle No. 5 goes to the heart of current debates about the individual vs society.

To clarify this principle, we must first define what we mean by the terms "the population served" and the "health of the population." In the context of these principles, the population served is the total population for which the organization has a responsibility to provide care. In the current system it is convenient to think of examples such as the members of an HMO or the people who qualify for a state Medicaid program. In the terms of health system reform, it is convenient to think of the population covered by a health plan. However, it is also important to recognize that providers can have a responsibility for people outside their particular organization—such as the uninsured who require emergency care.

Without trying to define precisely the outer boundaries of the population served, the important point is that it is much broader than the individual patients seen by an individual practitioner. It includes that practitioner's patients, plus the patients of all the other providers in the organization, plus all the well people for whom the health plan has responsibility.

Defining what is meant by the health of the population is more difficult and requires some concentration. However, it is important to work through the definition because it provides the foundation for resolving what is probably the most contentious issue we will face in the coming decade—setting priorities among treatments. The central point is easy to grasp: The health of the population is a "sum" of the health of all the individuals in the population. The justification for focusing on the sum across all the individuals is also easy to understand: If patients are going to be treated from a resource pool into which everyone in the population has contributed, then the distribution of resources from the pool should give equal and fair consideration to all the individuals who contributed. The more difficult concepts are how the benefits to an individual should be measured, and how the sum of benefits to a group of individuals should be calculated so as to maximize the total health of the population.

To help answer those questions and to distinguish principle No. 5 clearly from alternative principles that might be used to set priorities for treatments, I will pose a test question. This question requires that you think of a measure or scale that you can use to compare the benefits of different treatments. In this context the magnitude of a treatment's benefit should include both its benefits and harms (ie, its "net" benefit), and should incorporate both the importance of the outcomes (eg, survival from cancer vs relief from a headache) and the probabilities that they will occur (eg, a 50% vs a 2% increase in cancer survival). Although there are formal scales that can be used for this purpose, you can think of a common-sense scale such as a number from zero to 100 if you prefer. The scale should be cardinal in the sense that the score you assign to each treatment should reflect the relative magnitude of the benefit of that treatment compared with other treatments. Specifically, if you believe that the benefits of two treatments are such that one application of one treatment (ie, to one patient) is equally desirable as two applications of another treatment (ie, to two patients), you should assign the first treatment a score that is twice as high as the score you assign to the second treatment.

Some people—perhaps responding to a sense of egalitarianism—might object to the idea that treatments can be ranked in the manner I just described. To help think through this, you can ask yourself the following question. If you could choose to do only one of the following, which would you prefer to do: (1) prevent one 30-year-old mother of three from dying of cervical cancer, (2) treat a child who has noncyanotic tetralogy of Fallot (very debilitating, but not fatal), (3) repair a child's cleft lip, or (4) treat a person's tennis elbow? Unless you are truly indifferent about each of these four treatments, then a scale of benefits exists, and it is possible to rank treatments in order of their benefits. (If you are truly indifferent, then the principle for setting priorities should be to choose the least expensive treatment first. In this example, first priority would go to fixing all the tennis elbows, second priority would go to repairing all the cleft lips, and so forth.) A second possible objection is that even if it is possible to rank the benefits in their order of importance, you might not believe that it is possible to develop a cardinal ranking that implies a willingness to trade treatments across patients. To help think about that, try the following: I am going to assume that you assigned a higher benefit to treating a case of tetralogy of Fallot than to repairing one cleft lip. Now suppose you could either (1) treat one case of noncyanotic tetralogy of Fallot, or (2) repair 10 cleft lips, or 100 cleft lips, or every cleft lip there is in the world. If there is any number of cleft lip repairs that you would consider as desirable as treating one case of tetralogy of Fallot, then there is a measure of benefit that has the properties we want. Finally, you should not worry about whose values would be used to make choices like these. To help focus on the principles, you can assume that the country will use your values to score the treatments.

Now that we have clarified what we mean by the magnitude of benefit of a treatment, we can pose the test problem. To get right to the point, I am going to construct the problem so that it raises the most difficult and agonizing comparison. In reality, most decisions will be easier than this. Imagine that you have enough money to offer only one of the following two treatment programs. Program A provides 60 units of benefit to one person. Program B provides 30 units of benefit to five people (ie, each of the five people gets 30 units of benefit, for a total of 150 units). Given these definitions (and remember that the benefits of the treatments are based on your values), principle No. 5 says that, if you can do only one of these programs, you should give higher priority to program B than to program A. The reason is clear; program B does more to increase the health of the population than does program A.

This is a head-on collision in the debate about the individual (the one patient who would receive treatment A) vs society (the five who will receive treatment B), and resolves the debate in favor of society. It is also consistent with the maxim, "the greatest good to the greatest number." Astute readers will realize that if the values assigned for the benefit of each treatment have the cardinal property described, then there is no choice but to prefer program B. By assigning scores of 60 to treatment A and 30 to treatment B, you were expressing a willingness to trade one application of A for two applications of B. This test problem offered you an opportunity to trade one application of A for five applications of B, which would obviously be a desirable trade. Nonetheless, some might want program A because, on a patient-by-patient basis, it provides a greater benefit.

This principle will cause great discomfort to practitioners when one of their treatments receives a low priority. Because this discomfort will probably make this the most controversial principle, it is helpful to address it directly. We should begin by recognizing that the discomfort is caused by a noble instinct, which is to try to help any individual we see who is in trouble. We should also recognize that the instinct has many desirable qualities. The most obvious is that it helps ensure that the patients we see receive the best possible treatment. Having said this, however, it is also important to understand some of the drawbacks of the instinct and to contemplate some ways to alleviate the discomfort it causes.

The first point is that if we give in to the discomfort and follow our instincts, that will not solve the problem of how we should set priorities. That is, maximizing the care we provide to our personal patients is not really an alternative to principle No. 5. To the extent that it sets priorities at all, it sets priorities according to types of patients (eg, "my patients" vs "someone else's patients"), not types of treatments. Such a position is obviously difficult to defend. But beyond that, trying to maximize the care we give to our personal patients is not a successful method for achieving the requirement that we keep costs within a limited budget. In terms of the test problem, if each practitioner seeks to maximize the treatments of his or her personal patients, practitioners with patients who need treatment A will order treatment A for their patients, and practitioners with patients who need treatment B will order that treatment for their patients. The end result is that both program A and program B will be done, which exceeds the specified limit. This is just what is happening in our current health care system; our attempts to maximize the care we give to our individual patients have led to increases in costs that are unacceptable (the opening premise). This is occurring even though a large portion of the population is omitted from this strategy altogether, because it has no coverage at all. So the first point is that giving in to our discomfort and seeking to maximize the care we provide to our personal patients not only fails to solve the problem of resource limits, it makes it worse.

A second point is that applying principle No. 5 will not mean that patients will be denied treatments that have high value. To address a more specific fear, a treatment will not receive a low priority simply because it is expensive. An expensive treatment would receive a low priority only if its benefits were too small to justify its cost.

A third point is that we have already been making these types of choices for decades. That is, despite our perceptions that we are maximizing the care we give to personal patients, we already make choices that fail to do that. Medicine is filled with indications, thresholds, and limits that are based on an implicit judgment that some amounts of benefit are just too small to be worth the cost. Frequencies of screening tests and indications for imaging tests are just a few examples. Although the choices will become more explicit and intense in the future, appreciation of this long tradition should help relieve some of the discomfort.

A fourth point is that at least some of the discomfort of withholding program A from one patient, even your patient, should be soothed by realizing that five other patients will receive treatment B, which we have agreed will provide greater total benefit. Conversely, if your patient receives treatment A, you will have to deal with the fact that five patients will be deprived of treatment B. A final approach for dealing with the discomfort is to ask yourself which health plan you would want your newborn grandchild to join: one that offers program A or one that offers program B.

If you decide not to accept the principle I have proposed for setting priorities across treatments, then you will need to agree on some other principle for setting priorities. We have seen that trying to maximize the care we give to our personal patients is not an alternative, because it sets priorities across people, not treatments, and because it does not achieve the required objective of keeping costs within the required limits. Some other ways that are sometimes used to set priorities include family and friends over strangers (eg, physicians' spouses get special treatment); income and family status (as Medicaid now does); the prominence or visibility of an individual patient (eg, a politician or patient covered in the nightly news); the squeaking wheel (eg, patients who threaten to sue); political correctness; the lobbying power of a particular advocacy group; the visibility of a disease (eg, cancer); the technical appeal of a treatment (eg, transplantation); and fear of malpractice. Although all these are real and can sometimes be justified in special circumstances, and although each will undoubtedly continue to play some role in individual decisions, it is clear that none of them is suitable as a general principle.

There are, however, two other candidates for a principle for setting priorities that might receive serious consideration. One is to give priority to treatments in the order of the severity of the health problems they treat. For example, this approach might give first priority to treatments that address urgent, life-threatening problems; next priority to treatments that address problems that are life-threatening but more chronic; third priority to treatments for problems that are severely debilitating but not life-threatening; and so forth. Although this approach has a strong surface appeal—apply the most resources to the most serious problems—it has some very questionable implications. For example, application of this strategy would provide all possible treatments for an acute life-threatening disease no matter how futile the treatment, how low the probability of success, or how high the cost. Indeed, this principle does not even use information on the amount of benefit provided by different treatments. Rather, it is based on an assumption that if a treatment is used for an important problem, it must have an important benefit, which is clearly not always true. Here is a test question. If you could do only one, which would you prefer: a treatment that increased the chance of surviving a heart attack from 92% to 92.5%, or a treatment that would completely restore all function to a 12-year-old quadriplegic? This approach would require that you choose the former because it addresses an acute life-threatening problem.

The other possible principle for setting priorities across treatments that might receive serious consideration is to rank treatments by the amount of benefit they provide to an individual patient. This is preferable to the one just mentioned, because it does at least consider the actual benefits of a treatment. However, because this approach ignores the cost of the treatment, it does not take into account the number of patients who could actually be helped, within the available budget. In terms of the test problem, this strategy would give priority to program A over program B, because treatment A provides 60 units of benefit per patient, whereas treatment B provides only 30 units of benefit per patient. However, this strategy would miss the fact that for the same amount of money, treatment B could be given to five times as many patients as could treatment A. If you want to take into account the costs of a treatment (which affects the number of patients it can be used to help), and if you want to be consistent with the way you have determined the benefit of a treatment, then you need to choose principle No. 5, which maximizes the total benefit a treatment can provide to the population.

Principle No. 5 has many implications. One that has already been alluded to should be made explicit.

6. The Priority a Treatment Should Receive Should Not Depend on Whether the Particular Individuals Who Would Receive the Treatment Are Our Personal Patients.

In terms of the previous example, we should give priority to program B over program A, even if the individual helped by program A is our own patient, while the five people helped by program B are not. This principle resolves part of the debate about the difference between "statistical" vs "identifiable" lives; it says that a statistical life (a person who is not your patient) is just as real and important as an identifiable life (a person who is your patient). We need this principle to avoid the obvious contradictions that would arise from the fact that lives that are "identifiable" to one practitioner are "statistical" to another practitioner and vice versa. Those who disagree with this principle will have to justify a position that their patients are more important than the patients of their colleagues. They will also have to find some way to reconcile the conflicts that will constantly arise when their colleagues apply the same logic to shift resources back to their own patients.

This principle has important implications for the idea that the physician should serve as the advocate of his or her patients. It reminds us that in organizations that cover the costs of treatments from shared resources, physicians' responsibilities extend beyond their personal patients to affect all the patients in the population they help serve. When resources are limited, and when treatments are being paid for from a resource pool to which everyone contributed, a better maxim is that the physician should serve as an advocate of all the individuals in the population, not just their personal patients.

This principle also has implications for "rationing at the bedside." I interpret this term to mean requiring the practitioner to personally make a specific decision to withhold some beneficial treatment from a specific patient because of its cost. Principle No. 6 does imply that some beneficial treatments will be withheld from some patients, as has occurred in the past. However, there is nothing in this principle that forces the individual practitioner to make these decisions one-on-one at the bedside. A far better way to implement these decisions is to use the traditional approach of embedding them in guidelines, which the physicians and patients can then follow without having to suffer the anguish of making the decision themselves. A current recommendation for annual mammograms is an example—compared with 6-month examinations, it is rationing.

Before we leave this topic, it is useful to address the remaining part of the debate about statistical vs identifiable lives—the "rule of rescue."[2] The rule of rescue is based on the observation that many people place a very high value on attempts to rescue individual, identifiable people who face a desperate problem, provided that they fit certain criteria. A prototypical example is a child who falls down a well. Flying a child from Bosnia to the United States for surgery is a recent example. The main criteria are that the circumstances should be extraordinary (eg, relatively rare and very dire), that we can identify with the individual who is in distress, and that the incident has high symbolic value. For example, we do not apply the rule of rescue to a homeless man dying of pneumonia over a steam grate.

There is no denying the fact that the rule of rescue is real—both as individuals and as a society we do feel a strong instinct to help particular individuals who attract our attention like that. Fortunately, this instinct can be accommodated in the fifth principle. The key is in the measure of benefit. Imagine that treatment A is a long-shot heroic attempt to save the life of a particular individual at a cost of $400 000. If we place such a high value on trying to rescue this individual that we are willing to allocate the $400 000 to this treatment, even if that would mean withholding more mundane but more effective treatments from a larger number of patients, we can accommodate that by assigning an extremely high score to the treatment, "long-shot heroic treatment of this particular individual." If we set the score of this treatment high enough, it will always receive priority, no matter how many resources it might pull from other treatments. The point here is not to make a judgment about the appropriateness of the rule of rescue, but to say that, to the extent that society wants to allocate resources to trying to rescue particular individuals, the fifth principle can accommodate that.

If the principles I have proposed thus far are accepted, then several additional principles follow from them.

7. Determining the Priority of a Treatment Will Require Estimating the Magnitudes of Its Benefits, Harms, and Costs.

Although this is not really arguable, because it follows directly from the fifth principle, it has very important implications. Specifically, it will require a shift in medical decision making from qualitative thinking to quantitative thinking. Qualitative thinking looks only at the possibility of benefit. Representative phrases are that a treatment should be used if it "might be beneficial," if it provides "any hope of benefit," if it is "all we have to offer," or if it is "the patient's only hope." Elsewhere I have called this the "criterion of potential benefit."[3] In contrast, quantitative thinking requires that we do our best to determine that there actually is benefit, and that we estimate the magnitude of the benefit (the "criterion of actual benefit"). In terms of the test problem for principle No. 5, it is clear that we would have no basis for choosing between treatments A and B if all we could say about them is that they both have some benefit. To have any hope of allocating resources to the best treatments, we have to estimate the actual benefits of the treatments. The main objections to this principle will be the extra work involved to make the estimates and the prohibition of vague testimonials. However, seeking estimates of benefits, harms, and costs is clearly consistent with the time-honored concepts of intelligent decisionmaking and informed consent.

Applying this principle will mean that we will have to obtain the estimates of the benefits, harms, and costs from some source, which leads to principle No. 8.

8. To the Greatest Extent Possible, Estimates of Benefits, Harms, and Costs Should Be Based on Empirical Evidence. A Corollary Is That When Empirical Evidence Contradicts Subjective Judgments, Empirical Evidence Should Take Priority.

In the past, the most common method used to determine the values of different treatments has been to simply ask those who should know—to draw on clinical judgment, expert opinion, and professional consensus. Principle No. 8 says that we should first examine whatever actual evidence exists about the treatment and that we should use axiom-based methods to interpret that evidence. This principle obviously has important implications for the methods used to design guidelines.[4,5]

Although all the principles face methodological problems, applying this one will be especially difficult, which is why it begins with the qualifier, "to the greatest extent possible." Because the available evidence for a treatment is never perfect, it is rarely possible to rely entirely on empirical evidence, and some expert judgments will always be necessary. The intention of this principle is not to say that expert judgment will never play a role in evaluating a treatment. Rather, the intention is to ensure that there is a systematic search for evidence, that whatever evidence does exist is given priority, and that expert judgments are limited to specific "technical" questions for which medical expertise is required, rather than to global judgments about a treatment.

If there is agreement about the sources of information for making decisions about treatments, the next question is the actual criteria that a treatment must meet before it should be promoted. They are addressed in the next principle.

9. Before It Should Be Promoted for Use, a Treatment Should Satisfy Three Criteria.

- There should be convincing evidence that, compared with no treatment, the treatment is effective in improving health outcomes.
- Compared with no treatment, its beneficial effects on health outcomes should outweigh any harmful effects on health outcomes.
- Compared with the next best alternative treatment, the treatment should represent a good use of resources in the sense that it satisfies principle No. 5.

This is really a summary of the preceding principles in the sense that if a treatment satisfies the others it will automatically satisfy this, and vice versa. Nonetheless, it is convenient to have this type of checklist to apply to specific treatments. This principle also highlights some important issues.

First, the principle addresses the "promotion" of a treatment. Examples of guidelines or activities that actively promote a treatment are initiation of coverage (if the treatment is not already covered), guidelines that recommend its use, inclusion in quality improvement criteria or quality "report cards" that encourage high rates of use, advertising or marketing that promotes use, malpractice sanctions for nonuse, and so forth. Thus, this principle is fairly lenient in that it does not stipulate that a treatment cannot be used unless it satisfies the criteria. For example, a treatment such as radical prostatectomy for localized cancer that clearly has harms and costs, but that has not been documented to have benefit,[6] could still be used as an "option."[7] The principle says only that it should not be promoted through guidelines such as those just listed. An aggressive program to reduce waste and improve quality would have to tighten this principle to say that a treatment should be discouraged if it fails to satisfy the criteria.

Second, this principle works for treatments that are designed to be cost-saving, as well as for treatments that provide additional benefit at an additional cost. By the first and second criteria, a cost-saving treatment would still have to be effective and beneficial, and the third criterion would require that the amount of savings more than offsets any decrement in benefit, either by enabling the treatment of more patients with this health problem or by shifting resources to more cost-effective treatments for other health problems. Similarly, if a treatment increases benefit but at a higher cost, the third criterion requires that the increase in benefit from this treatment be large enough to make up for the loss of benefit caused by pulling resources from other treatments.

Third, the emphasis on health outcomes—outcomes that patients can experience and care about such as life and death, pain, suffering, disability, and appearance—is important. When the only available evidence addresses intermediate outcomes (eg, serum cholesterol, shrinkage of a tumor on roentgenogram, normalization of enzyme levels), the case for a treatment must include additional evidence that a change in intermediate outcomes caused by the treatment causes an improvement in health outcomes.

Fourth, the second criterion raises a new issue, which is the need to make comparisons between benefits and harms. The obvious question is this: Who should make those judgments?

10. When Making Judgments About Benefits, Harms, and Costs, to the Greatest Extent Possible, the Judgments Should Reflect the Preferences of the Individuals Who Will Actually Receive the Treatments.

The justification of this principle is obvious: Because it is patients who will actually live or die by the outcome and who will eventually pay the costs, it is they who should have the primary say in what is done to them (including having nothing done). Application of this principle will vary depending on the nature of the decision and the patient. The most obvious way to apply this principle is to present to each patient, one by one, with information about the benefits, harms, and costs of alternative treatments and let them choose. Unfortunately, this one-on-one approach is often not feasible, or is inappropriate because it omits other factors that are important to consider. For example, this approach would be infeasible if there were insufficient time; if the options were too confusing for the patient, despite every effort by the physician to make them understandable; if the patient were unconscious or incompetent; or if the patient simply did not want to participate actively in the decision. This approach would also be inappropriate if the alternative treatments had different costs, because it is unrealistic to expect patients who do not actually pay the costs to incorporate the costs accurately in their decisions. However, the presence of these problems does not change the principle itself, which is that to the greatest extent possible, the preferences applied should be the preferences of those who will actually receive the treatment.

For many treatments, the quality of the evidence and the relative magnitudes of benefits, harms, and costs will make it easy to apply the 9th and 10th principles. However, for many other treatments there will be real debates about whether they are effective, beneficial, or a good use of resources. To resolve these debates, it is necessary to determine who should bear the burden of proof. This is addressed in the last principle.

11. When Determining Whether a Treatment Satisfies the Criteria of Principle No. 9, the Burden of Proof Should Be on Those Who Want to Promote the Use of the Treatment.

Whichever way the burden is placed—on those who want to use the treatment before there is convincing evidence of effectiveness and benefit, or on those who want to wait for better evidence—there will be some mistakes made. Placing the burden on proponents will retard the use of some treatments that, although we might not be able to demonstrate it yet, are actually effective, beneficial, and a good use of resources. Conversely, placing the burden on skeptics to prove that a treatment is ineffective or harmful will allow some treatments to slip through that are actually ineffective, a poor use of resources, or even harmful. Based on an analogy with our court system, a case might be made that a treatment should be considered "innocent" (eg, effective, beneficial, cost-effective) until it is proven guilty. I have proposed the opposite, for the following reasons.

First, there are many precedents. Begin with the Hippocratic oath, which admonishes us to "first, do no harm," and with the fact that harm takes many forms, including the morbidity and cost of a treatment. I interpret the oath to mean that before we do things to patients, we should have good reason to believe that they will be benefited. This principle is also consistent with the Food and Drug Act and its amendments, which require evidence of safety and efficacy before drugs can be marketed. It is also consistent with the scientific tradition of the last several centuries, in which ideas progress in an orderly fashion from hypothesis through testing to implementation, not from hypothesis directly to implementation.

Second, if proponents of a cost-increasing or harmful treatment did not have to establish its effectiveness, there would be virtually no brake on what could be promoted. For an absurd example, suppose someone wanted to promote the placement of patches of tar pitch behind the left ear as a treatment for thalassemia. Because there is no evidence at all about this treatment, opponents would not be able to prove that it was ineffective, and proponents would be free to promote its use.

Third, although errors will occur no matter who bears the burden of proof, the errors are much easier to reverse if the burden is on the proponent. If the use of a treatment is retarded because the evidence of benefit is not yet convincing, that problem can be corrected by doing the necessary research. For a truly effective treatment, the "cost" is a delay, not the permanent elimination of the treatment. On the other hand, if a treatment of unknown benefit can be promoted without requiring evidence of effectiveness, then there is no need to do the necessary research. In most cases the research will never be done (indeed, such research might well be labeled by proponents as unethical), and no one will ever know if the treatment is effective, beneficial, or a good use of resources. The difficulty of finding funding for research complicates the implementation of this principle. However, that problem must be solved by increasing the funds for research, not by changing the principle and opening the gates to all treatments anyone wants to promote.

A final reason to require evidence of effectiveness and benefit before promoting a treatment is that patients and practitioners need the information this principle would require in order to make intelligent decisions.

❖ Next Steps

These principles raise many questions. One of the most important is this: Will it really be necessary to ration treatments? More specifically, even if it is agreed that financial resources are limited, will it be possible to achieve all the necessary savings from administrative and logistical efficiencies, without having to cut into the content of medical care?

❖ References

1. Eddy DM. Three battles to watch in the 1990s. *JAMA*. 1993;270:520-526 (Chapter 24).
2. Jonsen A. Bentham in a box: technology assessment and health care allocation. *Law Med Health Care*. 1986;14:172-174.
3. Eddy DM. Medicine, money, and mathematics. *Am Coll Surg Bull*. 1992;77:36-49 (Chapter 30).
4. Eddy DM. Practice policies: guidelines for methods. *JAMA*. 1990;263:1839-1841 (Chapter 5).
5. Evidence-Based Medicine Working Group. Evidence-based medicine: a new approach to teaching the practice of medicine. *JAMA*. 1992;268:2420-2425.
6. Fleming C, Wasson JH, Albertsen PC, Barry MJ, Wennberg JE, for the Prostate Patient Outcomes Research Team. A decision analysis of alternative treatment strategies for clinically localized prostate cancer. *JAMA*. 1993;269:2650-2658.
7. Eddy DM. Designing a practice policy: standards, guidelines, and options. *JAMA*. 1990;263:3077, 3081, 3084 (Chapter 8).

❖ Source

Originally published in *JAMA*. 1994;271:1792-1798.

❖ Chapter 26

Health System Reform

Will Controlling Costs Require Rationing Services?

Unfortunately, it will.

Because that is such an unpleasant thought, it is important to examine each link in the supporting chain of reasoning. As the case for rationing tightens, there will be a tremendous temptation to go back and question the underlying premise. Therefore the first question is:

❖ Do We Really Have to Control Costs?

Yes, we do.

Although virtually everyone agrees that health care costs are a problem, it is worthwhile to review a few of the facts that indicate just how bad the problem is. Begin with the fact that for the last few decades health care costs have been increasing at a rate of about 11.5% a year.[1] This is far faster than other sectors of the economy, with the result that health care has steadily grown as a proportion of the gross domestic product (GDP), from about 5% in 1960 to about 12% in 1990. And as the growth in the GDP has slowed, the proportion going to health care has accelerated, gaining almost 1% on the GDP each year for the last several years. From 12% in 1990, it went to about 13% in 1991, 14% in 1992, and is now more than 15%.[2]

These national figures take on a greater sense of urgency when we narrow the focus to individual components and programs. For example, the cost of public programs grew 300% in just 10 years from 1980 to 1990.[1] Just in the year 1990, Medicaid costs increased by 33.2%. Although this reflected changes in entitlements and the recession, in addition to the intrinsic growth in per capita costs, it is a dramatic demonstration of the growing pressure health care is placing on state and federal governments. At the corporate level, an indication of the growing magnitude of the problem is that between 1965 and 1991, real health care costs per worker grew 65 times faster than real wages and salaries.[3] In 1965 health care costs comprised about 12% of after-tax business profits; in 1991 it was 97.5%. At a more personal level, between 1980 and 1990, per capita expenditures for health care increased 160%, from a little over $1000 to about $2600.[1] Today, the per capita expenditures are about $3900, which amounts to about $15 600 for a family of four. Although a typical family pays "only" about $5000 a year directly in the form of out-of-pocket expenses, co-payments, deductibles, and health insurance premiums, people still pay the remainder indirectly through such things as federal and state taxes and the lower wages and higher prices that result from having employer-based insurance.

We would not be alarmed if these trends were the result of an efficient market with well-informed consumers weighing the value of each service against its cost and choosing to spend their money on health care services rather than on other things such as housing or shoes. But that is not the case; the medical market is notoriously not efficient. Individual consumers rarely know the value of a service (indeed, determining the value of a health service is usually a major research project even for analysts), consumers do not pay the costs, and providers have lots of incentives to promote the service. Thus, there is no assurance that the value society is receiving in return for the rapidly rising expenditures is growing in concert with the costs being paid. Indeed, the fundamental flaws in the medical market imply just the opposite.

The problem of course is that every dollar spent on health care is a dollar not spent on something else. As health care consumes a higher and higher proportion of budgets, it pushes other programs aside. The federal budget illustrates the problem well: In 1965, health care consumed less than 5% of the federal budget; by 1990 it had tripled to 15%, and by 2000 it is projected to double again to 30%.[2] The obvious consequence is that there will be less and less money to spend on other things, such as education, crime, Social Security, defense, energy, transportation, and welfare. Either programs such as these will have to be cut back or taxes will have to be raised. The story is similar for state, corporate, and family budgets.

Some might argue that we need not worry about how much money is being spent on health care, because it creates jobs. Although it is true that one person's costs are another person's income, that does not mean that the health care sector should keep consuming larger and larger parts of the pie. Money spent on education or crime prevention would also create jobs. The critical question is whether the additional services bought by the ever-expanding expenditures on health care provide concomitant value, compared with all the other aspects of federal, state, corporate, and personal budgets that need resources. Given that the main force behind the expansion in health care is the lack of any direct feedback that forces consumers to compare the value against the cost (not to mention provider-induced demand), it is very difficult to argue that health care "deserves" to keep pushing other programs aside because it provides greater value than, say, education. To determine whether people

really believe the value they are getting from health care is worth the continually increasing costs, the critical test is whether they would voluntarily pay all
the insurance premiums, Medicare and Medicaid taxes, out-of-pocket costs,
and other costs directly out of their personal budgets (as they do now for cars
and stereo sets). The effect would be to about triple the payments currently
made by the typical family. Every employer who has negotiated with employees over health benefits, and every politician who has talked to constituents
about raising taxes, knows that they would not. The popularity of employer-
based insurance, despite all the distortions and complexities it introduces, is
but one tangible sign. To the extent that people tolerate the rising costs of health
care at all, they do so only when they think someone else is paying them.

But whatever one believes about the appropriateness of our current
spending levels, it is clear that these increases in costs cannot be sustained.
Some notable examples are that the Medicare trust fund for hospital care is
scheduled to go bankrupt just 7 years from now.[4] Preventing this will require
either doubling payroll taxes or cutting the current level of benefits in half.
The supplementary medical insurance trust fund that covers physicians and
outpatient services for Medicare will require more than $125 billion in general
revenues by the year 2000. Although this program cannot go bankrupt because it is funded from general revenues and enrollee premiums, raising the
$125 billion will require almost doubling the premiums each enrollee must
pay by the year 2000 (to $700 per person).[2]

If the past trends and current problems are bad, the long-term projections
are disastrous. Even under optimistic assumptions that the annual rate of increase in health care costs will drop from the 11.5% level seen over the last
several decades down to about 8.3%, national health expenditures are projected to grow to 32% of the GDP by the year 2030.[2] By the year 2030 the cost
of health care for every man, woman, and child in the country will increase to
about $12 000 in 1994 dollars (or about $48 000 in 2030 dollars).

Fortunately, these projections are all wrong. They are correct in that if current trends continue, this is where we will end up. But they are wrong in that
the consequences of the trends are such that they simply cannot be allowed to
continue. No matter how many constituencies might benefit from rising health
care costs, there is no way that the nation can spend a third of its GDP on that
single sector of the economy. Even at today's levels of expenditures, the federal government is running huge deficits just trying to maintain other programs at constant levels, every state government is searching for a way to
control its health care costs, and families are complaining about even the small
fraction of insurance premiums they now pay. Doubling or tripling health
care expenditures would be intolerable.

The inescapable conclusion is that although no one can say precisely what
proportion of the GDP should go to health care, everyone knows that the proportion cannot grow forever. One way or another, sooner or later, health care
costs must be stabilized at a constant proportion of the GDP. It is also clear
that sooner is much better than later. The importance of prompt action to gov-

ernment budgets is illustrated by a recent estimate that delaying by just 1 year the date by which premium increases must be held to the general inflation rate would add approximately $470 billion to the federal budget deficit.[5] The importance of prompt action to health plans is survival. Providers who are the first to control their costs to the GDP will be the ones who will emerge from the turmoil of the next few years as winners. Those that delay in controlling costs will fail.

If it is agreed that one way or the other, sooner or later, health care costs must be controlled, the next question is:

❖ How Deep Will the Cuts Have to Be?

Pretty deep.

A reference point for determining how difficult it will be to control costs to the GDP is President Clinton's Health Security Act. It proposes to control health care costs by two main mechanisms—the marketplace and caps on per capita premiums. The Health Security Act contains a variety of structures, such as health care alliances, and incentives, such as consumer choice and competition, designed to control costs. But just in case those market forces do not work, the president's plan includes an explicit cap on the growth of per capita premiums, in essence limiting them to the consumer price index (CPI) by 1999, after a 3-year phase-in period. To gain an insight into how difficult this will be, we can use figures projected for 1994 and imagine that we had to meet the cap today. The president's plan projects that in 1994 the CPI will increase 2.7%, population will increase about 1%, and health care costs (averaged over both public and private programs) will increase about 10%. If the numbers in 1999 look at all like the administration's estimates for 1994, achieving the goal of controlling the increases in premiums to the CPI plus population will require reducing the annual rate of growth from about 10% to about 3.7% (2.7% for inflation plus 1% for population), or about a 6% decrease.

Fortunately, this estimate might be too high. Both the CPI and health care costs vary considerably from year to year, and in fact health care costs have grown less rapidly in the first half of 1994 than was expected. Furthermore, a requirement that annual per capita premium increases be held to the CPI is a bit more stringent than would be required to hold health care costs to the GDP, because the GDP includes increases in productivity. If the long-term target is to match the growth rate of the GDP rather than the CPI, and if instead of 1994 estimates we use the trends of the last 20 years to predict the future, then the growth rate of national health expenditures will have to be cut by about 3% rather than 6%. Let us be optimistic and use the 3% estimate. (But beware of the fact that virtually every estimate of future health care costs has been an underestimate.)

A reduction in the growth rate of 3% might seem like a fairly easy target, but in fact it will be quite difficult to achieve. First, consider the magnitude of the problem that will be faced in any particular year. At the national level, health care expenditures will be about $1 trillion in 1994. A 3% reduction amounts to about $30 billion (a 6% reduction implies $60 billion). To appreciate the size of this, consider that $30 billion is about what the nation will spend this year on all health research and construction.[2] It is more than we spend on all government public health programs.[2] It is about what the nation spends on prescription drugs. At the level of an individual health plan, a health maintenance organization with 500 000 members and an annual budget of about $1 billion would have to reduce its costs by about $30 million. Administrators and providers who work in managed care settings know the difficulty of cutting that amount from an annual budget. For one example, if a 500 000-member plan used ionic agents instead of nonionic agents for low-risk patients needing intravenous radiographic contrast agents, which is not an easy policy to implement, it would save about $800 000.[6]

Reductions of 3% might not be too difficult if they were required only once, and if we had several years over which to achieve them. Unfortunately, in order to hold health care costs to a constant proportion of the GDP, reductions of this magnitude will have to be found every year—year after year—for the foreseeable future. Furthermore, achieving these reductions will not feel like a minor austerity program in which there is a little bit less "extra" money to be spent each year ("We will be able to grow only 8% this year instead of our usual 11%"). The "usual" 11% growth rate is deeply embedded in long-term trends in wages, prices, clinical practice patterns, development of new technologies, aging of the population, and expanding public expectations. Our health care system is like a 100-car train rolling down an 11.5% grade. "Business as usual" means perpetual cost increases of about 11.5%. That rate of growth will not change without aggressive and unpopular actions; finding annual reductions of 3% will require painful cuts, which will have to be repeated year after year after year. To complete the analogy of the train, we will have to slam on the brakes, and hold them there, for the foreseeable future. So the next question is, how will we do it? Or more specifically:

❖ Can We Control Costs by Administrative Efficiencies Alone?

No.

This is perhaps the most discouraging news. Ideally, we would like to find all the savings from activities that have little or no direct effect on the content or quality of patient care. Places to look include managerial activities, such as reducing paperwork; logistics, such as smarter decisions about buying vs leasing or negotiating better prices for equipment; and processes, such as streamlining schedules and minimizing lost laboratory tests. Let us call this collection of activities "administrative efficiencies." The important point is to distinguish them from activities that do directly affect patient care, such as preventive services, diagnostic tests, treatments, and support care. Let us call the latter "treatments" or the "content" of care as opposed to the "processes" of care.

Ideally, we would like to find the required 3% savings every year in administrative efficiencies alone—the processes of care—without touching the content of care. There are many reasons to be optimistic. Improvements in information systems and administrative simplification should reduce managerial costs; vertical and horizontal integration should provide economies of scale and better negotiating power; and the flurry of continuous quality improvement programs should improve the efficiency of processes. Unfortunately, although these activities can certainly reduce costs and should be done, even the most aggressive and successful programs of these types will not solve the cost problem permanently; they will only buy time.

To see this, imagine that beginning January 1, 1995, we had to control growth to the GDP, which means we would have to find about $30 billion of savings from the natural growth rate in costs. Now consider some of the more prominent targets for savings (Table 26.1). Perhaps the favorite is drug company profits. A generous estimate is that in 1994 drug company profits will be about $10 billion, or about 1% of the total health care budget. Imagine that, without discouraging drug companies from producing all the drugs we want, we could miraculously eliminate all drug company profits forever. If we could do that, it would save us about a third of the $30 billion we would need for the first year's worth of savings, or about 4 months' worth of savings. At the end of the 4 months, or in May 1995, we would have to turn around and start finding more savings. We could not reduce drug company profits any further, because that item would be gone from the budget.

How about administrative costs? In 1995 they will be on the order of $56 billion. Suppose we could eliminate all administrative costs forever (without affecting the logistics or processes of care). That would buy us almost 2 more years' worth of time, which would last to about March 1997. But when that 2 years was up, we would again have to go out to find the next year's worth of

TABLE 26.1   The Effects of Reductions in Selected Components of Health Care Expenditures

Component	Reduction, %	Amount Saved, $ Billions*	Time Bought, mo†
Drug company profits	100	10	4
Administration‡	100	56	22
Defensive medicine§	100	25§	10
Medical nondurable goods‖	50	42	17
Physician services	20	40	16
Construction	100	12	5
Total	. . .	185	6 y 2 mo

*Data from Burner et al[2] (Table 8).
†Assumes a savings of $30 billion buys 1 year of time.
‡Includes net cost of private health insurance.
§Guesstimate.
‖Includes drugs and drug company profits.

savings. Table 26.1 shows the amount of time that would be bought if we could eliminate or reduce other components of the budget that might be targeted for savings. Even under the wildest assumptions about cutting components of the budget, we would save only about 6 years of time. But when that time was up we would have to go out once again and find next year's savings of 3%.

It is critical to understand why each of the cuts just described will provide only temporary savings, setting the clock back by a few months or years, but not providing any permanent solution to the excess growth rate in costs. For example, it might seem that if we eliminate an item that is 3% of the budget, then that 3% should be saved every year thereafter and the problem should be solved. However, that would be true only if the portion of health care costs that was growing faster than the GDP were contained completely in that item, which is not the case. The fact is that every component of health care costs is growing at a faster rate than the GDP. Even as successive components are re-duced or even eliminated, the remaining components continue to increase about 3% faster than the GDP. Ironically, both drug costs and administrative costs are projected to grow over the next decade at rates (8.7% and 8.2%, re-spectively) that are slower than the average rate for all health care expendi-tures (10.4%),[2] and eliminating these would actually increase the rate of growth of the remaining components. That is, eliminating them would set the clock back about 2 years, but from that point on would actually speed up the growth in costs. The fact is that as long as any of the remaining components in the budget are growing at a rate faster than the GDP, we will need to continue to find savings. And as the easier targets are eliminated, the savings will be-come more and more difficult to find.

We can test these thoughts by examining the growth of various compo-nents of the health care system over the last few decades. Table 26.2 shows the actual expenditures for various components of the health care system from 1970 to 1991.[2] Total expenditures increased from $74.4 billion to $751.8 billion, an annual growth rate of 11.6%. Now suppose that back in 1970 we had man-aged to institute an extreme austerity program that, without damaging the quality of care at all, (1) cut administrative costs in half, (2) cut the cost of both prescription and nonprescription drugs (including profits) as well as all other medical nondurable goods in half, (3) cut physician services by 20%, (4) elim-inated all government public health programs, (5) eliminated all construction, and (6) eliminated all research. The effect would have been as shown in Table 26.3. Costs in 1970 and 1991 would have been reduced to $59.2 billion and $623.6 billion, respectively.

Now compare the costs in 1991 under the austerity program ($623.6 billion) with the actual costs in 1989 ($604.3 billion). The austerity program would have set the costs back not quite 2 years. The reason this austerity program set the clock back less than 2 years, while similar cuts shown in Table 26.1 set the clock back about 6 years, is that for Table 26.1 we assumed only 3% had to be saved each year. The fact is that from 1970 to 1991 health care costs ex-ceeded the GDP by much more than that. But a more important point is that

TABLE 26.2   National Health Expenditures: Actual Amounts in
Billions of Dollars*

	1970	1980	1989	1990	1991
Hospital care	27.9	102.4	232.4	258.1	288.6
Physician services	13.6	41.9	116.1	128.8	142.0
Home health care	0.1	1.3	5.6	7.6	9.8
Drugs and other medical nondurables	8.8	21.6	50.5	55.6	60.7
Nursing home care	4.9	20.0	47.5	53.3	59.9
Other personal health care†	9.6	32.3	78.9	88.0	99.3
Program administration	2.8	12.2	33.8	38.9	43.9
Government public health programs	1.4	7.2	18.9	22.0	24.5
Research	2.0	5.4	11.0	11.9	12.6
Construction	3.4	5.8	9.7	10.8	10.6
Total‡	74.4	250.1	604.3	675.0	751.8

*Data from Letsch et al[1] (Table 14).
†Includes dental services, other professional services, vision products, and other medical durables, as well as "other personal health care."
‡Numbers may not add to totals due to rounding.

TABLE 26.3   National Health Expenditures: Austerity Program
Amounts in Billions of Dollars*

	1970	1980	1989	1990	1991
Hospital care	27.9	102.4	232.4	258.1	288.6
Physician services†	10.9	33.5	92.9	103.0	113.6
Home health care	0.1	1.3	5.6	7.6	9.8
Drugs and other medical nondurables‡	4.4	10.8	25.3	27.8	30.4
Nursing home care	4.9	20.0	47.5	53.3	59.9
Other personal health care§	9.6	32.3	78.9	88.0	99.3
Program administration‡	1.4	6.1	16.9	19.5	22.0
Government public health programs‖	0	0	0	0	0
Research‖	0	0	0	0	0
Construction‖	0	0	0	0	0
Total	59.2	206.4	499.5	557.3	623.6

*Data from Letsch et al[1] (Table 14).
†Reduced 20%.
‡Reduced 50%.
§Includes dental services, other professional services, vision products, and other medical durables, as well "other personal health care."
‖Eliminated altogether.

even under the extreme assumptions of the austerity program, the rate of growth from 1970 to 1991 would be virtually unchanged—an increase from $59.2 billion to $623.6 billion over 21 years is an annual rate of 11.9%. We would have achieved about 2 years' of savings, but we would not have curbed the rate of growth at all (in fact, it would be slightly worse) and we would still face the problem of cutting about 3% from the budget every year on into the future. Applying the same exercise to projections for the next 35 years reveals the same result. The basic fact is worth repeating: No matter how many components in the budget we reduce or cut, as long as any of the remaining components are growing at a rate faster than the GDP, we will need to continue to find savings every year. The solution to the cost problem is to identify the sources of expenditures that are growing faster than the GDP and cut them. So the next question is:

❖ Is the Content of Care Growing Faster Than the GDP?

Yes, it is.

To address this question we need to look at health care expenditures from a different angle. Instead of looking at the traditional components such as hospital care and physician services, we need to look at the causes of increases in costs. They are sorted into four categories: general inflation, increased population, medical price inflation in excess of general inflation, and increases in the volume and intensity of services. Figure 26.1 shows how each of these causes contributed to the increase in costs from 1960 to 1991.[7] On the right side of the pie are the "acceptable" causes of the increase—general price inflation and population. If our objective is to control health care costs to the per

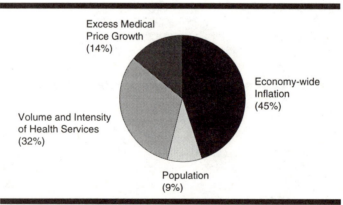

Data from Letsch.[7]

FIGURE 26.1   Components of Growth in Personal Health Care Expenditures, 1960-1991

capita inflation rate, then these are allowable increases. The left side of the pie describes the excess or "unacceptable" increases in costs. These are the factors that must be controlled. About 30% of the unacceptable increase in 1991 was medical price inflation in excess of general price inflation. An example of this would be a 15% increase in labor costs in a year when the general inflation rate would justify wage increases of only 5%. Holding health care costs to the GDP will require eliminating this factor. Averaged over the 30-year period from 1961 through 1991, this factor has caused health care costs to exceed the per capita CPI by about 1.6%.[7]

But even if we were spectacularly successful in curbing this part of the problem, that would gain less than one third of the savings we need. The residual was caused by what is commonly called the "volume and intensity of services." Setting aside increases in the size of the population and inflation in prices, the fact is that each year we do more to the average patient. The numbers fluctuate slightly from year to year, but between 1960 and 1991 the volume and intensity of services we provide to the average patient has grown about 3.6% each year, making it, on average, responsible for more than two thirds (70%) of the unacceptable growth.[7]

There are a variety of reasons for the high growth in the volume and intensity of services, including new technologies, more technologies per patient, aging of the population, and new diseases such as AIDS and Alzheimer's disease. We do not have to sort out the relative contributions of each of these factors, because all of them will have to be addressed if we are to eliminate the excess increase in costs. To summarize, controlling health care costs will require that we pay attention to two main factors: medical price inflation in excess of general inflation, and the growth in per capita volume and intensity of services. Holding medical price inflation to the CPI will require tough negotiations. Holding the increases in volume and intensity of services to a growth rate that matches the growth of the GDP will require tough decisions. Specifically, we will need to examine the value provided by particular services, decide which ones to keep, and decide which ones to drop. The obvious question this raises is:

❖ Is There Enough Waste in Health Care Practices That We Will Never Have to Actually Ration Effective Practices?

Alas, no.

Although no one would be proud to announce that there is a lot of waste in what practitioners do for their patients, for the purposes of controlling health care costs, everyone hopes there is. Whether we consider it bad news or good, studies of variations in practice patterns, inappropriate care, physician uncertainty, and the lack of good evidence of effectiveness for many practices suggest that there is a lot of waste. But that does not mean the job of finding and eliminating waste will be easy. Although the existence of waste should mean that there is room to cut costs without measurably reducing quality, the existence of waste will not eliminate the tough decisions, or the need to ration.

A discussion of waste must begin with a description of the different types of waste. One type, which we might call "harmful waste," consists of practices for which the harms outweigh the benefits. An example would be a carotid endarterectomy in an asymptomatic 60-year-old man with 20% occlusion. The next category includes practices for which the harms equal the benefits, but the practice has costs. An easy example would be use of a proprietary brand of a drug that is available generically at half the price. A more controversial example might be the choice of hydrochlorothiazide vs Captopril for particular indications. We might call this "equivocal but expensive care." The third category consists of practices that are known to have some harms and/or to increase costs, but for which there is no solid evidence of benefit. Examples of this category, which we might call "uncertain waste," are screening for prostate cancer with prostate-specific antigen in men older than 50 years, breast cancer screening in women younger than 50 years, and surgery for early-stage prostate cancer. Finally, there is the category of "relative waste"—practices that are known to have benefit, whose benefits outweigh their harms, but for which the magnitude of the benefit is too small to justify the cost. The intravenous use of non-ionic agents in low-risk patients[6] and routine annual cholesterol screenings are examples. Because most medical practices either have or are perceived to have at least some benefit, this is the largest category.

The critical question is whether we can find savings of about 3% each year by cutting waste without having to ration, which I will define here as not covering from public or shared resources some treatments that are acknowledged to have benefit.[8] There are three reasons we cannot. The first is that the last category of waste *is* "rationing," by virtually anyone's definition. That is, relative waste by the definition of the previous paragraph includes practices that people agree have some (albeit small) benefit, simply because their costs are considered too high relative to the magnitude of benefit. This immediately eliminates the largest category of waste as a target for avoiding rationing. So if we are to find all the savings we need each year, they will have to come from the first three categories of waste.

That brings up the second reason. Although an abstract case can be made that eliminating coverage of these practices is not rationing, we need to recall that every single instance of such practices occurs because some physician and patient believe that the treatment has value. Any attempt to block payment for these practices will be called rationing. Attempts to curb uncertain waste will be fought with cries of "But you can't prove the treatment is not effective," and "This is the patient's only hope." Attempts to limit coverage of the second category (equivocal waste) will encounter debates about whether the less expensive treatment really provides exactly the same benefit, and claims that the research results showing equivalent benefit between two treatments do not quite apply to this or that particular patient. And even for the first category where a technology assessment or expert panel finds a practice to be harmful, we have to remember that for every case of harmful waste there is a physician and patient who disagree with the evidence and the experts. We cannot expect physicians who have been using wasteful practices to come home one night and say to their spouses, "Honey, you know all those wasteful practices I've been doing for the last 15 years? Well, now that we have a health care cost crisis I won't be able to do them anymore, so we're going to have to switch to pasta on Thursday nights." The point is that there are honest disagreements about the values of different practices.

But suppose we could solve that problem. Imagine that we can push through the debates and eliminate all the practices in the first three categories of waste. That would still not eliminate the need to ration unless these categories of waste were solely responsible for the excess increase in volume and intensity of services every year. That is, to avoid having to ration truly effective services we would have to believe that each year health care costs are being increased about 3% by the first three categories of waste alone—that we are adding $30 billion of harmful, equivocal, and uncertain waste every year. Conversely, we would have to believe that there are no effective new technologies, and no nonwasteful treatments for new diseases, or aging populations that are driving up per capita costs. In short, no matter how tempting it is in the abstract to believe that we can solve our problem by eliminating waste, the practical steps we will have to take will walk like rationing and quack like rationing.

So here we are. Sooner or later, one way or another, we will have to make decisions about how we ration our resources. If that is granted, then the ultimate question is:

❖ Will This Harm Quality?

The answer to that depends critically on how we do it.

❖ References

1. Letsch S, Lazenby H, Levit K, Cowan C. National health expenditures: 1991. *Health Care Financ Rev.* Fall 1992;14:1-30.
2. Burner S, Waldo D, McKusick D. National health expenditures: projections through 2030. *Health Care Financ Rev.* Winter 1992;14:1-29.
3. Cowan C, McDonnell P. Business, households, and governments: health spending, 1991. *Health Care Financ Rev.* Spring 1993;14:227-248.
4. Board of Trustees, Federal Hospital Insurance Trust Fund. *Annual Report of the Board of Trustees of the Federal Hospital Insurance Trust Fund.* Baltimore, Md: Health Care Financing Adminstration; April 1992.
5. Senate Majority Leader George Mitchell (D-Me). Delaying Clinton plan's premium cap by one year could add $470 billion to deficit. *Health News Daily.* 1994;6(77):1.

6. Eddy DM. Applying cost-effectiveness analysis: the inside story. *JAMA*. 1992;268: 2575-2582 (Chapter 22).
7. Letsch S. Health spending in 1991. *Health Aff (Milwood)*. Spring 1993:94-110.
8. Eddy DM. Rationing by patient choice. *JAMA*. 1991;265:105-108 (Chapter 12).

❖ Source

Originally published in *JAMA*. 1994;272:324-328.

❖ CHAPTER 27

Rationing Resources While Improving Quality

How to Get More for Less

My last chapter concluded with a very unpleasant idea—that rationing services, refusing to cover a service from shared resources, is inevitable.[1] Although no one knows the correct proportion of the gross domestic product (GDP) that health care should consume, it is clear that one way or another, sooner or later, the growth must be stabilized. Ideally, we would like to find all the required savings in administrative and operational inefficiencies, without having to touch the content of care. Unfortunately, an analysis of the increases in health care costs over the last 30 years indicates that about two thirds of the excess increase—the portion of the increase that exceeds the general inflation rate and population growth—is caused by increases in the "volume and intensity of services." The other third is caused by medical price inflation that exceeds general price inflation. These two forces exist in large part because the cost consciousness that controls other types of expenditures, such as cars and stereo sets, is missing from decisions about medical practices. But that will have to change. To stabilize health care costs at or near a constant proportion of the GDP, we will have to limit the use of shared funds (eg, taxes, insurance premiums, and health maintenance organization dues) to cover some practices that have some value, because of their costs. That is, we will have to ration how we use those resources. The question is not whether, but how. The challenge is not to deny it, but to find a way to do it that not only avoids harming quality, but enhances it. That sounds impossible, but it can be done.

❖ Administrative Inefficiencies

We should begin with the obvious. Even though administrative and operational inefficiencies are not the root cause of the excess increases in costs, and even though eliminating them will not avoid rationing, it is still important to address these problems. Trimming administrative waste, buying smart, and improving the quality of processes will all help reduce costs, and many of them, especially improvements in processes, can improve the quality of outcomes at the same time. Thus, these activities should be pursued aggressively.

We should also aggressively pursue the second cause of the excess increase in costs—medical price inflation in excess of the general inflation rate. This will require very difficult negotiations, not only with the politically acceptable targets such as drug companies, device manufacturers, and various suppliers, but with labor—administrators, physicians, nurses, support personnel, and consultants.

These things should definitely be done. However, we have to recognize that all these activities put together will not be enough. There are two main problems. First, with the exception of the recent emphasis on continuous quality improvement, these are all things that good managers have been doing for a long time. They have been trying to buy smart, negotiate discounts, control utilization, trim administrative costs, and hold wages to inflation for decades. Because the obvious things have already been done, finding big savings here will not be easy. Second, to the extent we can find savings in administrative efficiencies, they will only buy time, and a surprisingly small amount of time at that. To repeat a previous illustration,[1] if back in 1970 we could have snapped our fingers and in that year and every year thereafter cut the use of all medical nondurables (including all drugs and drug company profits) by 50%, cut administrative costs in half, cut physician services (including not just their salaries, but all the services and tests they order in their offices and clinics) by 20%, completely eliminated all government public health programs, eliminated all construction, and eliminated all research, by 1991 we would have set our current expenditure levels back about 1 year and 9 months, but the rate of increase, which is the real problem, would not have changed. To the extent that there is waste in administration and operations, it should definitely be identified and eliminated. This will not only lower total expenses and buy some time, but will set the moral tone. However, these activities will not solve the problem. We will still have to ration, and we will still need to find a way to do it while simultaneously improving quality. So how can it be done?

❖ Inefficiencies in Practices

The key to getting more for less lies in the inefficiencies of health practices. The idealized view of health care is that health practices fall into one of two distinct categories. One category consists of those practices that are "medically appropriate," to draw a term from third-party payer benefit language. The other category consists of those that are not. This idealized view will admit that it is sometimes difficult to classify a particular practice because of incomplete evidence ("investigational"), but there is still a comforting perception that once the research is done, the appropriateness of a practice will become clear. Another idealized view is that practitioners do only those things that are medically appropriate and never do those things that are not medically appropriate. Again, there might be some exceptions, but the idealized perception is that our actions pretty much line up with the medical appropriateness of a practice.

Of course, neither of these views is true. First, health care services do not fall into two neat groups. Rather, they lie on a continuous spectrum with respect to many dimensions, such as the quality of the evidence of effectiveness, the amount of benefit, the amount of harm, the financial costs, and patient preferences for different outcomes. Some practices are very well documented and have extremely high value, providing a great deal of benefit at a low cost; other practices have extremely low value, providing little, no, or uncertain benefit, at a very high cost. The second point is that our current practice patterns do not correspond very well with the values of different practices on this spectrum. Many high-value practices are underused, and many low-value practices are overused.

These inefficiencies are both bad news and good. They are bad news in the obvious sense that they represent inappropriate care. They are good news in that they are the path to controlling costs while increasing quality. The strategy is to trade resources from the second category to the first category, from overused low-value practices to the underused high-value practices.

The concept is easy to follow with an abstract example. Imagine that in a health plan, 500 patients are receiving a treatment, call it Treatment A, that provides 5 units of benefit to each patient, at a cost of $1000 per patient. Imagine also that there are 500 patients who are candidates for another treatment, Treatment B, that provides 50 units of benefit at a cost of $100 per patient. These 500 candidates are not yet receiving Treatment B. If we stopped giving Treatment A to its 500 patients, we would free up $500 000 (500 patients × $1000 per patient), and lose 2500 units of benefit (500 patients × 5 units of benefit per patient). On the other hand, if we applied Treatment B to the 500 people who are not yet receiving it, the cost would be $50 000 (500 patients × $100 per patient), and we would gain 25 000 units of benefit (500 patients × 50 units of benefit per patient). Thus, by transferring resources out of Treatment A into Treatment B, we would cut costs by a factor of 10 (from $500 000 to $50 000) while increasing quality by a factor of 10 (from 2500 units of benefit to 25 000 units of benefit).

❖ Real Examples

Real examples require more work, but they are still easy to follow. Consider some projects currently under way in one health maintenance organization, Kaiser Permanente of Southern California (KPSC). Because I served as an adviser to KPSC for these projects, I will use the pronoun "we."

Breast Cancer Screening

The evidence on breast cancer screening is well known.[2] There are a dozen randomized controlled trials showing that for women between the ages of 50 and 70 years, biennial (every 2 years) examinations with various combinations of mammograms and breast physical examinations reduce 10-year breast cancer mortality by about a third. Unfortunately, these same studies fail to show that screening women under 50 years of age provides any benefit. Some studies suggest a benefit, while others suggest a harm, and many are in the middle. One meta-analysis of the data for younger women from Swedish trials indicates that after an 8-year delay there could be a 13% reduction in mortality, but there is a very wide range of uncertainty around that estimate that solidly straddles the null hypothesis of no effect.[3] Another larger meta-analysis that included more studies found that under one set of assumptions there was no effect at all, while under another set of assumptions there was an increase in mortality in screened women of 8%.[4] There is no direct evidence for women older than the age of 75 years; the best available evidence suggests a reduction in mortality of about 8% for women 70 to 74 years of age.[5]

Currently, KPSC does about 300 000 screening mammograms every year. About 50% of those are done for women between the ages of 50 and 75 years, 45% are done for women younger than 50 years (13.5% of them for women younger than 40 years), and 5% are done for women older than 75 years. Viewed another way, currently KPSC screens about 22% of women 30 to 40 years of age, 60% of women 40 to 50 years of age, 69% of women 50 to 75 years of age, and 57% of women 75 to 85 years of age. Using CAN*TROL,[6] we estimate that if this pattern of use continues, by the year 2010 KPSC can expect to prevent about 909 women from dying of breast cancer, at a cumulative (15-year) cost of approximately $707 million (or $500 million, discounted 5%).

Now consider a new strategy that strongly discourages the use of mammography for women younger than 50 years and older than 75 years, but expands its use annually for women between 50 and 75 years of age, to reach 95% of women in that age group. If such a strategy were implemented in January 1995, by the year 2010 KPSC could expect to increase the number of breast cancer deaths prevented from 909 to about 1206, at a cost of approximately $497 million (or $348 million discounted 5%), instead of $707 million. Thus, making the switch from the low-value mammograms in women younger than 50 years and older than 75 years to the high-value mammograms in women between the ages of 50 and 75 years would simultaneously decrease the number of breast cancer deaths by about 33% (preventing an additional 297 deaths) and reduce costs by about 30% (saving about $150 million). If mammograms were given biennially instead of annually, the results would be even more dramatic.

Cholesterol Treatment

One of the most visible national guidelines, issued in 1993 by the Second Adult Treatment Panel of the National Cholesterol Education Program (NCEP II), addresses the prevention, screening, and treatment of dyslipidemia.[7] The treatment portion of the guidelines recommended that individuals should be treated with drugs if, after a trial of diet, their low-density lipoprotein (LDL) cholesterol levels are higher than 4.9 mmol/L (190 mg/dL), or if they have two or more risk factors and an LDL cholesterol level higher than 4.1 mmol/L (160 mg/dL). Risk factors include being a man older than 45 years of age, being a woman older than 55 years of age and not on estrogen replacement therapy, smoking, hypertension, diabetes, family history of premature coronary heart disease (CHD), and a high-density lipoprotein (HDL) cholesterol level less than 0.9 mmol/L (35 mg/dL). An HDL cholesterol level of 1.6 mmol/L (60 mg/dL) or more is a "negative" risk factor that nullifies a positive risk factor when counting the total number of risk factors.

To prepare for the implementation of the treatment guideline, KPSC analyzed the expected outcomes for its population, focusing in particular on men 45 years and older and women 55 years and older without estrogen replacement therapy who had no personal history of a coronary artery disease event. Given KPSC's demographics and costs, and given the best available evidence on the epidemiology of different risk factors and the effectiveness of drug treatment, we estimated that the effect would be as shown in the first three lines of Table 27.1. Without any drug treatment, KPSC can expect to see about 40 600 sudden deaths or myocardial infarctions over the next 5 years (line 1). These events will generate treatment costs of approximately $887 million. If the guidelines recommended by NCEP II were implemented (lines 2 and 3), the number of sudden deaths and myocardial infarctions would be decreased by about 4800, to about 35 800. Unfortunately, gaining this benefit would have a high cost. The NCEP II guidelines target more than 16% of KPSC's adult population for treatment, and the drugs (including visits and monitoring) would cost approximately $151 million over 5 years. The reduction in the number of events would save approximately $105 million in treatment costs, leaving an increase in net cost of approximately $46 million over 5 years, or about $9 million a year.

When NCEP II developed its recommendations, it placed a high priority on simplicity—on the reasoning that that would improve acceptance by both physicians and patients. To apply the NCEP II guidelines, a physician need only look at a patient's LDL cholesterol level and count the number of risk factors. This simplicity, however, was achieved at a high price in efficiency. For example, consider two hypothetical patients. Mr Smith is a 65-year-old hypertensive smoker with a total cholesterol level of 5.8 mmol/L (225 mg/dL), an LDL cholesterol level of 4.0 mmol/L (155 mg/dL), and an HDL cholesterol level of 0.8 mmol/L (30 mg/dL). Mrs Brown is a 56-year-old woman

TABLE 27.1   Effect of the Second Adult Treatment Panel of the National Cholesterol Education Program (NCEP II) Guideline and the Optimal Guidelines on 5-Year Health and Economic Outcomes

| | People Treated, No. (%) | Sudden Deaths and Heart Attacks, No. | Costs, $ Millions* | | |
			Drugs	CHD Treatment	Net
Outcomes with no treatment	0 (0)	40 600	0	887	887
NCEP II guideline					
Outcomes	144 600 (16.4)	35 800	151	782	933
Difference	144 600 (16.4)	−4800	151	−105	46
Optimal guideline					
Outcomes	65 600 (7.4)	35 500	75	775	850
Difference	65 600 (7.4)	−5100	75	−112	−37

*CHD indicates coronary heart disease.

with a total cholesterol level of 7.0 mmol/L (275 mg/dL), an LDL cholesterol level of 5.1 mmol/L (195 mg/dL), and an HDL cholesterol level of 1.6 mmol/L (60 mg/dL). Under the NCEP II recommendation, Mr Smith would not be treated despite his tobacco use and hypertension because his LDL cholesterol level is below 4.1 mmol/L (160 mg/dL), whereas Mrs Brown would be treated because her LDL cholesterol level exceeds 4.9 mmol/L (190 mg/dL). But, based on epidemiological data from the Helsinki Heart Study[8] and the Framingham study,[9] Mr Smith has a much higher risk of dying suddenly or having a heart attack in the coming 5 years (4.7% chance of sudden death, 38% chance of myocardial infarction) than does Mrs Brown (0.15% chance of sudden death and 1.2% chance of myocardial infarction). Furthermore, Mr Smith would have much more to gain from treatment. For example, if drug treatment reduces cholesterol levels 20% and if the "1%, 2%" rule of thumb is used (a 1% decrease in cholesterol causes a 2% decrease in CHD events),[10,11] then Mr Smith's chance of a sudden death would be lowered from 4.7% to 2.8% (a difference of 1.9%) and his chance of myocardial infarction would be lowered from 38% to about 23% (a difference of 15%). By contrast, with treatment, Mrs Brown could expect a decrease in probability of sudden death from 0.15% to 0.09% (a difference of only 0.6%) and a decrease in probability of myocardial infarction from 1.2% to 0.7% (a difference of 0.5%). Another way to put this is that we would have to treat about 30 women like Mrs Brown to obtain the same benefit as treating one person like Mr Smith.

Although this comparison is extreme, it strongly suggests that if more detailed information about risk factors were used to select patients for drug treatment, it should be possible to design a guideline that produces greater benefit at a lower cost. To develop a more efficient guideline, we used a mathematical model to calculate the risks of CHD with and without treatment for 576 different risk categories based on the risk factors identified by the NCEP II. The model was then used to calculate an "optimal" strategy that would achieve at least as great a benefit as the NCEP II recommendations, but at the lowest possible cost. The model did this by ranking the risk categories by the magnitude of their risk and expected benefit from treatment, and then selecting risk categories off the top until the objective was reached.

The effects of the optimal strategy are shown in the last two lines of the table. The optimal strategy can be expected to prevent a larger number of sudden deaths and myocardial infarctions than would the NCEP II recommendation (5100 vs 4800), and to accomplish that result by treating less than half the number of people (7.4% vs 16.4%). Because the number of people under treatment would be smaller, drug costs would be lower ($75 million vs $151 million) and the increase in net costs that occurred with the NCEP would actually become a savings of about $37 million over 5 years. If the benefits and savings of preventing other CHD events, such as angina and coronary insufficiency, and of decreasing the use of special procedures such as angiograms were included, both the benefits and savings would be even greater.

The savings from this more efficient strategy could be used to help control the growth in KPSC's premiums (eg, keeping the growth rate even with the GDP), or the savings could be applied to fund other programs that would provide even greater benefit. For a dramatic example of what could be done with the money, $37 million applied to antitobacco education for pregnant women, even with a cost per person of $500 and a quit rate of only 5%, would prevent the loss of about 3700 woman-years of life to tobacco-related diseases (smoking lowers a person's life expectancy by about 8 years), and that does not include all the financial savings that would eventually accrue from preventing CHD, lung cancer, emphysema, and other health problems caused by smoking, or the benefits and savings from preventing low-birth-weight babies. However the savings are applied, the effect once again is to increase quality while decreasing costs.

Ionic vs Nonionic Contrast Agents

The previous two examples illustrated how transfers could be made within a particular intervention by selecting more carefully the particular patients who should receive the intervention. It is also possible to increase quality while controlling costs by making transfers across interventions. A previously described guideline for the use of contrast agents illustrates this method.[12] Each year approximately 50 000 radiographic procedures that require contrast agents are performed at KPSC. About 40 000 of those are for patients who are at low risk for a reaction (eg, no history of previous reactions or allergies, no cardiovascular or respiratory disease). Two types of agents are available. The traditional agents, high osmolar contrast agents (or HOCAs) are relatively inexpensive but can cause some reactions. A newer class of agents, low osmolar contrast agents (or LOCAs) has a lower risk of reaction, but costs about 10 to 20 times as much. Like every other health plan, KPSC had to decide which agent to use.

An analysis that has been described previously[12] indicated that if KPSC used LOCAs instead of HOCAs, it would prevent approximately 1000 mild reactions, 100 moderate reactions, and 40 severe but nonfatal reactions every year. On the other hand, that strategy would cost the organization approximately $3.5 million a year, even after taking into account the savings LOCAs could generate by reducing the costs of treating reactions.

To help decide whether to use LOCAs or HOCAs, we examined other uses to which the $3.5 million could be put. Putting $3.5 million into extending breast cancer screening for hard-to-reach women older than 50 years would prevent about 35 deaths from breast cancer. Alternatively, $3.5 million applied to cervical cancer screening would prevent about 100 deaths from cervical cancer, and $3.5 million put into antitobacco education for pregnant women would prevent the loss of about 350 woman-years of life. Compared with any of these three strategies, the use of nonionic agents is a low-value activity, and transferring resources from nonionic agents into any one of them would simultaneously improve quality while reducing costs.

There are innumerable other opportunities like these three. Every time we identify a no-value or low-value practice and develop a coverage policy or guideline that discourages its use, while simultaneously identifying a high-value practice that is underused and developing a coverage policy or guideline that encourages its use, we will simultaneously increase quality and reduce costs.

❖ What's the Catch?

The catch is that this strategy, depending on how strictly it is applied, will either discourage the use of or deny coverage for interventions that for some particular individuals might have benefit. That is where the rationing comes in. Whether it is "soft rationing" by discouraging use, or "hard rationing" through denial of coverage, from the point of view of patients and their physicians who cannot get covered something they want, the quality of care went down, not up. The fact that patients can always receive an uncovered service if they are willing to pay for it will not mollify their displeasure very much.

Each of the examples illustrates the problem. In the abstract example, each of the 500 patients who will no longer receive Treatment A lost 5 units of benefit. For breast cancer screening, many women younger than 50 years of age will feel deprived, despite the lack of evidence of benefit. For the drug treatment of dyslipidemia, many patients who are recommended for treatment by the NCEP II guidelines will not be treated by KPSC's optimal guidelines. And concerning contrast agents, the use of HOCAs instead of LOCAs will mean that there will be more reactions each year, a few of them severe.

The fact is that for every case where resources are transferred from no-value and low-value practices to high-value activities, there will be people who will not be covered for or who will be discouraged from using practices that they believe have value. Whether their loss is perceived or real, they will be on the short end of the rationing stick. If we focus on them, we have to conclude that we have not improved quality.

❖ Resolving the Paradox

Given this catch, it is important to be very clear about just how this strategy works. On the one hand, all the examples, both abstract and real, definitely delivered greater benefit and reduced costs. On the other hand, in each of the examples there were people who can claim they lost benefit and were harmed. Did quality go up or down?

The quality of care delivered by the health plan went up. To see this we need to establish the proper measure of quality for a health plan. The measure is determined by two facts. First, health plans are responsible for the health of a population. All the members paid into the resource pool that is being drawn on to provide care, and they all deserve to be counted in any measure of benefit or quality. Second, health plans are given finite resources for doing this: the dues, premiums, and payments provided by the members, businesses, and governments. These two facts—the broad, population-based responsibility and the financial constraints—converge to define the objective of a health plan and the proper measure of quality. The objective is to maximize the health of the population it serves, subject to the limits on its resources,[13] and the proper measure of quality is how well it does that. The critical points are that the measure of quality must span the entire population served by the plan and must allow for the limits on resources. The quality of care cannot be defined narrowly by the care a subset of selected individuals receives, without concern for the care received (or not received) by others in the plan whose care was not selected for measurement.

In terms of the examples, this means that the quality of a breast cancer screening program must consider all women, not just women younger than 50 years of age. Similarly, the quality of a cholesterol treatment program must encompass all adults, not just those originally targeted by a previous guideline. And the quality of care should count not just the small proportion of the population who have reactions to contrast agents (for KPSC, 40 severe reactions out of a population of 2.2 million), but must also count women who might die of cervical cancer. In short, the measure of quality should be very democratic.

Once we agree on that, it is easy to appreciate how the strategy of trading resources increases the quality of care delivered to the population as a whole, despite causing harm to smaller subsets of people. When resources are transferred from practices that have little or no value to practices that have high value, benefits are being transferred from one group of people to another. Each transfer represents a loss of benefit to some, which is a loss of quality, but also represents an increase in benefit to others, which is an increase in quality. To increase overall benefit and overall quality—the quality of care delivered to the entire population—the strategy must ensure that the amount of benefit gained with each transfer is greater, preferably much greater, than the amount of benefit lost. If that condition is satisfied, then the quality of care delivered by the health plan will go up with every transfer.

That is just what happened in the three examples. Some previously screened women younger than 50 years are discouraged from receiving mammograms, which they see as a harm, but some previously unscreened women older than 50 years gain mammograms, which provides much greater benefit. If all the women in KPSC are counted (as required by the democratic measure of quality), the new guideline saves more lives and costs less money. With cholesterol treatment, the optimal guideline caused Mrs Brown to lose some benefit (her 5-year chance of a sudden death or myocardial infarction went up 0.56%), but caused Mr Smith to gain much more benefit (his 5-year chance of a sudden death or myocardial infarction went down about 17%). Considering all adults in KPSC, the new guideline prevents more CHD events and either saves money, or if the savings are put into antitobacco education programs for pregnant women, adds 3700 woman-years of life otherwise lost to tobacco-related diseases. And while using HOCAs instead of LOCAs allows the possibility of 40 severe but nonfatal reactions, reallocation of the resources will prevent about 100 women from dying of cervical cancer. In each case the harm caused is much smaller than the benefit gained, and the total quality of the health plan's care goes up. The strategy works because, like the measure of quality, it too is democratic.

By itself this improvement in overall quality of care should justify the small amount of perceived or real harm that occurs with each transfer. But because we feel so uncomfortable about causing any harm at all, it is worthwhile to review three additional justifications. The first is that, whatever the harms caused by making the transfers, the harms would be even greater if we did not make the transfers. If KPSC continued to allocate 45% of its mammograms to women younger than 50 years instead of transferring the resources to older women where the benefit is undeniably greater, there would be no measurable increase in benefit to the younger women, and approximately 300 women older than 50 years would unnecessarily die of breast cancer. If KPSC adhered to the NCEP II guidelines to avoid harming Mrs Brown, Mr Smith would have a 20-fold greater chance of dying. If we did not save money by optimizing cholesterol treatment, we would miss the opportunity to prevent the loss of 3700 woman-years of life to tobacco. And if we tried to prevent the 40 severe but nonfatal reactions, 100 women would die of cervical cancer.

In a very real sense, this is a "zero-sum" game—when the resources are limited, resources given to one group are not available to someone else, and vice versa. To avoid this it is very tempting to say "do both." But that violates the premise that resources are limited. We could keep raising the limit, but that would require people to keep giving endlessly greater amounts of their money to the health system in a grand attempt to provide everyone with everything. As a nation, we cannot afford to do that forever.[1] As for individuals, stories appear every day about how people are not even willing to pay today's costs. As I write this chapter the newspaper reports the testimony of union representatives that not only should business pick up 80% of the tab for insurance premiums, but employees should not even pay taxes on the value of the employee benefit.[14]

The second justification for tolerating some harm in order to achieve greater benefit is more philosophical. When people decide to pool their resources to share the financial risks of health care, they must accept the fact that those resources will have to be shared in a way that maximizes the benefit to the entire group. Individuals cannot expect to draw without limit from the resource pool to maximize their personal care, regardless of the consequences to the other people who contributed to the pool. Individuals can increase the size of the pool, but they will have to agree to pay more money into it. When they balk at that and the size of the pool is fixed, health plans bear a deep responsibility for ensuring that the resources are allocated fairly—to maximize the health of the entire group, not just particular subsets.

Finally, there is the ultimate personal justification. Which health maintenance organization would you prefer to join, one that prevented 40 severe but nonfatal reactions to contrast agents, or one that prevented 100 women from dying of cervical cancer? One that prevented 4800 sudden deaths and myocardial infarctions, or one that prevented 5100 sudden deaths and myocardial infarctions and added 3700 woman-years of life otherwise lost to tobacco? One that prevented 33% more breast cancer deaths and cut costs 30%, or one that did not?

❖ Implementation

If the strategy for getting more for less is clear at a conceptual level, implementation of the strategy raises new issues. For a successful implementation, there are certain things we will need to do, and some we will not. First, consider what we will not need to do.

Things We Will Not Need to Do

We will not need to wait for economists to agree on the "correct" proportion of the GDP that health care expenditures should comprise. All that a health plan needs to know is that, sooner or later, costs have to be stabilized, and sooner is better than later. The practical implication is that we should start now.

Similarly, we will not have to wait for either the marketplace or national legislation to declare an explicit cap on the rates at which per capita premiums can rise. Whatever happens with health system reform—pure managed competition, caps, or both, or nothing—we know that we will have to hold the growth in health care costs at or very near to the GDP. If Congress does not address that today, it will tomorrow. Thus a practical strategy for any health plan is to target the increase in its rates each year to the increase in the GDP.

We will not need to tackle all practices at once, as Oregon tried. A beauty of the strategy described here is that it can be applied in piecemeal fashion—one practice at a time. Every time a health plan identifies a low-value or no-value practice that is overused and a high-value practice that is underused, it should make the switch. Every time it needs to find savings to meet a budget target, it can identify another inefficiency and correct it. This piecemeal approach enormously simplifies the methodologic problems and brings this strategy within reach of any health plan.

We will not need to have perfect information about either the health or economic outcomes of every practice, or even of the particular practices across which resources are to be transferred. As the examples illustrate, if we choose our practices well, there is a lot of room for uncertainty without destroying the essential validity of the transfer. For a specific example, the estimates of Mrs Brown's and Mr Smith's chances of a sudden death or myocardial infarction in 5 years (1.4% and 43%, respectively) were estimated from the Framingham study data coupled with data from the Helsinki Heart Study (because the Helsinki study contained a treatment variable). If only Framingham study data had been used, the estimates would have been 2.8% and 26%, respectively.[9] The two estimates differ by quite a bit, and we will never know which is more applicable to KPSC's population, but it does not matter; even if the estimates are based on the Framingham study data alone, Mr Smith still would derive about 10 times as much benefit from treatment as would Mrs Brown. Or consider the antitobacco education program for pregnant women. My analysis assumed a cost of $500 per patient and a quit rate of 5%. Suppose the cost to deliver the program to a woman is $1000 (or $100) instead of $500, and suppose the quit rate is 3% (or 10%) instead of 5%. Under these assumptions we would save 1110 woman-years of life (or 37 000) instead of 3700. The program is still a great buy. The reason this strategy can tolerate so much uncertainty is that, when well chosen, the trades involve practices that vary enormously in their value—leaving considerable room for imperfect information and uncertainty.

We will not have to get bogged down in debates about statistical significance, P values, or experimental biases. For an example, consider what is probably the most contentious of the examples—breast cancer screening for women younger than 50 years of age. The arguments are about whether the evidence shows an effect. Suppose we set issues of statistical significance aside and assume that breast cancer screening in younger women is effective and decreases mortality by the 13% indicated by the most optimistic meta-analysis.[3] If that were true, the number of breast cancer deaths prevented by KPSC's current practice patterns (with 45% of mammograms being done for women younger than 50 years) would be 1045 instead of 909. That is an increase of 136 women, but still far short of the 1206 prevented by focusing on women age 50 to 75 years. Compared with concentrating resources on older women, the strategy that includes younger women still causes both greater harm and higher costs.

We will not need to wait for the methodologists to reach agreement on the ideal measure of quality or other academic points. As these examples illustrate, when the practices are well chosen, the comparisons are obvious. Both the breast cancer screening and cholesterol treatment examples involved transfers across patient indications, so the outcomes are already directly comparable—breast cancer deaths vs breast cancer deaths, and CHD events vs CHD events. Clearly, no abstract measures such as quality-adjusted life-years are needed for these problems. However, for contrast agents the outcomes that were compared are quite different—severe reactions vs cancer deaths or CHD events. But no one needs to survey the von Neuman-Morgenstern utilities of 1000 randomly selected people to decide that preventing 100 women from dying of cervical cancer is better than preventing 40 people from having a severe but nonfatal reaction (or even preventing one fatal reaction). As before, when there are wide differences in the values of the interventions being compared, the comparisons are easy.

We will not have to resolve every problem that we set up. If a potential transfer is identified, but the analysis gets too complicated, the trade-offs get too close, or the debate gets too contentious, there is no need to pound the problem into the ground. Frequently, the easiest strategy is to drop that problem and move on to another. For example, mammography screening in women *older* than 50 years might not be a very good use of resources. In the Canadian randomized controlled trial, adding mammography to breast physical examinations had virtually no effect on survival,[15] and a rigorous analysis might well recommend against using mammography at all, in any age group. However, given the extreme controversy and ill will such a recommendation would create, and given that there are other more obvious and powerful trades to be made, there is no need to press this point. Plans can save the energy and use the goodwill to implement other transfers that are more obvious and less contentious.

We will not necessarily have to target high-cost treatments with all the social trauma that that evokes. The issue is not a treatment's cost, but its value. If a high-cost treatment addresses important outcomes, such as life and death, and provides high benefits, it will not be cut. Conversely, however, the mere fact that a treatment addresses a life-threatening disease and is the patient's only hope should not protect it from this strategy.

We will not need advanced clinical or financial accounting systems to make the transfers. Although it would be nice to be able to transfer resources from contrast agents to cervical cancer screening the way a corporation might transfer funds from the marketing department to the research department, that is not necessary to begin applying this strategy. Even without such accounting systems, the transfers can be made by creating complementary coverage policies or guidelines, one that turns off or discourages the low-value practice, and another that turns on or encourages the high-value practice. To be sure, the transfers will not be as rapid or complete as when executed through a formal accounting system, but they will be good enough to begin.

Finally, there is no need to break new conceptual ground regarding rationing. Although this strategy does draw lines that will allow some harm to some individuals, we have already been doing that for centuries. The cholesterol guidelines illustrate this point well. Even if we followed the NCEP II guidelines for cholesterol treatment, we would be depriving some individuals of benefit. For example, the NCEP II guideline recommends treatment for people who have two or more risk factors and LDL cholesterol levels of 4.1 mmol/L (160 mg/dL). What about someone with three risk factors and an LDL cholesterol level of 4.0 mmol/L (155 mg/dL)? Such a person has about a 25% probability of a sudden death or myocardial infarction, and treatment could be expected to reduce that chance by about 30%. But such a person is omitted from NCEP II. That is rationing. Medical practices are riddled with thresholds like this; neither the idea nor the implementation of rationing is new.

Things We Will Need to Do

Although this strategy has some desirable properties that will simplify its implementation, there are several things that we will have to do, some of which will be difficult.

First, we will need to analyze practices at the level of specific indications. "Mammography" does not have a value. Nor does "cholesterol treatment" or even "LOCAs." The differences in value appeared when we zoomed in on different age groups and risk factors. This makes sense; if we have to ration resources, we should do it at the level of clinical detail that is meaningful to practitioners.

Second, we will need to accept once and for all that resources are limited. It is the limitation on resources that both necessitates and justifies this strategy for getting more for less. If there is disagreement about that, that disagreement must be resolved before this strategy can be used. If the disagreement cannot be resolved by reviewing the facts,[1, 13] ask those who pay the premiums if they will pay more.

Third, when determining the appropriate use of an intervention, we will need to change our way of thinking from qualitative reasoning to quantitative reasoning. To a great extent, the predicament we face today is the result of qualitative reasoning that assumes that if a practice might have any benefit it should be done—the "criterion of potential benefit." Because this type of reasoning does not try to determine the amount of value a practice provides—separating those with high value from those with small value—it has left us with the large inefficiencies that we see in our practices today. To take advantage of these inefficiencies, we will have to develop better skills for quantitative reasoning. It is no coincidence that every example in this chapter was studded with numbers; it is not possible to determine how much benefit will be gained or how much cost will be saved by a transfer without estimating the benefits or the costs.

Fourth, we will need to change from focusing on individuals to focusing on populations—from "individual-based" decision making to "population-based" decision making. In particular, practitioners need to develop an allegiance to the entire membership of the health plan. This will be difficult for those who see themselves as serving as their patients' advocate in a struggle with administrators and insurers. That perception is incorrect. When physicians hoard resources for their own patients, they are not taking from administrators or insurers; they are taking from other patients. If each practitioner is concerned only about his or her individual patient, without concern for the impact of his or her decisions on other patients, the result will not be lower costs and higher quality, but higher costs and lower quality.

Fifth, we will need to help patients understand the consequences of a limited resource pool and the need to be fair. Patients' expectations (and demands) play an extremely important role in determining the use of interventions. But to a great extent, those expectations are shaped by physicians. How well patients accept a new coverage policy or guideline will depend to a large extent on how it is presented to them. For an obvious example, it will not do to have a practitioner say, "I'd like to give you this low-osmolar agent because it has lower risks, but I can't because the administrators are forcing me to save money at the expense of your life." The choice of a contrast agent should be handled the same way a practitioner would handle the individual who does not fit the criteria for NCEP II cholesterol guidelines. In most cases there will be no need to say anything at all. In other cases, the explanation might be, "Well, for patients like you the appropriate approach is. . . ."

Sixth, we will need to ensure that the measures used to judge the quality of health plans support this strategy for increasing quality while decreasing costs. In particular the specific measures must be population-based and as highly aggregated as possible, without losing validity. If the proportion of myocardial infarction patients who are put on the latest monitoring equipment is chosen as a measure, health plans will be forced to buy the latest monitoring equipment, even though that might not be the best way to reduce morbidity and mortality from CHD. A measure such as survival of myocardial infarction would at least enable plans to optimize across different treatments for myocardial infarction, finding the most effective mix of better monitoring equipment, β-blockers, aspirin, thrombolytic agents, percutaneous transluminal coronary angioplasty, and helicopters. But the best measure would be a risk-adjusted rate of myocardial infarctions and sudden deaths in the population. This would expand the interventions over which plans could optimize to include antitobacco education, diet, and exercise. Fortunately, most of the measures used in current report cards are properly population-based. But as these measures are implemented and new measures are developed, the population-based perspective and the need to give plans room to optimize across an entire spectrum of interventions will have to be recognized. Indeed, the best approach is to determine the best transfers first, and then design the measures of quality to reinforce them.

❖ What You Can Do

The most important single thing any individual practitioner can do to improve the quality of health care in the era of cost constraints is self-restraint or, "When in doubt, don't." It is impossible to overemphasize the importance of this step. Perhaps the sweetest carrot to hold out is that if practitioners systematically applied this maxim, we might, just might, be able to avoid the type of explicit and controversial rationing this chapter describes. This is not to say that we will not have to cut back on the content of care—on the volume and intensity of services. The economic evidence on the causes of excess increases in costs is clear that that will be necessary. But it is to say that we might be able to achieve the required reductions by eliminating practices that are truly discretionary in the sense that they have little or no value and individual practitioners can control them on a procedure-by-procedure basis, without restrictive coverage policies or guidelines. For one example, which I hope is extreme, a recent article in *US News and World Report* on home infusion treatment described how a physician ordered long-term home infusions of antibiotics for a patient with Lyme disease, at a cost of $5000 a week, not because it is known to benefit the patient (indeed, the American College of Rheumatology recently issued a guideline saying that antibiotic infusions for Lyme disease should be limited), but because, to quote, "You've got to come up with something."[16] Everything we have done in the past "because there is nothing else to offer," or "just to be on the safe side," or "because the patient is pressuring me," or "because I might get sued" should be reevaluated. Unless there is good reason to believe that the patient will truly benefit, leave it out "just to be fair to other patients." Through their day-to-day decisions, physicians can determine whether the need to control costs will improve quality or will harm it. They can also determine whether the process will be relatively painless, or chaotic and bitter. The coming decade will reveal which they choose.

❖ Next Steps

If health plans and individual practitioners are to succeed in making transfers that increase quality while reducing costs, they will need both guidance and protection. Guidance will be needed to ensure that decisions are consistent and have the desired effects. Protection will be needed to defend both plans and practitioners when they make and implement controversial decisions. The best way to address both those needs is to develop explicit criteria that will sort out high-value practices from those that have little or no value and will support transfers from one to the other. Currently, the closest we get to such criteria are through vague and variable terms such as "medically necessary" and "medically appropriate." But these are far too vague and variably interpreted. If we are to control costs while preserving quality, the first need is to develop better criteria for benefit language.

❖ References

1. Eddy DM. Health system reform: will controlling costs require rationing services? *JAMA.* 1994;272:324-328 (Chapter 26).
2. Fletcher SW, Black W, Harris R, Rimer RK, Shapiro S. Report of the International Workshop on Screening for Breast Cancer. *J Natl Cancer Inst.* 1993;85:1644-1656.
3. Nystrom L, Rutqvist LE, Wall S, et al. Breast cancer screening with mammography: overview of Swedish randomised trials. *Lancet.* 1993;341:973-978.
4. Elwood JM, Cox B, Richardson AK. The effectiveness of breast cancer screening by mammography in younger women. *Online J Curr Clin Trials [serial online].* 1993; Doc 32.
5. Tabar L, Fagerberg G, Duffy SW, Day NE, Gad A, Grontoft O. Update of the Swedish two-country program of mammographic screening for breast cancer. *Radiol Clin North Am.* 1992;30:187-210.

6. Eddy DM. A computer-based model for designing cancer control strategies. *NCI Monogr.* 1986;2:75-82.

7. Expert Panel on Detection, Evaluation, and Treatment of High Blood Cholesterol in Adults. Summary of the second report of the National Cholesterol Education Program (NCEP) Expert Panel on Detection, Evaluation, and Treatment of High Blood Cholesterol in Adults (Adult Treatment Panel II). *JAMA.* 1993;269:3015-3023.

8. Manninen V, Elo MO, Frick MH, et al. Lipid alterations and the decline in the incidence of coronary heart disease in the Helsinki Heart Study. *JAMA.* 1988;260:641-651.

9. Anderson KM, Wilson PWF, Odell PM, Kannel WB. An updated coronary risk profile: a statement for health professionals. *Circulation.* 1991;83:356-362.

10. Lipid Research Clinics Program. The Lipid Research Clinics Coronary Primary Prevention Trial results, I: reduction in incidence of coronary heart disease. *JAMA.* 1984;251:351-364.

11. Tyroler HA. Review of lipid-lowering clinical trials in relation to observational epidemiologic studies. *Circulation.* 1987;76:515-522.

12. Eddy DM. Applying cost-effectiveness analysis: the inside story. *JAMA.* 1992;268: 2575-2582 (Chapter 22).

13. Eddy DM. Principles for making difficult decisions in difficult times. *JAMA.* 1994; 271:1792-1798 (Chapter 25).

14. Pear R. Taxing health benefits gets poor reception at hearing. *New York Times.* April 27, 1994:A-12.

15. Miller AB, Baines CJ, To T, Wall C. Canadian National Breast Screening Study, 2: breast cancer detection and death rates among women 50 to 59 years. *Can Med Assoc J.* 1992;147:1477-1488.

16. Lord M. A high-priced hookup. *US News World Rep.* May 9, 1994:63-69.

❖ Source

Originally published in *JAMA.* 1994;272:817-824.

❖ PART II

❖ CHAPTER 28

Clinical Policies and the Quality of Clinical Practice

The quality and cost of medical care depend heavily on the decisions made by physicians. In turn, one of the most important factors influencing physicians is the collection of clinical policies that guide their actions.

To appreciate the roles of clinical policies, or guidelines, consider how a physician selects a diagnostic or therapeutic plan for a patient. Perhaps the most obvious approach would be to weigh consciously the consequences of different choices. A physician might identify the possible courses of action, estimate the outcomes that might occur with each action, weigh the value of each outcome by the probability that it would occur, and select the action that had the highest expected value. The model is so simple and natural that it is tempting to conclude that this is how most clinical decisions must be made.

Brief consideration of even a trivial medical problem, however, reveals that the number of actions and outcomes, the need to assign and compare values explicitly, the difficulties of probability estimation and manipulation, and the sheer size of the computation all place this method beyond the capacity of the human mind, making it impractical and unusable in everyday practice.

A better description of clinical decisionmaking would assign a prominent role to clinical policies or guidelines that tell one what to do when certain situations occur. These policies usually take the form of a simple "if . . ., then . . ." instruction: "If A, then do B." These types of policies most often appear as simple statements in textbooks or articles. Some may be codified as indications, contraindications, drugs of choice, essentials of diagnosis, and a wide variety of other principles, axioms, dictums, and maxims. More formally, they can appear as FDA regulations, third-party reimbursement rules, correct answers to examination questions, and policy statements of national organizations. The distinguishing feature of a clinical policy or guideline is that it

297

makes an unambiguous recommendation about the management of a specific clinical problem for a specific group of patients.

Consider an example: A physician trying to decide whether to perform a biopsy in a 30-year-old woman with a solitary breast mass may sort through pages of descriptions of fibroadenomas, cancers, mastitis, fat necrosis, and half a dozen other conditions; compare the features of each with the findings in the patient; estimate the probability that the patient has each condition; weigh the pros and cons of an unnecessary biopsy versus a delayed diagnosis of cancer; mull over the ethical, legal, and economic implications of each option; discuss all the facts with the patient; and then decide. Or the physician can simply apply an accepted policy: "If a dominant lump develops, it should be removed and examined microscopically."[1] With this single sentence, an extremely complicated problem is reduced to a simple rule.

Well-designed policies can be a tremendous aid to physicians who lack the time or expertise to perform their own analyses of difficult clinical problems. On the other hand, a poorly designed policy can result in the mismanagement of hundreds of thousands of patients and in the misallocation of billions of dollars. Unfortunately, there is reason to believe that there are flaws in the process by which the medical profession currently generates clinical policies. This chapter explores some of the sources of errors and biases in the policymaking process and suggests some steps to improve the quality of clinical policies.

❖ The Origins of Clinical Policies

Although some clinical policies are produced by organizations that have direct legal or economic control over their implementation, such as the FDA, the Occupational Safety and Health Administration, or third-party payers, the overwhelming majority are not produced by a recognizable group but are produced by hundreds of physicians, all acting individually. These policies are not made; they flow. The main stream is the literature—reports of research results, conclusions of articles, editorial comments, and letters to editors. Other tributaries range from comments at meetings and grand rounds to conversations in x-ray reading rooms and hospital cafeterias. Over a period of years, hundreds of comments can converge to form a policy, which if widely accepted, will become "standard and accepted practice." For these purposes, a policymaker is anyone who makes an unambiguous public recommendation about the management of a particular clinical problem.

❖ Errors and Biases in the Policymaking Process

It is easy to appreciate that errors can occur in any of the steps that transform a research idea into a clinical recommendation. The literature on virtually any clinical problem contains numerous examples of poorly designed experiments, inaccurate presentations of data, incorrect interpretations of results, unjustified conclusions, and outright errors in reasoning.[24] The potential harm caused by such errors is obvious; no one wants a clinical decision to be based on faulty reasoning. However, the sources of the errors and the ways to prevent them are less obvious and require a discussion of the forces and biases that affect the policymakers.

Oversimplification

Perhaps the most important factor that affects the quality of clinical policies is that most medical problems are extremely and deceptively complicated. A cardinal principle of rational decision making is to try to estimate what would happen if various actions were taken, but in clinical medicine such an analysis is simply beyond the training and experience of most policymakers.

Consider a comparatively simple problem: the use of a screening test to detect breast cancer. The important outcomes that we would want a policymaker to consider include any discomfort caused by the test; any risks of the test (eg, the radiation hazard of mammography); the chance of a false-positive test result and any risks, side effects, or discomfort caused by its workup; the costs; the chance of finding a cancer; any change in the extent of therapy required; and, perhaps most important, any change in the chance that a woman would die of the disease. Factors that affect these outcomes include age-specific and sex-specific incidence and mortality rates; risk factors; the natural history of the disease; the effectiveness of the screening test; the effectiveness of any other tests that are available to detect the same condition; the order and frequency with which the tests are given; the rates of any risks, complications, side effects, or false-positive test results; the effectiveness of treatment and how it varies with the earliness of detection; and the costs (both financial and nonfinancial) of the test, initial care, continuing care, and terminal care.

Faced with this number of factors and the complexity of their relations, policymakers may limit their attention to one or two outcomes. Even then, the problem may be too difficult and may need further simplification. Suppose a policymaker tried to estimate only one of the outcomes in the problem just described: the effect of the test on the chance that a woman would die of breast cancer. Any policymaker who tried to analyze explicitly just this one outcome would still have to consider the chance that the woman had an asymptomatic but potentially detectable cancer, which would be a function of her age, risk factors, and the results of previous screening tests; the stage of any cancer that might be present; the chance that the test would detect a cancer in that stage; the effectiveness of treatment for a cancer detected in that stage, taking into account any lead time in diagnosis; and the probability that the woman would die of another cause. The results of these calculations would then have to be compared with what would happen if the woman were not screened.

It is no surprise that virtually no one who makes a recommendation for cancer screening has actually thought through all of this, and that extremely few policy statements are backed up by any explicit estimate of even one outcome, much less by an analysis of the full set of important outcomes. As a consequence of this complexity the great majority of recommendations are based on far simpler questions. For example, "Is the test capable of detecting cancer in asymptomatic people?" or "Is there a shift in the stage at time of detection?" or "Is the test convenient?" We tend to be satisfied with documenting one or two very simple features of the tests or intermediate measures of outcomes, apparently taking for granted that this will imply a benefit for the real outcomes of interest, such as longer life, decreased suffering, and decreased disability.

Oversimplification can have serious effects. Three of the most obvious are that a medical activity that appears worthwhile when seen from an oversimplified point of view might actually provide little or no real benefit to patients; an activity that might truly affect an important outcome in a beneficial way can be outweighed by other outcomes that have not been examined, such as side effects, costs, and risks; and that if one does not estimate all the important outcomes of an activity, it is virtually impossible to compare the relative values of different activities or the effectiveness of different ways of achieving an objective.

Two other consequences of the fact that many policy recommendations are based on oversimplified reasoning are that this opens the policymaking process to a wide variety of biases and that there is no detailed rationale that fully describes the expected consequences of the policy.

Empiricism

Because they are untrained in the analytical methods needed to estimate the consequences of a recommendation explicitly, some policymakers may overemphasize empirical sources of knowledge. The persistence of empiricism in medicine may be a legacy of the ancient Greek Empiric school of medical thought, which based all knowledge on experience alone and had a deliberate disregard for theoretical study. Whatever the source, an excessive reliance on empirical observations that minimizes the role of abstract analysis can have some bad consequences.

One of the most important is a tendency to draw sweeping conclusions from a few observations. The fallacies of this approach are obvious. The number of cases in a single practice is too small, the possibility of confounding factors too great, and our memories too poor to permit valid conclusions. People tend to overemphasize factors that can be easily observed, that have occurred recently, or that have a high emotional impact, and to underemphasize factors that are not easily observed, are difficult to measure, or are difficult to identify with. An inability to see beyond one's immediate experience can bias an analysis, restrict options, and leave a policymaker poorly prepared to deal with the complexity of the issues faced.

Case-Selection Biases

Many of the most active policymakers practice in teaching institutions and tertiary-care hospitals. Although this has some benefits, it also introduces some very important potential biases because these settings see a high proportion of referral cases, which in turn distorts the experiences of the policymakers, compared to practitioners in more typical settings. Policies that are designed to have teaching value in addition to patient-care value and policies that are designed in a setting where there is a higher than ordinary proportion of cases that are rare or difficult to diagnose may be inappropriate for other settings in which education is not as important, where diagnostic problems are more straightforward, and where rare diseases rarely occur.

Incentives

The failures of the medical marketplace are well known. Unfortunately, most of them lead to the overuse of procedures. One way for a clinical investigator to succeed is to contribute to the development of a new test, device, or treatment, and careers can rise or fall with the fate of the procedure. Industry has obvious financial motives to introduce new tools, and equally strong motives to retain old ones. Hospitals need to have the latest and best. Clinicians want to do anything that might help. They also collect fees for the procedures they perform, and they fear lawsuits about the ones they do not. Sick patients and their families are not in a good position to question whatever is being offered; rarely do they have the information, the background, or the emotional stamina. The rationing power of price is lost when third-party payment spreads the costs over thousands of people. The effect of these incentives on the policymaking process is clear: Policies that promote procedures, even procedures that might have little or no value, are more likely to survive than policies that restrict them.

The Advocacy System

Ideally, a policymaker will consider all the important consequences of a policy before drawing a conclusion, and will present the evidence for both sides of a case before making a decision or issuing a recommendation. But when policymakers contribute to a clinical policy, they often do so not as judges but as advocates, focusing on only a small part of the problem and making the best case they can for their point of view. Arguments in favor of a personal conviction may be made forcefully. Counterarguments may go unmentioned.

The implicit assumption behind the advocacy system is that if each policymaker makes the strongest argument possible, then by some competitive process all the important issues will be raised and the best policies will emerge.

In medicine this system fails for several reasons. First, it enables policymakers to focus on narrow objectives that may be detrimental from a larger point of view. Second, there is nothing to ensure that anyone will challenge a claim made by an advocate. Existing incentives do not usually lead to a full debate, and a recommendation may well be accepted simply because no one is motivated to argue against it, or because some accommodation can be reached by which all parties get their proposals accepted. The debates that do occur often appear to be over territory rather than the merit of an issue. Third, there are no ground rules or judges to ensure that all the issues are raised and that the debate is rational.

Expertise

When third-party payers, the government, or other organizations want advice about a policy, they may call in experts. Unfortunately, with expertise often comes bias. Experts who have spent years studying a subject often have personal, professional, or financial commitments to it. People tend to recommend what they know best.

The problems raised by a dependence on experts are especially tenacious. An outsider—someone who does not have a previous commitment—might be needed to perform an unbiased evaluation. However, such outsiders are by definition not recognized as experts in the subject. Furthermore, unless they are specifically asked their views, they do not have the same inherent motivation to study the problem, and they may be reluctant to challenge the experts. Finally, if an outsider does challenge an expert, who is to be believed?

Policy by Consensus

The achievement of a consensus about a clinical recommendation is often interpreted as evidence that the recommendation is correct. Unfortunately, a consensus can be determined as much by the *number* of statements that advocate a certain position as by the *quality* of those statements. When we are unable to evaluate critically the rationale for a policy, we tend to believe what we hear most frequently, and if a recommendation is repeated often enough it will be accepted. A consensus may do no more than identify the point at which all the errors, oversimplifications, and biases converge; it does not necessarily identify what is best.

The Burden of Proof

The burden of proof is on anyone who wants to change an existing policy. The reason for this is straightforward: If policies are carefully constructed, and if we can assume that they are correct, then there must be good reason before they should be changed. Any other rule would bring chaos.

However, in many cases these assumptions do not hold. Initial policies are usually set when experience with a new procedure is limited, and these policies are often arbitrary. For example, when a screening test is being introduced, it is not unreasonable to set the frequency at one test per year. When a surgical treatment for cancer is being developed, it is reasonable to try to extract as much of the cancerous tissue as possible. Problems arise when a policy that was admittedly arbitrary when it was created becomes time-honored, standard and accepted—so comfortable that it cannot be changed. It took more than half a century to reexamine the frequency of the Pap smear or to modify the surgical approach to breast cancer.

Decentralization

Most policies emerge from hundreds of statements made by hundreds of individual physicians. The importance of this decentralized process is that the formation of a policy depends on the perspectives, objectives, and values of the policymakers. If a policy were designed by a formally constituted group, that group could be instructed to take a comprehensive view—to examine all the evidence, compare the benefits with the risks and costs, and consider alternative uses of resources. On the other hand, when a policy is the result of statements made by individual people, there is much less opportunity for a comprehensive view, and much more vulnerability to personal biases.

This individualistic perspective can bias recommendations. In his or her personal clinical practice a physician may spare no effort to improve the health of an individual patient, ignoring questions of cost, feasibility, quality control, alternative uses of resources, small risks, or even evidence of effectiveness—all factors that must be considered when a policy is recommended for a larger population. Unfortunately, what is done to the population at large is the sum of what every clinician does in the office and on the wards. If every physician orders a "routine" chest film, not because it is appropriate for a national program but because it is acceptable for an individual patient, then the effect is virtually identical to a national policy calling for routine chest films. The current decentralized system by which clinical policies are developed can reinforce this by spreading and formalizing the patterns of practice that occur in individual offices. Such individualistic practices, in turn, establish national practice.

Other problems with a decentralized system are the difficulties in taking the large view, coordinating policies, setting standards, ensuring quality, or identifying responsibility.

Utilization Review

Many of the methods currently used to review utilization or assess the quality of care can inhibit the modification of bad policies. A common assumption is that the policies that are current at any time are correct and that the task of quality control is to identify and investigate cases that deviate too much from those policies. This approach does not reevaluate the policies themselves; it evaluates only whether current policies are followed. This tends to lock existing policies in place; it may threaten anyone who applies a different policy, even though the new one may be correct; it misses an opportunity to improve the policies themselves; and it institutionalizes the assumption that the current process for setting policies is adequate.

Tradition

The most basic factor that affects the quality of clinical policies is that medicine has not yet developed a tradition of conducting a comprehensive analysis before implementing a policy. The profession has placed a high value on developing the basic science of medicine, but it has not emphasized at all the process by which the science is translated into practice. This creates a self-perpetuating problem. Because such a tradition does not exist, the data needed for an analysis are not collected, the methods needed to analyze the data are not well developed, and the procedures needed to ensure that analyses are conducted and outcomes are monitored are not in place. In turn, the lack of data, methods, and procedures inhibits those who attempt analyses, and the tradition of conducting comprehensive analysis remains dormant.

❖ Discussion

This brief list is not intended to imply that no one ever estimates outcomes, that all policymakers are biased, or that all policies are wrong. There exist examples of excellent analyses, and many individuals and organizations are pressing for better evaluation of medical practices. The purposes of identifying sources of errors and biases in the policymaking process are to expose the vulnerability of the existing process, to document the need for improvement, and to suggest how that might be accomplished.

The reliance on clinical policies has great strengths. It is impossible for a physician to analyze explicitly all the decisions he or she faces in a typical day. The existence of clinical policies eases this burden. Because policies evolve from hundreds of sources, the treatment of an individual patient benefits from the judgments of many physicians instead of being determined by the abilities and values of a single physician. The use of policies resists sudden changes by unproved bursts of enthusiasm or disfavor. The use of policies also has the potential for producing a higher quality of care. In theory, policies that are analyzed explicitly can take all the important factors into account. Policies can be constructed by the best minds and the authors can employ aids that are generally unavailable to individual physicians. These include consultants skilled in experimental design, economics, statistics, and decision analysis; tools such as computers; and information from specially designed surveys or experiments. Finally, a system based on clinical policies is alive and can adapt to local skills and values as well as to changes in opportunities, expectations, and costs.

Clinical policies also offer a powerful means for guiding the practice of medicine. They form a network that reaches every physician. They are an integral part of the nervous system by which information is passed and the actions of practitioners are controlled. As such, clinical policies present a natural and effective way to direct the collective behavior of clinicians. It is not possible to modify the analytic skills, perspective, and values of each practitioner. It is possible, however, to modify a clinical policy, and through that policy to modify what is taught and accepted as good medical practice.

However, with these potential benefits and uses come costs. The most obvious is that poor policies have tremendous power to spoil the quality of medical care. A policy can affect the behavior of many physicians, and if a policy is bad, having thousands of physicians follow it will be very bad. Its influence can extend far beyond individual practitioners to dictate the standards of care formally through malpractice decisions, quality-of-care determinations, and third-party payment rules. Finally, the inertia inherent in the process by which clinical policies evolve can be undesirable, impeding the modification of bad policies or the acceptance of good ones.

In all, it appears that the use of practice policies is a good system for helping practitioners to make decisions, but the policies must be set carefully. Some changes in the process by which we set policies would be worthwhile.

Policymakers

Anyone who makes a policy statement has a responsibility to be as accurate, complete, and fair as possible. As a first step, policymakers should state explicitly the outcomes that they have considered when making a recommendation, and for each outcome they should try to estimate what would occur if the recommended policy were followed. To the greatest extent possible, the expected outcomes should be quantified; we should not be satisfied with easy predictions like "It will reduce death," "The risks are negligible," or "The two tests complement one another." Analyses should not only include the consequences for an individual patient but should also estimate the costs and effects that would ensue if the policy were adopted by others, and applied broadly to all similar patients. As much as possible, the outcomes examined should be the health outcomes of interest rather than intermediate measures of these outcomes.

A corollary to the suggestion that policymakers explain their recommendations is that they limit their statements to those for which a detailed and convincing rationale can be presented. This may limit the number of statements that can be made, but it is a more responsible approach to policymaking and should stimulate efforts to document the true effect of a recommendation on ultimate health outcomes.

These suggestions are not to say that no one should be permitted to draw any conclusions unless there is perfect information and the outcomes can be predicted with certainty. We will always be plagued with complexity, uncertainty, and incomplete information. The intent of these suggestions is to encourage policymakers to conduct as full and careful an analysis as possible with the available information and methods, and to describe their reasoning, including the uncertainties and assumptions. If one of the consequences of trying to implement these suggestions is a cry for better data and analytic techniques, one of the main purposes of these suggestions will have been served.

Editors

Most editorial policies now require that authors describe their experimental methods so that interested readers can evaluate the results. It is no less important to ask anyone who makes a policy recommendation to document the rationale for the recommendation.

Educators

Medical education does not adequately prepare physicians for analyzing clinical problems. Over the past several centuries, methods have been developed to solve complicated problems in other fields, but even the simplest of these tools has barely dented clinical decision making. Medical students and physicians who want to help set clinical policies can learn these techniques. It is neither necessary nor desirable to make every physician a decision analyst, but a reasonable objective would be to give physicians enough experience in quantitative reasoning that they will know how to solve simple problems themselves, when and how to consult an analyst, and how to interpret the advice.

Clinicians

Clinicians who interpret and implement policies should withhold judgment on any recommendation that is not supported by a convincing rationale. Practitioners should also understand that a policy is not necessarily correct, simply because it is repeated frequently and is "time-honored." To take advantage of improvements in knowledge and technology, we must be prepared to modify our clinical policies. When a change is proposed, we would be wise to study the rationale for the original policy as well as the arguments for the proposed change.

These steps may represent a great deal of work but they are essential if we are to develop our policies and care for our patients rationally. When one considers the work involved in deciphering a complicated biochemical process, in designing a CT scanner, or in conducting a good clinical trial, it makes little sense to take such care in all the other steps that carry a medical procedure from idea to practice and not work as hard to analyze the last and most important step: determining how the procedure should be put to use. In the coming years, the profession will have to make many difficult choices as it seeks to improve the quality of medical care without increasing costs. To do this successfully, we will have to improve the process by which we set our clinical policies.

❖ References

1. Ackerman LV, del Regato JA. *Cancer: Diagnosis, Treatment, and Prognosis*. 4th ed. St. Louis, Mo: CV Mosby, 1970:861.
2. Eddy DM. *Analysis of a Clinical Policy: A Case Study of Mammography*. Durham, NC: Duke University, 1981. Center for Health Policy Research and Education. Report 81-15.
3. Eddy DM. Variations in physician practice: the role of uncertainty. *Health Aff*. 1984; 3:74-89 (Chapter 29).
4. Eddy DM. Medicine, money, and mathematics. *Bull Am Coll Surgeons*. 1992;77:36-49 (Chapter 30).

❖ Source

Originally published in *N Engl J Med*. 1982;307:343-347. Reprinted by permission of *The New England Journal of Medicine*. Copyright 1982, Massachusetts Medical Society.

Variations in Physician Practice

The Role of Uncertainty

Why do physicians vary so much in the way they practice medicine? At first view, there should be no problem. There are diseases—neatly named and categorized by textbooks, journal articles, and medical specialty societies. There are various procedures physicians can use to diagnose and treat these diseases. It should be possible to determine the value of any particular procedure by applying it to patients who have a disease and observing the outcome. And the rest should be easy—if the outcome is good, the procedure should be used for patients with that disease; if the outcome is bad, it should not. Some variation in practice patterns can be expected due to differences in the incidence of various diseases, patient preferences, and the available resources, but these variations should be small and explainable.

The problem of course is that nothing is this simple. Uncertainty, biases, errors, and differences of opinions, motives, and values weaken every link in the chain that connects a patient's actual condition to the selection of a diagnostic test or treatment. This chapter describes some of the factors that cause decisions about the use of medical procedures to be so difficult, and that contribute to the alarming variations we observe in actual practice. It examines the components of the decision problem a physician faces, and the psychology of medical reasoning, focusing in particular on the role of uncertainty. Finally, it suggests some actions to reduce uncertainty and encourage consistency of good medical practice.

Uncertainty creeps into medical practice through every pore. Whether a physician is defining a disease, making a diagnosis, selecting a procedure, observing outcomes, assessing probabilities, assigning preferences, or putting it all together, he is walking on very slippery terrain. It is difficult for nonphysicians, and for many physicians, to appreciate how complex these tasks are, how poorly we understand them, and how easy it is for honest people to come to different conclusions.

❖ Defining a Disease

If one looks at patients who are obviously ill, it is fairly easy to identify the physical and chemical disorders that characterize that illness. On the other hand, a large part of medicine is practiced on people who do not have obvious illnesses, but rather have signs, symptoms, or findings that may or may not represent an illness that should be treated. Three closely related problems make it difficult to determine whether or not a patient actually has a disease that needs to be diagnosed or treated.

One problem is that the dividing line between "normal" and "abnormal" is not nearly as sharp as a cursory reading of a textbook would suggest. First, the clues on which we base the diagnosis of many diseases can be very difficult to see, with frequent errors in both directions (missing an existing disease, and "finding" a nondisease). Second, even if the diagnosis were correct and a disease were acknowledged to be present, the "disease" might not actually cause the patient any harm. Dysplasia of the cervix is a good example of both problems. It is an abnormal finding in the sense that most women do not have it, and it is associated with the development of cancer of the cervix. On the other hand, it is notoriously difficult to diagnose with certainty because dysplastic cells are only slightly different in appearance than normal cells (see the example to follow under "Making a Diagnosis"), and in the majority of cases it disappears spontaneously (assuming it was there in the first place). Obesity, hyperplasia of the tonsils, fibrocystic disease of the breast, and dozens of other conditions pose similar dilemmas.

A second problem is that many "diseases," at least at the time they are diagnosed, do not by themselves cause pain, suffering, disability, or a threat to life. They are considered diseases only because they increase the probability that something else that is truly bad will happen in the future. This raises two more sources of uncertainty:

1. If a condition presages a bad outcome, one must judge the probabilities. Most conditions of this type do not always cause a "real" disease, and the "real" disease can usually occur without the condition. In situ lobular carcinoma of the breast presages a future invasive breast cancer less than 50% of the time, and the great majority of invasive breast cancers occur without a history of in situ lobular carcinoma.

2. Just because a condition can precede a "real" disease and can indicate a higher probability that the disease will develop does not necessarily mean that it causes the disease, or that treating the condition will prevent it from occurring. Ocular hypertension and glaucoma are good examples; loss of visual field and blindness appear to occur whether or not the ocular pressure is lowered.[1]

The difficulty of defining a disease is compounded by the fact that many of the signs, symptoms, findings, and conditions that might suggest a disease are extremely common. If a breast biopsy were performed on a random sample of senior citizens, fully 90% of them could have fibrocystic disease. If obesity is a disease, the average American is diseased. By the time they reach 70, about two thirds of women have had their uteruses removed. Because the average blood pressure increases with age, some physicians feel a need to relabel "hypertension" to keep the majority of older people from having this disease.

And the ambiguities grow worse as medical technology expands. More and more diseases are being defined by an abnormal result on some test, leaving uncertainty about its real meaning to a patient, and about the appropriate treatment. Silent gallstones were silent until the oral cholecystogram was introduced, dysplasia of the cervix did not exist before the Pap smear, and many people's coronary artery disease showed up only on a treadmill test. Finding "diseases" early may be worthwhile, but it is difficult to know what else is being scooped up in the net.

Given these uncertainties about what constitutes a disease, it should not be surprising that there are debates about the definitions of many diseases, and when there is agreement about a definition, it is often blatantly and admittedly arbitrary. A quick review of the literature reveals multiple definitions of glaucoma, diabetes, fibrocystic disease of the breast, coronary artery disease, myocardial infarction, stroke, and dozens of other conditions. Morbid obesity is defined as 100% above the ideal weight. But what is "ideal," and why 100%? The lesson is that for many conditions a clinician faces, there is no clear definition of disease that provides an unequivocal guide to action, and there is wide room for differences of opinion and variations in practice.

❖ Making a Diagnosis

Suppose everyone agreed that a particular collection of signs, symptoms, and test results constituted an unequivocal definition of a disease. Would this eliminate the uncertainty? Unfortunately, even when sharp criteria are created, physicians vary widely in their application of these criteria— in their ability to ask about symptoms, observe signs, interpret test results, and record the answers. The literature on "observer variation" has been growing for a long time. To cite some of the classics:

> Cyanosis, or blueing of the face and fingers, is considered a sign of low oxygen content in the blood. One investigator compared the abilities of twenty-two doctors to note cyanosis in twenty patients, the true diagnosis of cyanosis being confirmed by oximeter under controlled conditions. Only 53 percent of the physicians were definite in diagnosing cyanosis in subjects with extremely low oxygen content. And 26 percent of the physicians said cyanosis existed in subjects with normal oxygen content.[2]

Perhaps the error rates are less severe if the physician can study "hard" evidence like x-rays, electrocardiograms, or laboratory procedures:

A set of 1807 photofluorograms containing thirty "positive" and 1760 "negative" films (as defined by unanimous agreement of seven experts), were read independently by ten physicians. As many as 32 percent of the positive films were missed, and 2 percent of the negative films (thirty-five films) were incorrectly called positive. When individual readers read the same films on two separate occasions, they disagreed with themselves about 20 percent of the time.[3]

A group of experts compiled 100 electrocardiogram tracings, fifty of which showed myocardial infarctions, twenty-five of which were normal, and twenty-five of which showed some other abnormality (according to the experts). These EKGs were then given to ten other cardiologists to test their diagnostic abilities. The proportion of EKGs judged by the ten cardiologists to show infarcts varied by a factor of two. If you had an infarct and went to physician A, there would be a 28 percent chance the physician would have missed it. If you did not have an infarct and went to physician B, there would be a 26 percent chance that physician would have said you had one.[4]

How much confidence can we have in taking a person's medical history?

Four physicians interviewed 993 coal miners about several common symptoms, including cough, sputum, shortness of breath, and pain. After each physician completed all his interviews, he was asked to record the proportion of miners who reported each symptom (for example, to state the proportion of miners who answered yes to the question, "Do you have a cough?") The proportion of miners reported to have various symptoms varied from 23 percent to 40 percent for cough, 13 percent to 42 percent for sputum, 10 percent to 18 percent for shortness of breath, and 6 percent to 17 percent for pain.[5]

Perhaps the hard eye of the microscope can yield definitive answers.

Thirteen pathologists were asked to read 1001 specimens obtained from biopsies of the cervix, and then to repeat the readings at a later time. On average, each pathologist agreed with himself only 89 percent of the time (intraobserver agreement), and with a panel of "senior" pathologists only 87 percent of the time (interobserver agreement). Looking only at the patients who actually had cervical pathology, the intraobserver agreement was only 68 percent and the interobserver agreement was only 51 percent. The pathologists were best at reading more advanced disease and normal tissue, but were labeled "unsatisfactory" in their ability to read the precancerous and preinvasive stages.[6]

Similar studies have been reported for the presence of clubbing of the fingers, anemia, psychiatric disease, and many other signs, symptoms, and procedures.[7-10] Even if there were no uncertainty about what constitutes a disease and how to define it, there would still be considerable uncertainty about whether or not a patient has the signs, symptoms, and findings needed to fit the definition.

❖ Selecting a Procedure

The task of selecting a procedure is no less difficult. There are two main issues.

First, for any patient condition there are dozens of procedures that can be ordered, in any combination, at any time. The list of procedures that might be included in a workup of chest pain or hypertension would take more than a page, spanning the spectrum from simply asking questions, to blood studies, to x-rays. Even for highly specific diagnostic problems, there can be a large choice of procedures. For example, if a woman presents with a breast mass and her physician wants to know its approximate size and architecture, the physician might contemplate an imaging procedure. The choice could include mammography, ultrasonography, thermography, diaphanography, computed tomography, lymphography, Mammoscan, and nuclear magnetic resonance imaging. A physician who chose mammography would still have to decide between xeromammography and film mammography, with several brands being available for the latter. There are about a dozen procedures that apply the principles of thermography. And why should a diagnostic workup be limited to one test? Why not follow a negative mammogram with a computed tomogram (or vice versa)?

For the detection of colorectal cancer, a physician can choose any combination of fecal occult blood tests (and there are more than a dozen brands), digital examination, rigid sigmoidoscopy, flexible 30 cm sigmoidoscopy, flexible 60 cm sigmoidoscopy, barium enema (either plain or air contrast), and colonoscopy. These choices are not trivial. Most procedures have different mechanisms of action and a long list of pros and cons. Different brands of fecal occult blood tests have very different sensitivities and specificities, and film mammography and xeromammography differ in their radiation exposure by a factor of about four. These procedures are for relatively well-defined diseases; imagine the problems of selecting procedures to evaluate symptoms like fatigue, headache, or fever that can have about a dozen causes.

Second, adding to the uncertainties of defining and choosing a procedure is the fact that the value of any particular procedure depends on who performs it, on whom it is performed, and the circumstances of performance. The potential for variability in the people who perform procedures can be appreciated by considering one of the simplest procedures, the Pap smear. A gynecologist reviewed the technique used by 60 of his colleagues to take a Pap smear, and found that only 15 of them performed the test properly. With this amount of slippage in such a simple test, one can only imagine the variation in quality that occurs with a more complicated procedure like coronary artery bypass surgery. With respect to who receives the procedure, the outcome of a test will depend on the probability the patient has the disease in question, on the physical condition of the patient (for example, young breasts absorb x-rays differently than older breasts), and on the patient's psychological condition (some people can tolerate passing a colonoscope all the way to the cecum, while others cannot). Finally, the circumstances under which a procedure is performed can have a dramatic effect on its value. Blood pressures go up for insurance examinations. Ocular pressures fluctuate by several millimeters of mercury every day. An IQ test can be a joy for a person with a good night's sleep, and a tragedy for a person with a head cold. The message is that a "procedure" is not a procedure. Each procedure has many faces, and many factors influence the quality and consequences of its use.

❖ Observing Outcomes

In theory, much of the uncertainty just described could be managed if it were possible to conduct enough experiments under enough conditions, and observe the outcomes. Unfortunately, measuring the outcomes of medical procedures is one of the most difficult problems we face. The goal is to predict how the use of a procedure in a particular case will affect that patient's health and welfare. Standing in the way are at least a half dozen major obstacles. The central problem is that there is a natural variation in the way people respond to a medical procedure. Take two people who, to the best of our ability to define such things, are identical in all important respects, submit them to the same operative procedure, and one will die on the operating table while the other will outlive his grandchild. Because of this natural variation, we can only talk about the probabilities of various outcomes—the probability that a diagnostic test will be positive if the disease is present (sensitivity), the probability that a test will be negative if the disease is absent (specificity), the probability that a treatment will yield a certain result, and so forth.

One consequence of this natural variation is that to study the outcomes of any procedure it is necessary to conduct the procedure on many different people who are thought to represent the particular patients we want to know about, and then average the results. This in turn raises additional problems. First, many of the diseases are fairly rare, and it is necessary to average over many people to get a sample large enough to yield reliable results. This usually requires using many physicians, drawing patients from many settings, and performing the experiments at different times. Each of these elements introduces additional variation. Some diseases are so rare that, in order to conduct the ideal clinical trials, it would be necessary to collect tens of thousands, if not hundreds of thousands, of participants. A good example is the frequency of the Pap smear. One might wonder why the merits of a 3-year versus 1-year frequency cannot be settled by a randomized controlled trial. Because of the low frequency of cervical cancer, and the small difference in outcomes expected for the two frequencies, almost 1 million women would be required for such a study.

An additional problem is that most procedures have multiple outcomes and it is not sufficient to examine just one of them. For example, a coronary artery bypass may change the life expectancy of a 60-year-old man with triple-vessel disease, but it will also change his joy of life for several weeks after the operation, the degree and severity of his chest pain, his ability to work and make love, his relationship with his son, the physical appearance of his chest, and his pocketbook. Pain, disability, anxiety, family relations, and any number of other outcomes are all important consequences of a procedure that deserve consideration. But the list is too long for practical experiments and many of the items on it are invisible or not measurable at all. We either lack suitable units (for example, for anxiety or pain), or the units exist but no experiments are fine enough to detect a change (for example, the increased incidence in breast cancer due to radiation from mammography).

Beyond this, many of the outcomes needed to evaluate a medical procedure take years to observe. There is no way to measure the 10-year survival of a patient following a portocaval shunt without waiting 10 years. To pursue the example of the Pap smear, the long duration of the preinvasive stages of the disease means that if the study with one million women were initiated, it would have to be continued for more than two decades to learn the results.

Finally, even when the best trials are conducted, we still might not get an answer. Consider the value of mammography in women under 50, and consider just one outcome—the effect on breast cancer mortality. Ignore for the time being the radiation hazard, false-positive test results, inconvenience, financial costs, and other issues. This is one of the best-studied problems in cancer prevention, benefiting from the largest (60 000 women) and longest (more than 15 years) completed randomized controlled trial, and an even larger uncontrolled study involving 270 000 women screened for 5 years in 29 centers around the country. Yet we still do not know the value of mammography in women under 50. The first study showed a slight reduction in mortality, but it was not statistically significant after 14 years of follow-up. The larger study suggested that mammography has improved since the first study, and that it is now almost as good in younger women as in older women, but the study was not controlled and we do not know if "almost" is good enough. Even for women over 50 years of age, where the first study showed a statistically significant reduction in breast cancer mortality (of about 40% at 10 years), there is enough uncertainty about the results that no fewer than four additional trials have been initiated to confirm them. These trials are still in progress.

Unable to turn to a definitive body of clinical and epidemiological research, a clinician or research scientist who wants to know the value of a procedure is left with a mixture of randomized controlled trials, nonrandomized trials, uncontrolled trials, and clinical observations. The evidence from different sources can easily go in different directions, and it is virtually impossible for anyone to sort things out in his or her head. Unfortunately, the individual physician may be most impressed by observations made in his or her individual practice. This source of evidence is notoriously vulnerable to bias and error. What a physician sees and remembers is biased by the types of patients who come in, by the decisions of the patients to accept a treatment and return for follow-up, by a natural desire to see good things, and by a whole series of emotions that charge one's memory. On top of these biases, the observations are vulnerable to large statistical errors because of the small number of patients a physician sees in a personal practice.

The difficulty of measuring outcomes has three important implications: We are uncertain about the precise consequences of using a particular procedure for a particular patient. We cannot, over the short term at least, resolve this uncertainty. And whatever a physician chooses to do cannot be proved right or wrong.

❖ Assessing Preferences

Now assume that a physician can know the outcomes of recommending a particular procedure for a particular patient. Is it possible to declare whether those outcomes are good or bad? Unfortunately, no. The basic problem is that any procedure has multiple outcomes, some good and some bad. The expected reduction in chest pain that some people will get from coronary artery bypass surgery is accompanied by a splitting of the chest, a chance of an operative mortality, days in the hospital, pain, anxiety, and financial expense. Because the outcomes are multiple and move in different directions, trade-offs have to be made. And making trade-offs involves values.

Just as there is a natural variation in how each of us responds to a medical procedure, there is a variation in how we value different outcomes. The fact that General Motors alone produces more than 50 distinct models of automobiles, not to mention dozens of options for each model, demonstrates how tastes about even a single item can vary. Imagine the variation in how different people value pain, disability, operative mortality, life expectancy, a day in a hospital, and who is going to feed the dogs.

In fact, for the outcomes of medical procedures, variations in the values of different people can be huge. Consider a single outcome of a fairly simple procedure—the scar from a breast biopsy. One of the ingredients to a physician's decision to recommend a biopsy for a woman with a breast mass is the physician's assessment of how the woman values the cosmetic effects of the surgery. How important is it to her not to have a small scar on her breast? While it is difficult to know precisely, one can pose questions such as the following to women.

Pretend that you have just had a breast biopsy. You have already received the results of the biopsy and know that you do not have cancer. There is no more medical information to be obtained from further studies. However, following the biopsy, you have on the upper outer quadrant (at about 3 o'clock) of your left breast a small one-inch scar that is slightly indented from the removal of a piece of tissue about the size of a pecan. I am a wizard and I can snap my fingers and make that scar disappear without a trace. I cannot erase the memory of your hospitalization, any anxiety you had prior to surgery, or any of the other events surrounding your biopsy, but if I snap my fingers, your scar will disappear. How much will you pay me to snap my fingers?

When about 20 women were asked this question in an informal setting, the answers ranged from less than $100 to $10 000. In addition to the wide variation in the answers, it is pertinent that husbands typically gave lower numbers than their wives, and physicians gave the lowest numbers of all.

To the inherent variation in values individual patients place on different outcomes must be added two additional sources of uncertainty and variation in assessing values. First, because decisions about procedures are typically made by physicians on behalf of their patients, the physicians must infer their patients' values, and keep them distinct from their own personal preferences. This raises the second problem, communication. It is difficult enough to assess one's own values about the outcomes of a complicated decision (think about switching jobs); consider having someone else try to learn your thoughts and do it for you. The room for error in communication can be appreciated by returning to the experiment in which four physicians asked 993 coal miners about cough, shortness of breath, pain, and sputum. The variation in their reports of responses to a simple question like, "Do you have a cough?" was large; imagine a question like, "How do you feel about operative mortality?"

❖ Putting It All Together

The final decision about how to manage a patient requires synthesizing all the information about a disease, the patient, signs and symptoms, the effectiveness of dozens of tests and treatments, outcomes, and values. All of this must be done without knowing precisely what the patient has, with uncertainty about signs and symptoms, with imperfect knowledge of the sensitivity and specificity of tests, with no training in manipulating probabilities, with incomplete and biased information about outcomes, and with no language for communicating or assessing values. If each piece of this puzzle is difficult, it is even more difficult for anyone to synthesize all the information and be certain of the answer. It would be an extremely hard task for a research team; there is no hope that it could occur with any precision in the head of a busy clinician. Hence the wide variability in the estimates physicians place on the values of procedures.

Two final examples document how difficult it is to combine information from many sources to estimate the value of a particular procedure. The fecal occult blood test can be used to detect blood in the stool of asymptomatic people for the early detection of colorectal cancer. Flexible sigmoidoscopy (60 cm) can detect precancerous adenomas and cancers. At a recent meeting of experts in colorectal cancer detection, all of whom were very familiar with fecal occult blood testing (and most of whom had participated in two previous meetings on cancer detection in the previous four years), the attendees were asked the following question: "What is the overall reduction in colorectal cancer incidence and mortality that could be expected if all men and women over the age of 50 were tested with fecal occult blood tests and 60 cm flexible sigmoidoscopy every year?" The answer to this question is obviously central to any estimate of the value of fecal occult blood testing and sigmoidoscopy, and it is pertinent that the experts were unanimous in their belief that the fecal occult blood test was valuable and should indeed be recommended annually to men and women over 50. The answers were distributed as shown in Figure 29.1. It is tempting to say that nonexperts, or people who did not share the belief that the fecal occult blood test is valuable, would have shown a wider variation, but the variation expressed by this group could hardly be any wider. As startling as the degree of variation in the estimates is that the attendees were surprised by the results; they had never communicated this number to each other, and had no idea they had such differences of opinion.

The second example is a classic. A survey of 1000 11-year-old schoolchildren in New York City found that 65% had undergone tonsillectomy. The remaining children were sent for examinations to a group of physicians and 45% were selected for tonsillectomy. Those rejected were examined by another group of physicians and 46% were selected for surgery. When the remaining children were examined again by another group of physicians, a similar percent were recommended for tonsillectomy, leaving only 65 students. At that point, the study was halted for lack of physicians.[11]

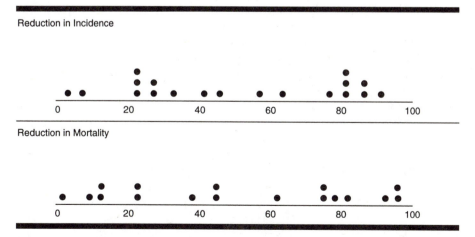

FIGURE 29.1   Effect of Screening Annual Fecal Occult Blood Test and Annual Flexible Scope

❖ Consequences

The view of anyone who wants a close look at the consequences of different medical procedures is, at best, smoky. Some procedures may present a clear picture, and their value, or lack of it, may be obvious; putting a finger on a bleeding carotid artery is an extreme example. But for many, if not most medical procedures, we can only see shadows and gross movements. We usually know the direction in which various outcome measures can move when a medical activity is undertaken, but we typically do not know the probabilities they will move in those directions, or how far they will move. We certainly do not know how a particular individual will respond. Words like "rare," "common," and "a lot" must be used instead of "One out of 1000," or "seven on a scale of one to ten."

There is also a strong tendency to oversimplify. One of the easiest ways to fit a large problem in our minds is to lop off huge parts of it. In medical decisions, one option is to focus on length of life and discount inconvenience, pain, disability, short-term risks, and financial costs. A physician can also draw on a number of simplifying heuristics. Anyone uncomfortable dealing with probabilities can use the heuristic, "If there is any chance of (some disease), (some procedure) should be performed." If one cannot estimate the number of people to be saved, one can use the heuristic, "If but one patient is saved, the entire effort is worthwhile." If one cannot contemplate alternative uses of resources that might deliver a greater benefit to a population, there is the heuristic, "Costs should not be considered in decisions about individual patients." There is a general purpose heuristic, "When in doubt, do it." Or as one investigator wrote, "An error of commission is to be preferred to an error of omission." Unfortunately, a large number of incentives encourage simplifications that lead to overutilization. It is time-consuming, mentally taxing, and often threatening to colleagues for a physician to undertake a deep analysis of a confusing clinical problem. A physician is less likely to be sued for doing too much than too little. Most physicians' incomes go up if they do more, and go down if they do less. Hospitals get to fill more beds and bill for more procedures, laboratories collect more money for services, and companies sell more drugs, devices, and instruments. The more that is done, the more the providers win. The losers are patients, consumers, and taxpayers—anyone who has to undergo a valueless procedure or pay the bill.

In the end, given all the uncertainties, incentives, and heuristics, a physician will have to do what is comfortable. If it is admitted that the uncertainty surrounding the use of a procedure is great, and that there is no way to identify for certain what is best, or to prove that any particular action is right or wrong, the safest and most comfortable position is to do what others are doing. The applicable maxim is "safety in numbers." A physician who follows the practices of his or her colleagues is safe from criticism, free from having to explain his or her actions, and defended by the concurrence of colleagues.

This tendency to follow the pack is the most important single explanation of regional variations in medical practice. If uncertainty caused individual physicians to practice at random, or to follow their personal interpretations and values, without any attempts to match the actions of their neighbors, the variations in practice patterns would average out, and no significant differences would be observed at the regional level. Differences between regions are observed because individual physicians tend to follow what is considered standard and accepted in the community. A community standard evolves from statements published in national journals and textbooks, from the opinions of established physicians, and from new ideas brought to the community by new physicians. The community standards themselves exist because enough is known to enable the leaders of a community to develop opinions which, when followed by their colleagues, become community standards. The differences between community standards exist because not enough is known to establish which opinion is correct. We call the community standards for a particular practice clinical policies, and anyone who makes an unambiguous recommendation about a medical practice is a policymaker.[12]

❖ What Harm Is Done?

First, it should be clear that some variation in practice is appropriate. The differences in patients' risks, signs and symptoms, responses to treatment, and values are real. Differences in physicians' talents and the available facilities are also real. If physicians were able to tailor their practices to take these individual differences into account, variations would be both inevitable and desirable. The problem is that uncertainty so clouds every aspect of this problem that many of the appropriate variations cannot occur, and many of the variations we see are not motivated by logic or a deep understanding of the issues.

There is no doubt that uncertainty about the consequences of different medical activities can harm both the quality and cost of medical practice. It is also true, however, that most of the simplifications and heuristics point in one direction, toward overutilization. When this happens the price is paid in terms of inconvenience, pain, distress, days in the hospital, unnecessary risks, and money.

❖ Conclusions

Many of the problems described in this chapter are insurmountable. There is no way to shorten the time needed to observe 10-year survival rates, and there is no way to increase the frequency of rare diseases, reduce the number of outcomes that are important to a patient, or decrease natural variations in response to treatment. Nor do we want to suppress the differences that exist in patients' preferences.

However, while we cannot eliminate uncertainty, we can decrease the amount of it and develop strategies to minimize its damage. In fact, the profession and society have not begun to exploit the available techniques for reducing uncertainty and maximizing expected outcomes. The evaluation of medical practices and the development of clinical policies deserve much more attention and a higher priority than they currently get. Wennberg and others have described how databases and other techniques can improve the available information. The next task is to improve our ability to process the information we get. This calls for several actions, all designed to develop a tradition that insists on the collection and evaluation of information to understand and describe the consequences of medical practices.

First, physicians can do more to admit the existence of uncertainty, both to themselves and to their patients. Although this will undoubtedly be unsettling, it is honest, and it opens the way for a more intensive search for ways to reduce uncertainty.

Second, people who want to promote policies regarding the use of medical procedures can learn the necessary languages. Over the past few hundred years languages have been developed for collecting and interpreting evidence (statistics), dealing with uncertainty (probability theory), synthesizing evidence and estimating outcomes (mathematics), and making decisions (economics and decision theory). These languages are not currently learned by most clinical policymakers; they should be.

Third, physicians who follow existing policies can examine more carefully the supporting evidence and logic. The mere fact that a policy or guideline is established and accepted does not make it correct.

Fourth, to encourage and assist the two previous actions, any policy statement or guideline, whether it be made by an individual physician at a hospital conference, or a third-party payer considering reimbursement, should be accompanied by (1) a list of medical and economic outcomes that were considered in making the policy, (2) the policymaker's estimates of what can be expected to happen with respect to each of the listed outcomes if the policy is followed, and (3) the supporting evidence for those estimates. Any policymaker unable or unwilling to supply that information should not be making policies.

Fifth, editors and reviewers of journals can encourage the publication of good papers that synthesize existing information, estimate the outcomes of different policies, and present the rationales for different actions. Such work, while not traditional, is both difficult and important.

Sixth, editors and reviewers can require that any author who recommends a policy supply the information listed in the fourth action. No good journal today will report the results of an experiment without a description of the design and methods; it is no less important to describe the reasoning behind a policy statement.

Seventh, the government can support far more evaluation research to analyze medical practices. The National Institutes of Health spend more than $5 billion each year to learn more about diseases and develop tests and procedures. The budget of the major federal unit [in 1984] charged with determining how medical procedures should be used, the National Center for Health Care Technology (NCHCT), was $4 million, less than one thousandth as large. Even that was considered too much, and the budget was cut to zero. Not only should the NCHCT be revived, it should be expanded by a factor of 10 to 100. Research to evaluate medical practices is like the windows in a car; without them there is little way to know where you are going.

Finally, patients can push the process by asking questions. If informed of an operative mortality rate, they can ask, "What percent?" If told about the discomfort of a particular procedure, they can ask how it compares to having a tooth pulled under novocaine, or some other event they can identify with. If a procedure is recommended, a patient can ask why? what might be found? with what probability? what difference will it make? and so forth. Many physicians will be uneasy and some even angry when asked questions of this type, because they may not know the answers. But there are few things better than asking questions to force research to get the answers.

I believe these actions should be taken. Some of the uncertainty and the resulting variations in practice patterns that exist are unavoidable, but much of the uncertainty can be managed far better than is done now. The problems that exist today are not the fault of any individuals; the fault lies with the profession and society as a whole for not developing the traditions and methods needed to assess medical practices. Today the problem is bad; 5 years from now, if not improved, it will be a tragedy.

❖ References

1. Eddy DM, Sanders LE, Eddy J. The value of screening for glaucoma with tonometry. *Surv Ophthalmol*. 1983;28:194-205.
2. Comroe JH, Botelho S. The unreliability of cyanosis in the recognition of arterial anoxemia. *Am J Med Sci*. 1947;214:1-6.
3. Yerushalmy J. Reliability of chest radiography in the diagnosis of pulmonary lesions. *Am J Surg*. 1955;89;23:1-240.
4. Davies LO. Observer variation in reports on electrocardiograms. *Br Heart J*. 1958; 20:153.
5. Cochrane AL, Chapman PJ, Oldham PD. Observers' errors in taking medical histories. *Lancet*. 1951;1:1007-1009.
6. Ringsted J, Amtrup E, Asklund C, et al. Reliability of histo-pathological diagnosis of squamous epithelial changes of the uterine cervix. *APMIS*. Section A: Pathology 1978;86:273-278.
7. Pyke DA. Finger clubbing: validity as a physical sign. *Lancet*. 1954;2:352-354.
8. Fairbanks VF. Is the peripheral blood film reliable for the diagnosis of iron deficiency anemia? *Am J Clin Pathol*. 1971;55:447-451.
9. Ash P. The reliability of psychiatric diagnoses. *J Abnorm Social Psychol*. 1974;44:272-276.
10. Beck AT, Ward CH, Mendelson M, Mock JE, Erbaugh JK. Reliability of psychiatric diagnoses, 2: A study of consistency of clinical judgments and ratings. *Am J Psychiatry*. 1962;119:351-357.

11. American Child Health Association. *Physical Defects: The Pathway to Correction*. New York, NY: American Child Health Association; 1934:80-96.
12. Eddy DM. Clinical policies and the quality of clinical practice. *N Engl J Med*. 1982; 307:343-347 (Chapter 28).

❖ Source

❖ CHAPTER 30

Medicine, Money, and Mathematics

Medicine today is in the middle of a major intellectual transition. Indeed, it is not going too far to say that it is in the middle of an intellectual revolution. All the elements of a revolution are present. It is a major change. It is important. The stakes are high. And people are vigorously arguing both sides.

For centuries, the practice of medicine has been based on one huge assumption. The assumption is that physicians instinctively know the right thing to do. We call it "clinical judgment," or the "art of medicine." Somehow, the assumption goes, physicians are able to assimilate all they have learned from their medical education, their training, research, their personal experiences, and conversations with their colleagues, as well as all the information about their patients—their signs, symptoms, hopes, and fears—to determine the right thing to do. The assumption is that, in our heads, by some wonderful instinct that is either selected for by medical schools, or taught through medical training, each of us can process all this information to make the right decisions and choose the right actions for our patients. This assumption is the foundation of your patients' trust in you as their individual physician. This assumption is also the basis for our claims that as physicians we ought to be left alone to practice medicine as we see fit.

Note: This article is an edited version of the American Urological Association Lecture, which was presented on October 21, 1991, during the annual meeting of the American College of Surgeons in Chicago, Ill.

❖ The Intellectual Problem

In the last few years, the assumption has been severely challenged. There are four lines of weakness: observations of variations in practice patterns, studies of inappropriate care, variations in physicians' perceptions of outcomes, and exposés of poor evidence.

Variations in Practice Patterns

The research on variations in practice patterns is well known. In Vermont, the chance of having one's tonsils removed as a child range from 8% in one community to 70% in another. In Iowa, the chance a man will undergo prostate surgery by age 85 varies from 15% to more than 60%. A comparison of utilization rates across four states found more than threefold differences in rates of heart bypass, thyroid, and prostate surgeries; fivefold differences for back and abdominal surgeries; sevenfold differences for knee replacements; and almost 20-fold differences for carotid endarterectomies.

These findings are not limited to surgery. No matter what type of intervention is examined—from the use of laboratory tests to hospital admissions for medical conditions—variations like these are found. While some of the variations might be explained by differences in demographics and patient preferences, it is not possible to explain all of them away. When similar patients are treated in such different ways, there is a strong implication that the decisionmaking process is loose—that there is a wide range of uncertainty and a good chance that at least some of the decisions are arbitrary. With so many *different* things being done, it is absolutely impossible that everyone is doing the *right* thing.

Inappropriate Care

These observations of variations in practices raise several questions. "Which end of the range is correct? Are patients getting too much or too little?" Partial answers can be gained by examining some research on the appropriateness of the care we are delivering. These studies are also well known. A panel of experts determined the appropriateness of different indications for various procedures, such as coronary angiography, coronary artery bypass surgery, gastroscopy, and carotid endarterectomy. The investigators then reviewed the charts of thousands of patients to determine the actual indications for which the procedures were being performed. They found that only about half the procedures were being performed for indications that had been judged by the experts to be appropriate. In about one fourth of the cases, the indications were clearly inappropriate, and in one fourth they were considered equivocal. As might be expected, this research was controversial—both for its methods and its results. But it did raise serious questions about whether all physicians are doing the right thing.

Variations in Perceptions

One of the more important methodological issues raised by the research on appropriateness of care concerns the experts. How do we know that *their* judgments were correct? Unfortunately, there is startling evidence that physicians, whether small-town practitioners or big-city experts, have vastly different perceptions of the outcomes of different practices. Because this line of research is less well known, I will give a few specific examples.

A group of physicians in a surgical subspecialty was asked to describe their beliefs about the effect of one of their most common procedures on one of its most important outcomes. A specific patient was described, and each physician was asked to imagine the patient asking the following question. "Doctor, if I have this procedure, what is the chance that this outcome will occur?" The specialists' answers ranged from 0% to 100%. In the room were people who thought the outcome would never occur, would occur 1 out of 500 times, 1 out of 200 times, 1 out of 100 times, 1 out of 20 times, 10%, 20%, 50%, 75%, and 100% of the time. For reasons that should be obvious, I will not reveal the name of the specialty. However, no group should feel smug. Wherever we look, we find these types of variations in physicians' perceptions of the outcomes of their procedures.

For another example, let's look at the results of a survey conducted by a task force of the American Urological Association (AUA). They asked 140 urologists to describe the chance that a 65-year-old man with moderate symptoms of benign prostatic hypertrophy (BPH) (defined as a Qmax of less than 12 ml/sec) would develop complete urinary retention within the next 5 years. The estimates ranged almost evenly from a 10% chance to an 80% chance.

One of the tightest ranges of answers I have seen concerned cardiac surgeons' estimates of the outcomes of two different types of heart valves—xenographs and mechanical heart valves. The surgeons were asked to estimate the probabilities of valve failure, death at reoperation, hemorrhage, and embolization. The answers ranged from about 3% to 95% for the chance of valve failure with xenographs to a range of estimates from 0% to 25% of valve failure with mechanical grafts. For most of the outcomes, the estimates ranged from 0% to 50%.

This line of research is especially impressive because it looks inside the heads of physicians. Remember the fundamental assumption. It is that every practitioner can instinctively know the right thing to do. But how can we possibly all be right if we are each thinking such different things? Before we leave these examples, consider the implications for informed consent, expert testimony, and the use of consensus methods to develop practice guidelines.

Poor Evidence

Why is there such a wide range of uncertainty? It is not because physicians are stupid. It is because the information base for medical practice is extremely poor. I can quote general findings, such as that by the Congressional Office of Technology Assessment, that only about 10% to 20% of medical practices are backed up by well-designed, randomized controlled trials. But a more impressive way to make the point is to examine the actual evidence that exists for specific procedures.

Again I will choose an example from urology. A panel cosponsored by the AUA is currently developing guidelines for the management of benign prostatic hypertrophy. This disease is extremely common; more than 300 000 men are operated on each year for BPH. Developing a guideline for the treatment of this disease requires retrieving all the evidence that exists about the effectiveness of different treatments. A MEDLINE search identified hundreds of papers. It is one of the best-studied problems in urology. The panel sorted through the articles to select the randomized controlled trials. In fact, there is not a single randomized controlled trial, or even a nonrandomized well controlled study that compares any pair of treatments for benign prostatic hypertrophy.

As you can imagine, this type of evidence on variations in practice patterns, inappropriateness of care, physician uncertainty, and poor evidence has drastically changed our perceptions of medical practice. The overwhelming impression is that medicine doesn't have its act together.

The perception we all want to have is that medicine is firmly based on reality: Hospitals are tightly run operations, with patients coming in sick, and leaving completely well and filled with happiness. Our research enterprise systematically identifies important problems, and works like a seismograph, returning clear, crisp information about the reality below the epidemiology and pathophysiology of diseases, and the effectiveness of interventions. That information is transmitted speedily to practitioners, who apply it unerringly. A Mercedes-Benz automobile is parked in front of the hospital, but that's okay because the system is working beautifully.

Unfortunately, that image is being shattered. The truth is that the practice of medicine is not based firmly on reality. In fact, it is more like a bowl of Jell-o, quivering above reality, held in place by a few sticks and bandages. The hospital is crumbling, with administrators hanging on for dear life. Our research enterprise is not a seismograph. It looks more like a few buckets being lowered down to gather tidbits of information about what's really happening. Furthermore, the transmission of research information into practice is precarious and the results are used selectively by practitioners. But there is still a Mercedes-Benz in front of the hospital.

❖ Financial Problems

Strangely, the information I have just described about uncertainty and variations, by itself, would not have caused an intellectual revolution. Indeed, studies of variations in practice patterns have been published for almost a century. It is easy enough to ignore everything I have just related—to write it off as the product of health services researchers who do not understand the realities of clinical practice. We could search for some methodological flaws in each of the studies (if you are picky enough, every study has *some* flaw), and ignore the findings.

What, then, converted these revelations into a revolution? One factor is the leadership of a few extraordinary people who recognized these problems for what they are—a severe threat to the quality of care. I'll single out as examples people like the surgeons in Maine and Iowa, who have helped pioneer the modern era of research on practice variations. I'll also single out the AUA, which has led the way not only in pursuing variations, but in designing guidelines and calling for controlled trials of BPH treatment.

But there is another force that has pushed the issue into the public eye—and brought in government and business. That is *costs*. Studies of uncertainty, poor evidence, and variations could have remained merely an intellectual exercise, without really affecting the practice of medicine, were it not for the extraordinary and inexorable increase in health care costs.

You all know the numbers. In 1990, our country spent approximately $670 billion on health care. The number is certainly more than $700 billion today. Health care consumes about 12% of the GNP. It is the largest component of state budgets; in 1988 most states spent 15% of their general revenues on Medicaid. Because of the way we spread costs around, health care costs affect every aspect of our economy. For example, about $700 of every automobile goes toward the health care costs of automakers' employees. The number that impresses me the most is that for every man, woman, and child in the country, we spend more than $2500 each year. Consider that in the context of the median family income, which is approximately $30 000 for a family of four. At $2500 per person, a family of four is spending approximately $10 000 on health care costs; that represents about one third of the median family income.

Even more distressing is the fact that health care costs are out of control. Health care costs have been rising almost twice as fast as the general inflation rate for decades, despite massive efforts to control them.

A final point about costs is that they are unacceptable. As you well know, federal and state governments are taking more and more drastic actions to control costs. Employers have drawn the line and are implementing stronger and stronger steps to manage the care they are paying for. Health care costs are the most common cause of strikes between unions and management. And national health insurance promises to be the major domestic issue for the 1992 elections.

❖ Sources of the Problem

So, why are we in this pickle? The intellectual and financial problems I have just described are the symptoms of a deeper problem. There are two main forces at work.

One is well known: Third-party payment has cut the feedback loop that usually determines the balance between quality and cost. For other goods and services, such as shoes and stereo sets, we can rely on the marketplace not only to bring demand for services into alignment with costs, but also to press providers for information about the quality or outcomes of their products. In a real market, people will examine the quality of a product or service, examine its cost, and determine whether the quality is worth the cost.

Because of third-party payment, however, that connection has been cut. Patients do not see directly the costs of services, and you, who advise them on their decisions, know that. Both you and your patients have an extremely strong and understandable desire to maximize quality, and your choices are not restrained by the usual market forces of costs. The result is what we see—costs that are out of control.

But that is only a partial explanation of the pickle we are in. It explains a lot about costs. But it does not explain the uncertainty, wide ranges in perceptions of outcomes, wide variations in practices, and poor research. Doctors are not the Keystone Kops; how did we get this far, knowing so little? The reason is the second problem, the one I want to focus on most in this speech. The second problem is that medical decisions are complicated, and they are getting more complicated every day.

The complexity of medical decisions can be appreciated by reviewing the two main steps that are involved in every decision (Figure 30.1). Suppose you are faced with a choice between two treatments. To make that choice, you must first estimate the outcomes of the two treatments—that is, you must first determine the benefits, harms, and costs of each treatment. To the greatest extent possible, you should base those estimates on hard evidence, but because there are always gaps in the research, you will also have to apply some subjective judgments. Once you have done this, you can proceed to the second step, which is to compare the benefits, harms, and costs associated with the two treatments. These comparisons are not questions of science; they are value judgments based on personal preferences. There is no right or wrong answer, and different people can have different preferences. Ideally, the preferences should be those of our patients because they are the ones who will actually receive the benefits and harms, and who will eventually pay the costs.

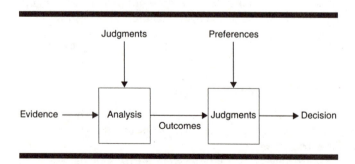

FIGURE 30.1   Two Main Steps of a Decision Process

Now let us focus on the first step. There are two main ways to learn the outcomes of different treatments. One is from experience—observing the outcomes of your patients and your colleagues' patients. A slightly more modern version of this is the uncontrolled clinical series. The other way to learn the outcomes of a treatment is through clinical research, the systematic assignment of treatments and observation of outcomes, with proper controls to ensure that any differences in outcomes are due to the different treatments, not to other miscellaneous factors. The first method—simple observation—and its big brother, the uncontrolled clinical series, work well if three conditions hold: the outcomes are obvious, the outcomes are immediate, and the treatments cause dramatic changes in the outcomes, so dramatic that the changes cannot be explained by any other factors.

In the past, say when my grandfather was practicing medicine, decisions tended to be more clear-cut. Setting a fracture, suturing a laceration, lancing an abscess, or relieving acute urinary obstruction are good examples. The outcomes were fairly immediate and obvious, and the desirability of the outcomes was clear. To be sure, he had a bottle of *Nux Vomica* on his shelf and I'm sure he unnecessarily took out some tonsils, but in general the choices were clear. For these types of practices, it was relatively easy for physicians to determine the outcomes and choose the right thing to do.

In the modern era of medicine, however, there has been a definite shift in the types of outcomes of medical practices. As our procedures have become more complicated and pushed further and further against the frontiers, the outcomes have been more and more difficult to track. They tend to be *long-term, probabilistic*, and *indirect*. The difference between simple and radical treatments for breast cancer is a good example. The decision rests on comparing 5-year survival rates that might differ by only a few percentage points. The outcomes are long-term (5 years) and probabilistic. It is safe to say that a practitioner could *never* learn with any accuracy the relative effectiveness of these two procedures from his or her personal experiences, or even by comparing clinical series.

The problem is that our clinical research has not kept pace with the growing complexity of outcomes. We are still relying on personal observations and uncontrolled clinical series, mixed together with heavy doses of clinical judgment, to learn the outcomes of our practices. These methods are simply not up to the task of evaluating modern medical practices. Our ability to develop new procedures that squeeze out another few percentage points of effectiveness has far outstripped our ability to determine the role of those procedures in practice.

This point is important enough to reinforce with an example. Suppose you have just treated a patient for colorectal cancer and are wondering whether you should ask the patient to come back in, say, 6 months for some follow-up. Perhaps you are considering some surveillance procedure such as colonoscopy, barium enema, carcinoembryonic antigen, or even a computed tomography (CT) scan to look for liver metastases. How would you make such a decision? Indeed, how *do* you make such decisions?

Let's think about the use of a CT scan for liver metastasis, a surveillance practice that is recommended by many experts. I can assure you that there are no randomized controlled trials that compare the effects of different surveillance strategies on survival or any other outcome. How then do you proceed? Somewhere in the back of your mind is a sense of the chance that if you used the test, you would actually find a metastasis. You then must think about what you would do if you did find a metastasis—about how you would treat it. Finally, you would have to determine how the treatment might affect outcomes such as survival.

If that is the broad structure, let's think harder about each of those factors. The chance you would find a metastasis is determined by two things: the chance that the patient *has* a metastasis, and the probability that the test will detect a metastasis if it is present. The first is controlled by the nature of the primary cancer, such as its size, location, and cellular characteristics; by how effective you thought your treatment was; and perhaps by some risk factors, such as the patient's age, concurrent diseases, and so forth. The chance that the test will detect a metastasis, if one happens to be present, is determined by the surveillance tests you decide to use, the frequencies you choose, and the sensitivities of the tests. The sensitivities in turn are determined by the properties of the tests and the technical skills of the person conducting them. If a metastasis *is* found, it could be in different stages of development, depending on the nature of the primary cancer, your treatment, the surveillance strategy, and the sensitivity of the test. The stage of the metastasis in turn affects the choice and possible outcomes of treatment.

I could add another layer of complexity to this example, but the main point has been made. It is *impossible* for any human brain to keep track of all these factors. The fact is that *no one* knows the outcomes of different surveillance strategies for metastasis from colorectal cancer. Right now, there is no rational basis for choosing between different strategies. If you feel comfortable with your current decision it is probably because you are following someone else's recommendation, and you have assumed that he or she has figured it all out. Trust me, they haven't. Unfortunately, this example is typical of hundreds, if not thousands of decisions that are made every day. It is no wonder that everywhere we look we find wide variations in perceptions of outcomes and wide variations in practice—we are really only guessing.

Those are some problems with estimating the outcomes of different patient management strategies. Unfortunately there are also problems with the second step of the decision-making process—the value judgments. Even if we knew the benefits, harms, and costs of different diagnostic tests and treatments, the value judgments are enormously difficult.

❖ Dealing With Complexity

I have just made the case that medical decisions are enormously complex. For most medical practices, it is virtually impossible to estimate the outcomes with any certainty, and when physicians are asked to describe their personal estimates, they vary across the board. It is no wonder then that practices vary widely and that people disagree about which practices are appropriate. I have also argued that the reason for this uncertainty is that the evidence base for medicine is poor. Finally, even if we had information on outcomes, the value judgments required to complete a decision are enormously difficult.

How, then, do we deal with this complexity? Indeed, medicine *does* go on. Every day, every one of you makes decisions, despite your uncertainty and despite the poor evidence. Obviously, the answer to this question—how we deal with the complexity—has tremendous implications for the quality and cost of medical care.

We deal with complexity in two main ways. First, we simplify the problem. Second, we tend to think qualitatively. On the first point, one of the more prominent ways we simplify questions is to ignore financial costs. We can rationalize that stand by claiming that it is unethical to consider costs and/or that it is someone else's responsibility (although we bristle when others actually try to do it). That single maneuver immediately lifts an enormous burden from the decision-making process. For example, all the value judgments I have mentioned become moot.

Another simplification we make is to settle for intermediate outcomes, without pressing on to document the relationship between the intermediate outcome and the health outcome of real interest. For example, if it takes too long to observe the effect of a glaucoma treatment on the long-term chance of blindness, we might settle for observing how the treatment affects intraocular pressure. The problem with this, of course, is that intermediate outcomes are imperfect proxies for long-term outcomes. The intermediate outcome can occur when the long-term outcome does not, and vice versa. Use of intermediate outcomes just adds one more probabilistic element to the guessing game about outcomes.

The other major mechanism we use to deal with complexity is to think qualitatively. The effect of this is summarized in what I call the *criterion of potential benefit*. That criterion says that a treatment is appropriate if it *might* have some benefit. The beauty of this criterion is that it is very easy to apply. You do not have to know the actual magnitudes of benefits, harms, or costs. Nor do you even need to have good evidence of benefit. All you need to establish is that the treatment *might* have benefit. The maxims I learned in medical school are, "an error of commission is to be preferred to an error of omission," or "when in doubt, cut it out," or "if but one patient is helped, then the treatment is worthwhile."

Unfortunately, the criterion of potential benefit has major problems. They all stem from the fact that, because the criterion of potential benefit does not require any information about the actual outcomes of procedures, it allows us to go through life without ever estimating or knowing those outcomes. If a patient asks "What is the chance of such and such an outcome?" we will not know the answer. Two doctors can look the patient straight in the eye and give answers that can vary from 10% to 90%. Another problem is that without information about the magnitudes of benefits and harms of different treatments, there is no rational basis for choosing between them. The criterion of potential benefit also leaves us helpless in dealing with costs. If we do not know the magnitudes of benefits, harms, or costs, it is impossible to determine whether the health outcomes are worth their costs. Indeed, the criterion of potential benefit does not even ask about costs. A final problem is that the criterion of potential benefit provides no basis for making the tough decisions that are required when resources get tight.

The ultimate consequence of relying on the criterion of potential benefit is the set of problems that I described previously. We are uncertain about outcomes, there are wide variations in practice patterns, a large proportion of practices appear to be inappropriate, the evidence for most procedures is poor, and there are uncontrollable increases in costs. In short, the criterion of potential benefit leads to lower-quality care and higher costs.

❖ The Solution

What's the solution? The solution, as you can gather from the title of this chapter, has two parts. One is to explicitly incorporate costs in our decisions and practice guidelines. The other is to think *quantitatively*, not *qualitatively*. These two ideas can be captured in what I call the *criterion of actual benefit*.

This criterion says that whether a treatment is appropriate depends on the *magnitudes* of its benefits, harms, and costs. It is not sufficient to simply say that a treatment *might* have benefit. Rather, it is necessary to say that it *does* have benefit; that the benefit is documented by good evidence; that we can estimate the magnitudes of the benefits, harms, and costs with reasonable certainty; and that the benefits outweigh the harms and justify the costs. I will emphasize the last point. The criterion of *actual* benefits calls for a conscious, explicit comparison of health outcomes and costs.

With the possible exception of my claim that costs should be included, I believe everyone would agree with the criterion of actual benefit. Who would say that we should recommend procedures for which the benefits do not outweigh the harms? If there is a sticking point, it is costs.

Incorporating Costs in Medical Decisions

Let us examine what is probably the most contentious issue, whether costs should be incorporated in medical decisions. I will argue that they should be, for four main reasons: First, costs are real. You charge for your services. Hospitals charge for their services. So do pharmaceutical companies, medical supply companies, and everyone else in this industry. Thus, charges are made, costs are incurred, and someone, sooner or later, will have to pay them.

The second point is that people care about costs. They are not willing to spend any amount of money, no matter how large, to get any amount of benefit, no matter how small. To document this, we can not only examine our own personal behavior, but the empirical and political evidence as well. The empirical evidence comes from studies such as the Health Insurance Study, where it was found that patients who had to pay out-of-pocket costs chose to receive less care than did people who had health insurance.[13] The political evidence is everywhere. Hardly a day goes by without a newspaper article on health care costs. If costs were not of concern, we would not be talking about them. Perhaps the most obvious clue that people care about costs is that we could immediately solve the cost problem by simply raising insurance premiums, HMO dues, and taxes. Our studious avoidance of this most obvious solution indicates that people care about costs.

The third point is extremely important, because many people fail to see it. The fact is that, despite our heroic attempts to make someone else pay our health care costs, eventually all the costs are paid by real people. This point is especially puzzling, because when you see patients in your offices, you know that those patients will not actually pay the costs of the particular services you are about to give them. However, you can be absolutely certain that they *will* end up paying the costs eventually. We have raised the laundering of health care costs to a very high art. Indeed, we have so many launderers, we make BCCI look like amateurs. But you can be certain that after all the laundering has been completed, all the costs will still be there—to be paid by real people.

This point is best illustrated with an example. As you know, many states have passed laws that require health insurance companies to cover the costs of screening mammograms. That sounds wonderful. A woman, let us call her Mrs Jones, can go into a screening center, get a mammogram, and not have to pay for it. The actual cost to her will be a tiny increase in her insurance premium next year, about $0.0000002. But how can that be? How can a mammogram that costs $100 to $200 on the marketplace end up costing only $0.0000002? Who will actually pay for that mammogram?

You can be sure that the screening center will send a bill to the insurance company. But the insurance company is just a launderer. It will pass the costs on to the people who pay the premiums, which will cause all the other subscribers to pick up part of the cost of Mrs Jones' mammogram. But it doesn't end there. Most of Mrs Jones' and other subscribers' costs are paid by their employers, through group contracts. The employers, who are also launderers, will pass the costs on to their employees through lower benefits and salaries, or to their customers through higher costs of products and services, or to the stockholders through lower profits. But the buck does not stop there either. Employers' health care costs are deductible, which means the government will end up receiving lower tax revenues. But the government is also a launderer. To cover the lost tax revenues, it can raise taxes, which sends the costs back to people, or it can cut back on other services, which hurts the people who would have benefited from those services, or it can add the cost to the national debt. But even that does not make it disappear; increases in the national debt are paid by real people through higher interest rates, higher inflation, lower investment rates, recessions, and so forth. You can be sure that after mother nature has completed all the bookkeeping, all the costs of that mammogram will be paid by real people, like Mrs Jones.

Now, if Mrs Jones were the only person taking advantage of the "free" mammogram, the impact of that particular mammogram would be spread out over 250 million people and would be minuscule. However, *everyone* is taking advantage of similar good deals for *every* procedure. When we take into account *all* the services received by *all* the people, we discover—much to our surprise—that every man, woman, and child is paying on average $2500, for a total of $700 billion. In our feverish attempt to make someone else pay the costs of our health care, we all end up paying for each other, and we all end up paying more than we want.

My last point about costs is that if we do not address them, someone else will. One way or another, costs *will* be taken into account. Mechanisms already in place are prospective payment; relative value scales; performance volume standards; "priority-setting" such as that going on in Oregon; a variety of managed care techniques, such as precertification, utilization review, second opinions, and capitation; practice guidelines; and attempts to define "essential services" and "basic care." If you are wondering why you have to telephone someone to get permission to perform a tonsillectomy, it is because we failed to develop mechanisms for controlling costs within the profession. The problem with these external mechanisms is that, depending on how they are done, they can be onerous, disruptive, insulting, and might not work. Corporations, insurance companies, and the government are only using them in a desperate attempt to solve a problem that we have not solved for ourselves.

Quantitative Reasoning: An Example

Now let's return to the idea of quantitative thinking. We have seen the problems with qualitative thinking; *quantitative* thinking goes a long way toward correcting these problems.

Rather than make abstract arguments, I will illustrate the differences between qualitative and quantitative thinking with an example. For convenience, I will use a story published in the *Washington Post* when I was developing this chapter. The story was criticizing the recommendations of the National Cholesterol Education Program (or NCEP) for the management of hypercholesterolemia. As you read this example, understand that my intention is not in any way to denigrate the NCEP or its members. In fact, that panel had on it some of the best epidemiologists, statisticians, and clinicians in the country. The NCEP was simply using the time-honored approach to designing policies, which looks for *potential* benefit, and does not require estimating the *actual consequences* of the policy. My point will be not that the NCEP did anything wrong, but that it is time to change the time-honored approach.

As you know, in 1988 the NCEP recommended a fairly aggressive strategy: after a trial of diet, patients with two or more risk factors should be treated with drugs if their LDL cholesterol levels exceed 160 mg/dL. Patients with only one or no risk factor should be treated if their LDL cholesterol levels exceed 190 mg/dL. Incidentally, being male is a risk factor, so many of us immediately have one strike. Other risk factors are use of tobacco, hypertension, diabetes, and low levels of high-density lipoprotein (HDL).

On the face of it, this seems like a reasonable strategy. It has been well documented that high cholesterol levels are associated with a higher risk of cardiovascular events, and randomized controlled trials have demonstrated that drugs can not only reduce cholesterol levels but can actually decrease the chance of cardiac events. Furthermore, because cardiovascular disease is one of the most common causes of death, the magnitude of the problem appears to justify the magnitude of the strategy. By the criterion of potential benefit, this recommendation is a winner.

So, what's the problem? The article in the *Post* was citing charges that in fact, the NCEP had cast too broad a net, that the strategy would require treating large numbers of people, most of whom would never benefit from the treatment. The article went on to ask whether there might be a more focused strategy, and described narrower treatment criteria proposed in Canada.

How do we address these charges? One obvious approach is to look at the original NCEP report to see what they said about the effects of their strategy. An encouraging clue is that an accompanying editorial said that the NCEP recommendations were "cost-effective" and "would have a major impact on coronary artery disease." So how cost-effective is the NCEP's plan? Let us examine the report for the information that would settle the argument.

Unfortunately, there is no such information. Despite the claims of the editorial, and despite lots of numbers in the report, the panel never estimated the costs, or the effectiveness, or the effect of the strategy it was recommending. Why not? Because the policy itself and the accompanying editorial were products of qualitative reasoning. With qualitative reasoning, you can issue recommendations and make statements about costs and benefits, without *ever actually knowing* the costs or benefits.

Now let us see how quantitative reasoning would approach this problem. Let us try to answer three questions. First, are the NCEP guidelines consistent? That is, do they selectively choose people for treatment who are at the highest risk of cardiac events and who have the most to gain from treatment? Second, what are the actual chances of cardiac events in the people who are selected for treatment, and the actual benefits of treatment? We can also ask about the effects of implementing this strategy in a population. The third question is whether there is a better strategy.

To address the first two questions, I present you with two patients, both of whom have tried diet. Mrs Smith is 42 years old and has a high LDL cholesterol level (195 mg/dL), but no other risk factors for coronary heart disease. Mr Brown, who is 67 years old, has an LDL cholesterol level that is only moderately elevated (155 mg/dL), but he has a number of other risk factors such as tobacco use, hypertension, and low HDL. How should they be treated? The NCEP guidelines say that Mrs Smith should be treated. Although she has no other risk factors, her cholesterol level exceeds the threshold for treatment. The guidelines say that Mr Brown should *not* be treated. Even though he has several risk factors, his cholesterol is below the 160 mg/dL threshold for treatment. Presumably, his risk of a cardiac event is lower than Mrs Smith's, and he has less to gain from treatment.

With that as background, let us now determine the actual probabilities that Mrs Smith and Mr Brown will have a cardiac event in the next 5 years. We can determine this from large studies such as the Framingham project and the Helsinki Heart Study. Based on these studies, Mrs Smith's chance of an event in the next 5 years is about 1.2%, or 120 in 10 000. Mr Brown's is about 40%, or 4000 in 10 000. Despite the fact that Mr Brown was not selected for treatment, his risk of a sudden death or heart attack is almost 40 times higher than Mrs Smith's. Furthermore, the benefit that Mr Brown would have received from treatment, a reduction in probability of death of about 10%, was approximately 250 times the benefit that Mrs Smith would get, about 0.4%. Why in the world would the NCEP recommend treating Mrs Smith but not Mr Brown? The answer is because they were thinking qualitatively, and qualitative reasoning is not powerful enough to determine the actual effects of an intervention—even if they differ by a factor of 25. The NCEP reasoned that because Mrs Smith has a higher cholesterol level than Mr Brown, she should benefit more. To determine the effect of the other risk factors would have required quantitative reasoning, which was not applied.

Now let us examine the problem from the point of view of a population. For convenience, I'll discuss calculations for the Kaiser Foundation Health Plan of Southern California, an HMO with which I am currently working. Imagine that you are the chief of cardiology. The NCEP recommendations have just come out, and you must recommend whether they should be implemented. The stakes are high—this HMO has more than 2 million members.

What would you like to know before recommending the NCEP guidelines? Reasonable factors to consider are the number of people who would be targeted for treatment, the number of events that could be expected to occur in that population without treatment, the number of events that would be prevented by treatment, the financial costs of the drugs and any tests required to monitor the drugs, and any savings that might accrue from preventing cardiovascular events. We have already seen that the NCEP itself didn't estimate the answers to any of these questions, because qualitative reasoning and the criterion of potential benefit do not require them.

However, using a fairly simple model that combines information on the demographics of the Kaiser population, the epidemiology of risk factors as determined from the Framingham and Helsinki Heart studies, the effectiveness of treatment as determined by the Helsinki Heart Study, and some simple economic analyses of the cost of drugs and treatment for coronary artery disease, we can estimate the answers to the questions I just posed (Table 30.1).

In the absence of treatment, we can expect about 100 000 cardiac events to occur during the next 5 years. The events will be of various types. Approximately 4% will be sudden death, 30% will be myocardial infarctions, 8% will be coronary insufficiency, 30% will be angina, and 28% will be "atherosclerosis." These events will cost the health plan well over $1 billion over 5 years. If cholesterol treatment were implemented according to the NCEP guidelines, the number of events could be expected to go down to about 90 000, or about 10 000 events would be prevented. However, it would cost more than $300 million over 5 years to pay for the drugs and monitoring. About $140 million would be saved by preventing cardiovascular events, leaving a net 5-year cost of about $190 million. Applying the NCEP guidelines would involve treating approximately 18% of the adult population in the HMO, or more than 140 000 people. In case you are wondering, nationally the impact would be to prevent about 1.2 million events over 5 years at a 5-year cost of approximately $37 billion for drugs, or a net cost of $20 billion after reduced treatment costs are taken into account. Now you have the numbers you need to make an informed decision about implementing the NCEP recommendations.

But before you do that, let's use quantitative reasoning to go a step further. For example, you might wonder whether there is a better strategy. From our analysis of Mrs Smith and Mr Brown we have already seen that the NCEP guidelines are very inconsistent. They do not systematically treat the people who have the highest risk. We can use the epidemiological information on risk factors to do a better job of selecting the highest-risk people for treatment.

For example, we can identify a strategy that achieves the same benefit as the NCEP but at a minimal cost. Table 30.2 shows the results of such a strategy. Notice that the effect is still to prevent about 10 000 events, because that was our objective. However, by doing a better job of targeting the highest-risk patients, that objective can be achieved by treating only 7% of the population instead of 18%—that is, treating only 60 000 people instead of 140 000. Because fewer people have to be treated, the drug costs are cut more than in half, to about $140 million. We continue to save about $140 million from reducing the

TABLE **30.1** Implications of NCEP Guidelines for a Large HMO*

	Events Prevented, No.	Economic Outcomes, $ (Billions)		
		Drug and Screening Costs	Treatment of Cardiac Events	Net Costs
No treatment	102 066	0.000	1.370	1.370
Treatment	91 962	0.322	1.234	1.557
Effect	−10 104	0.322	−0.136	0.187

*Number (%) treated: 142 797 (18.09).

TABLE 30.2   Implications of Optimal Strategy for a Large HMO*

	Events Prevented, No.	Economic Outcomes, $ (Billions)		
		Drug and Screening Costs	Treatment of Cardiac Events	Net Costs
No treatment	102 066	0.000	1.370	1.370
Treatment	91 962	0.138	1.234	1.372
Effect	−10 104	0.138	−0.136	0.002

*Number (%) treated: 59 603 (7.55).

costs of treating coronary artery disease events, so this strategy turns out to be virtually free. In summary, the two strategies both have the same effect, but the optimal strategy ends up costing approximately 1/200th as much as the NCEP recommendations.

Before I close the example, I want to quote from a physician who was criticizing the critics. He was complaining about the use of quantitative methods, and his statements reflect a common misconception about quantitative methods. When asked by the reporter to comment on the criticisms of the NCEP, a cardiologist from George Washington University said, "The fundamental issue is that they (the critics of the NCEP) are dealing with models. They are not dealing with facts. They are not dealing with patients."[4] He went on to say that economists' computer models contain many unverifiable assumptions and cannot be trusted as the basis for making decisions about patients.

In fact, models are not built out of thin air. That would be dumb. Models use the same "facts" that physicians use. Indeed, they use many more facts. In this case, the facts came from large epidemiological studies and randomized controlled trials of drug treatments. The difference between the model and the physician's head is that the model is far more powerful and accurate in keeping track of and processing the facts. In essence, this cardiologist has made an appeal to the fundamental assumption that we began with—that somehow, through some wonderful, mysterious instinct, physicians can process all the information in their heads and come up with the right answer. Unfortunately, we have seen that that assumption is very difficult to accept. In this particular example, to the extent that the large epidemiological studies and randomized controlled trials represent the "facts," the instincts of the experts on the panel came up with a very wrong answer when they recommended treating Mrs Smith instead of Mr Brown.

❖ Conclusions

Medicine is indeed in the middle of an intellectual revolution. Methods of reasoning and problem solving that might have worked well in the past are not sufficient to handle today's problems. Given the enormous complexity of medical decisions, it is no longer reasonable to assume that we can process in our heads all the relevant information and always come up with the correct answers. Indeed, that myth has been shattered. We are *all* coming up with *different* answers, and it is absolutely impossible for all of us to be correct.

Compared with the complexity of the problems we face, the techniques that we are currently using to make decisions and to design practice guidelines are primitive. They might have been sufficient for the 1930s and 1940s, and maybe even for the 1950s and 1960s, but not for the 1990s, and certainly not for the next century. Heuristics, such as ignoring costs and asking only if a practice might have some benefit, are wholly inadequate for today's realities. Depending on personal experiences, anecdotes, and clinical series is no longer appropriate. The thought of designing national guidelines that affect millions of people and billions of dollars without ever estimating their actual consequences is unacceptable. In short, our ability to unveil the mysteries of health and diseases and to develop ingenious interventions has far outstripped our ability to use that information. Our practices are way out in front of our intellectual lines of supply.

❖ The Future

Let me close by telling you the future. First, the process I have described is irreversible. Medicine is too large, too complex, and too important an enterprise to be run by clinical judgment and qualitative reasoning. Those individuals who prefer the good old days might be able to stall for a few more years, but the forces are too strong and the stakes are too high to hold out forever.

What will all this mean to you? You'll be thinking and talking in more quantitative terms. When you want to be precise with colleagues and patients, you'll use numbers and probabilities, not fuzzy words like "many," "most," or "rare." When Mrs Smith asks you a question, you will have the answer. If Mrs Smith asks three cardiologists the same question, she will get the same answer from all three.

There will also be changes in your day-to-day routine. The most visible change will be that there will be a computer terminal on your desk. (Many of you already have them.) Don't worry, you won't have to learn how to type. All you will need to do is point and touch. But you *will* use the computer. You will use it to bring up information on patients when they enter your offices. You will use it to access information on the patient's problem, its outcomes, and its treatments. And you will *enter* information about the patient's current problem, what you found, what you did, and the outcomes that occurred. In return, the computer will make your life much easier by writing your notes and keeping your charts. It will give you the information you need for decisions such as the chance that Mrs Smith will have a cardiac event in 5 years. It will also offer you guidelines derived by your colleagues for how to manage patients like the one you are seeing.

That is what you will see in your daily practice. But many more things will be happening behind the scenes. The information you provide on your patients will be used to learn much more than we ever dreamed possible about who our patients are, what diseases they get, what we do to them, what outcomes occur, and what it all costs. This information will be available to you at the touch of a screen, but will also be used by the expert panels of the future to analyze the pros and cons of different strategies and to develop practice guidelines. The days of recommending a $10 billion program without ever estimating its consequences will be over. That approach will seem as strange as buying a new house without asking its price, or taking a job without asking its salary.

How do I know all this will happen? Because it *has* to. We're using 19th-century methods to make decisions about 21st-century medical practices. It's almost silly, when you step back and think about it. It would be like a modern bank trying to keep its records by hand, using only pen and ink. No, even worse—it's like not keeping records at all. You could compare it to a loan officer trying to estimate *subjectively* your monthly mortgage payment, or five loan officers coming up with five different rates for the *same* loan for five different people. It's time to change!

I can see all that very clearly. The one thing I am uncertain about is *who* will make the decisions about costs. Notice that I did not say *whether* costs will be considered. I know that that will happen. Indeed, it is already happening. The only question in my mind is *who* will take costs into account. Will *we* do it, within the profession, primarily through practice guidelines? Or will it be done by outsiders, by business and the government, primarily through the meat axe approaches of prospective payment, volume performance standards, precertification, and utilization review?

If I had to guess now, I would say that *we* will do it because as obnoxious as that might seem now, and as much of a break in tradition that it represents, doing it ourselves is much more desirable than having others do it. We are the ones with the clinical knowledge. We are the ones who best understand our patients' desires. And we are in the best position to tailor decisions about costs for individual patient indications. We will probably do it, because it is the right thing to do.

In closing, let me say that there are two ways to view the changes that I have just described. One is as a *threat*. The other is as a *privilege*. I prefer the latter. We are the ones who are witnessing—no, we are the ones who are *creating*, the most important advancement to date in the intellectual infrastructure of medicine. The changes that are under way today are as inspiring and important as genetic engineering, transplantation, imaging, or any of the other advances in medical science.

It is an exciting challenge, and we're up to it.

❖ References

1. Manning WG J, Wells KB, Duan N, et al. How cost sharing affects the use of ambulatory mental health services. *JAMA*. 1986;256:1930-1934.
2. Newhouse JP, Manning WG, Morris CN, et al. Some interim results from a controlled trial of cost sharing in health insurance. *N Engl J Med*. 1981;305:1501-1507.
3. O'Grady KF, Manning WG, Newhouse JP, Brook RH. The impact of cost sharing on emergency department use. *N Engl J Med*. 1985;313:484-490.
4. John LaRosa, in Gladwell M: "Putting a Price on Each Life. Economics Cuts to Heart of Cholesterol Program." *Washington Post*. October 15, 1991.

❖ Source

Originally published in *Am Coll Surg Bull*. 1992;77:36-49. Reprinted by permission from the *Bulletin of the American College of Surgeons*. Copyright 1992, American College of Surgeons.

CHAPTER 31

A Conversation
With My Mother

You have already met my father.[1] Now meet my mother. She died a few weeks ago. She wanted me to tell you how.

Her name was Virginia. Up until about 6 months ago, at age 84, she was the proverbial "little old lady in sneakers." After my father died of colon cancer several years ago, she lived by herself in one of those grand old Greek revival houses you see on postcards of small New England towns. Hers was in Middlebury, Vermont.

My mother was very independent, very self-sufficient, and very content. My brother and his family lived next door. Although she was quite close to them, she tried hard not to interfere in their lives. She spent most of her time reading large-print books, working word puzzles, and watching the news and professional sports on TV. She liked the house kept full of light. Every day she would take two outings, one in the morning to the small country store across the street to pick up the *Boston Globe*, and one in the afternoon to the Grand Union across town, to pick up some item she purposefully omitted from the previous day's shopping list. She did this in all but the worst weather. On icy days, she would wear golf shoes to keep from slipping and attach spikes to the tip of her cane. I think she was about 5 feet 2 and 120 pounds, but I am not certain. I know she started out at about 5 feet 4, but she seemed to shrink a little bit each year, getting cuter with time as many old people do. Her wrinkles matched her age, emphasizing a permanent thin-lipped smile that extended all the way to her little Kris Kringle eyes. The only thing that embarrassed her was her thinning gray hair, but she covered that up with a rather dashing tweed fedora that matched her Talbots' outfits. She loved to tease people by wearing outrageous necklaces. The one made from the front teeth of camels was her favorite.

To be sure, she had had her share of problems in the past: diverticulitis and endometriosis when she was younger, more recently a broken hip, a bout with depression, some hearing loss, and cataracts. But she was a walking tribute to the best things in American medicine. Coming from a family of four generations of physicians, she was fond of bragging that, but for lens implants, hearing aids, hip surgery, and Elavil, she would be blind, deaf, bedridden, and depressed. At age 84, her only problems were a slight rectal prolapse, which she could reduce fairly easily, some urinary incontinence, and a fear that if her eyesight got much worse she would lose her main pleasures. But those things were easy to deal with and she was, to use her New England expression, "happy as a clam."

"David, I can't tell you how content I am. Except for missing your father, these are the best years of my life."

Yes, all was well with my mother, until about 6 months ago. That was when she developed acute cholelithiasis. From that point on, her health began to unravel with amazing speed. She recovered from the cholecystectomy on schedule and within a few weeks of leaving the hospital was resuming her walks downtown. But about 6 weeks after the surgery she was suddenly hit with a case of severe diarrhea, so severe that it extended her rectal prolapse to about 8 inches and dehydrated her to the point that she had to be readmitted. As soon as her physician got her rehydrated, other complications quickly set in. She developed oral thrush, apparently due to the antibiotic treatment for her diarrhea, and her antidepressants got out of balance. For some reason that was never fully determined, she also became anemic, which was treated with iron, which made her nauseated. She could not eat, she got weak, her skin itched, and her body ached. Oh yes, they also found a lump in her breast, the diagnosis of which was postponed, and atrial fibrillation. Needless to say, she was quite depressed.

Her depression was accentuated by the need to deal with her rectal prolapse. On the one hand, she really disliked the thought of more surgery. She especially hated the nasogastric tube and the intense postoperative fatigue. On the other hand, the prolapse was very painful. The least cough or strain would send it out to rub against the sheets, and she could not push it back the way she used to. She knew that she could not possibly walk to the Grand Union again unless it was fixed.

It was at that time that she first began to talk to me about how she could end her life gracefully. As a physician's wife, she was used to thinking about life and death and prided herself on being able to deal maturely with the idea of death. She had signed every living will and advance directive she could find, and carried a card that donated her organs. Even though she knew they would not do anyone much good (*"Can they recycle my artificial hip and lenses?"*), she liked the way the card announced her acceptance of the fact that all things must some day end. She dreaded the thought of being in a nursing home, unable to take care of herself, her body, mind, and interests progressively declining until she was little more than a blank stare, waiting for death to mercifully take her away.

"I know they can keep me alive a long time, but what's the point? If the pleasure is gone and the direction is steadily down, why should I have to draw it out until I'm 'rescued' by cancer, a heart attack, or a stroke? That could take years. I understand that some people want to hang on until all the possible treatments have been tried to squeeze out the last drops of life. That's fine for them. But not for me."

My own philosophy, undoubtedly influenced heavily by my parents, is that choosing the best way to end your life should be the ultimate individual right—a right to be exercised between oneself and one's beliefs, without intrusions from governments or the beliefs of others. On the other hand, I also believe that such decisions should be made only with an accurate understanding of one's prognosis and should never be made in the middle of a correctable depression or a temporary trough. So my brother, sister, and I coaxed her to see a rectal surgeon about having her prolapse repaired and to put off thoughts of suicide until her health problems were stabilized and her antidepressants were back in balance.

With the surgeon's help, we explored the possible outcomes of the available procedures for her prolapse. My mother did not mind the higher mortality rates of the more extensive operations—in fact, she wanted them. Her main concern was to avoid rectal incontinence, which she knew would dampen any hopes of returning to her former lifestyle.

Unfortunately, that was the outcome she got. By the time she had recovered from the rectal surgery, she was totally incontinent "at both ends," to use her words. She was bedridden, anemic, exhausted, nauseated, achy, and itchy. Furthermore, over the period of this illness her eyesight had begun to fail to the point she could no longer read. Because she was too sick to live at home, even with my brother's help, but not sick enough to be hospitalized, we had to move her to an intermediate care facility.

On the positive side, her antidepressants were working again and she had regained her clarity of mind, her spirit, and her humor. But she was very unhappy. She knew instinctively, and her physician confirmed, that after all the insults of the past few months it was very unlikely she would ever be able to take care of herself alone or walk to the Grand Union. That was when she began to press me harder about suicide.

"Let me put this in terms you should understand, David. My 'quality of life'—isn't that what you call it?—has dropped below zero. I know there is nothing fatally wrong with me and that I could live on for many more years. With a colostomy and some luck I might even be able to recover a bit of my former lifestyle, for a while. But do we have to do that just because it's possible? Is the meaning of life defined by its duration? Or does life have a purpose so large that it doesn't have to be prolonged at any cost to preserve its meaning?

"I've lived a wonderful life, but it has to end sometime and this is the right time for me. My decision is not about whether I'm going to die—we will all die sooner or later. My decision is about when and how. I don't want to spoil the wonder of my life by dragging it out in years of decay. I want to go now, while the good memories are still fresh. I have always known that eventually the right time would come, and now I know that this is it. Help me find a way."

I discussed her request with my brother and sister and with her nurses and physician. Although we all had different feelings about her request, we agreed that she satisfied our criteria of being well informed, stable, and not depressed. For selfish reasons we wanted her to live as long as possible, but we realized that it was not our desires that mattered. What mattered to us were her wishes. She was totally rational about her conviction that this was "her time." Now she was asking for our help, and it struck us as the height of paternalism (or filialism?) to impose our desires over hers.

I bought *Final Exit*[2] for her, and we read it together. If she were to end her life, she would obviously have to do it with pills. But as anyone who has thought about this knows, accomplishing that is not easy. Patients can rarely get the pills themselves, especially in a controlled setting like a hospital or nursing home. Anyone who provides the pills knowing they will be used for suicide could be arrested. Even if those problems are solved and the pills are available, they can be difficult to take, especially by the frail. Most likely, my mother would fall asleep before she could swallow the full dose. A way around this would be for her to put a bag over her head with a rubber band at her neck to ensure that she would suffocate if she fell asleep before talking all the pills. But my mother did not like that idea because of the depressing picture it would present to those who found her body. She contemplated drawing a happy smile on the bag, but did not think that would give the correct impression either. The picture my mother wanted to leave to the world was that her death was a happy moment, like the end of a wonderful movie, a time for good memories and a peaceful acceptance of whatever the future might hold. She did not like the image of being a quasi-criminal sneaking illegal medicines. The way she really wanted to die was to be given a morphine drip that she could control, to have her family around her holding her hands, and for her to turn up the drip.

As wonderful as that might sound, it is illegal. One problem was that my mother did not have a terminal condition or agonizing pain that might justify a morphine drip. Far from it. Her heart was strong enough to keep her alive for 10 more years, albeit as a frail, bedridden, partially blind, partially deaf, incontinent, and possibly stroked-out woman. But beyond that, no physician would dare give a patient access to a lethal medicine in a way that could be accused of assisting suicide. Legally, physicians can provide lots of comfort care, even if it might hasten a patient's death, but the primary purpose of the medicine must be to relieve suffering, not to cause death. Every now and then my mother would vent her frustration with the law and the arrogance of others who insist that everyone must accept their philosophy of death, but she knew that railing at what she considered to be misguided laws would not undo them. She needed to focus on finding a solution to her problem. She decided that the only realistic way out was for me to get her some drugs and for her to do her best to swallow them. Although I was very nervous at the thought of being turned in by someone who discovered our plan and felt it was their duty to stop it, I was willing to do my part. I respected her decision, and I knew she would do the same for me.

I had no difficulty finding a friend who could write a prescription for restricted drugs and who was willing to help us from a distance. In fact, I have yet to find anybody who agrees with the current laws. (*"So why do they exist?"*) But before I actually had to resolve any lingering conflicts and obtain the drugs, my mother's course took an unexpected and strangely welcomed twist. I received a call that she had developed pneumonia and had to be readmitted to the hospital. By the time I made contact with her, she had already reminded her attendants that she did not want to be resuscitated if she should have a heart attack or stroke.

"Is there anything more I can do?"

Pneumonia, the old folks' friend, I thought to myself. I told her that although advance directives usually apply to refusing treatments for emergencies such as heart attacks, it was always legal for her to refuse any treatment. In particular, she could refuse the antibiotics for the pneumonia. Her physician and nurses would undoubtedly advise her against it, but if she signed enough papers they would have to honor her request.

"What's it like to die of pneumonia? Will they keep me comfortable?"

I knew that without any medicine for comfort, pneumonia was not a pleasant way to die. But I was also confident that her physician was compassionate and would keep her comfortable. So she asked that the antibiotics be stopped. Given the deep gurgling in her throat every time she breathed, we all expected the infection to spread rapidly. She took a perverse pleasure in that week's cover story of *Newsweek*, which described the spread of resistant strains.

"Bring all the resistant strains in this hospital to me. That will be my present to the other patients."

But that did not happen. Against the odds, her pneumonia regressed. This discouraged her greatly—to see the solution so close, just to watch it slip away.

"What else can I do? Can I stop eating?"

I told her she could, but that that approach could take a long time. I then told her that if she was really intent on dying, she could stop drinking. Without water, no one, even the healthiest, can live more than a few days.

"Can they keep me comfortable?"

I talked with her physician. Although it ran against his instincts, he respected the clarity and firmness of my mother's decision and agreed that her quality of life had sunk below what she was willing to bear. He also knew that what she was asking from him was legal. He took out the IV and wrote orders that she should receive adequate medications to control discomfort.

My mother was elated. The next day happened to be her 85th birthday, which we celebrated with a party, balloons and all. She was beaming from ear to ear. She had done it. She had found the way. She relished her last piece of chocolate, and then stopped eating and drinking.

Over the next 4 days, my mother greeted her visitors with the first smiles she had shown for months. She energetically reminisced about the great times she had had and about things she was proud of. (She especially hoped I would tell you about her traveling alone across Africa at the age of 70, and surviving a capsized raft on Wyoming's Snake River at 82.) She also found a calming self-acceptance in describing things of which she was not proud. She slept between visits but woke up brightly whenever we touched her to share more memories and say a few more things she wanted us to know. On the fifth day it was more difficult to wake her. When we would take her hand she would open her eyes and smile, but she was too drowsy and weak to talk very much. On the sixth day, we could not wake her. Her face was relaxed in her natural smile, she was breathing unevenly, but peacefully. We held her hands for another 2 hours, until she died.

I had always imagined that when I finally stood in the middle of my parents' empty house, surrounded by the old smells, by hundreds of objects that represent a time forever lost, and by the terminal silence, I would be overwhelmingly saddened. But I wasn't. This death was not a sad death; it was a happy death. It did not come after years of decline, lost vitality, and loneliness; it came at the right time. My mother was not clinging desperately to what no one can have. She knew that death was not a tragedy to be postponed at any cost, but that death is a part of life, to be embraced at the proper time. She had done just what she wanted to do, just the way she wanted to do it. Without hoarding pills, without making me a criminal, without putting a bag over her head, and without huddling in a van with a carbon monoxide machine, she had found a way to bring her life gracefully to a close. Of course we cried. But although we will miss her greatly, her ability to achieve her death at her "right time" and in her "right way" transformed for us what could have been a desolate and crushing loss into a time for joy. Because she was happy, we were happy.

"Write about this, David. Tell others how well this worked for me. I'd like this to be my gift. Whether they are terminally ill, in intractable pain, or, like me,

just know that the right time has come for them, more people might want to know that this way exists. And maybe more physicians will help them find it."

Maybe they will. Rest in peace, Mom.

My mother wants to thank Dr Timothy Cope of Middlebury, Vermont, for his present on her 85th birthday.

❖ References

1. Eddy DM. Cost-effectiveness analysis: a conversation with my father. *JAMA*. 1992; 267:1669-1672, 1674-1675 (Chapter 19).
2. Humphry D. *Final Exit*. Secaucus, NJ: Carol Publishing Group; 1991.

❖ Source

Originally published in *JAMA*. 1994;272:179-181.

❖ Index

DATE DUE			